A COMPLETE GUIDE TO FAMILY SAFETY AND FIRST-AID

A COMPLETE GUIDE TO FAMILY SAFETY AND FIRST-AID

By

ASHWANI BHARDWAJ

GOODWILL PUBLISHING HOUSE

B-3, RATTAN JYOTI, 18, RAJENDRA PLACE
NEW DELHI-110 008 (INDIA)

Published by:

GOODWILL PUBLISHING HOUSE®

B-3 Rattan Jyoti, 18 Rajendra Place
New Delhi–110 008 (INDIA)
Tel: 25820556, 25750801, 25755559
Fax: 91-11-25764396
Email: goodwillpub@vsnl.net
ylp@bol.net.in
goodwillpub@gmail.com
Website: www.goodwillpublishinghouse.com

Printed at Kumar Offset Printers, Delhi-110092

Contents

Introduction

"Prevention is better than cure" and "a stitch in time saves nine" sums up the entire concept of safety. Home is a vital component of safety network because we feel most safe in our homes, but our laziness and "take-it-easy" attitude results in most items of our daily use lying haphazardly, which sometimes results in serious accidents. Just a small effort at the right time can take care of most of our household injuries. A slipper left in the middle of the room or a water spill on the floor or on the stairs can cause someone to trip or slip badly with nasty consequences.

Though tremendous technological advancement has made our lives simpler but at the same time rapid over-crowding and ever-rising pollution levels have led to a sharp increase in accident rate and fatal diseases, so some basic knowledge of family safety (including first-aid) has became a vital necessity for everyone including children, adults and the aged, to save precious lives, hard-earned money, valuable time and undue agony and pain.

The sole objective of this self-help book is "FAMILY WELFARE" and it covers all the important aspects in a wide range of situations and occasions presented in a simple, easy-to-understand manner with vivid illustrations. Even if a single mishap is prevented by reading this book, our purpose will be more than served.

So wish you all a SAFE AND HAPPY life.

CHAPTER

1

General Safety Measures for A 'Safe' Home and Workplace

A razor, a knife, a knitting needle or a pair of scissors mishandled can pierce or cut the skin, eyes, or any other part of the body and may result in fatal injury too, especially if the item happens to be rusty which may lead to deadly tetanus. All these things should be strictly kept out of the reach of children, the aged, the infirm and those who are mentally unfit, depressed or prone to violent anger

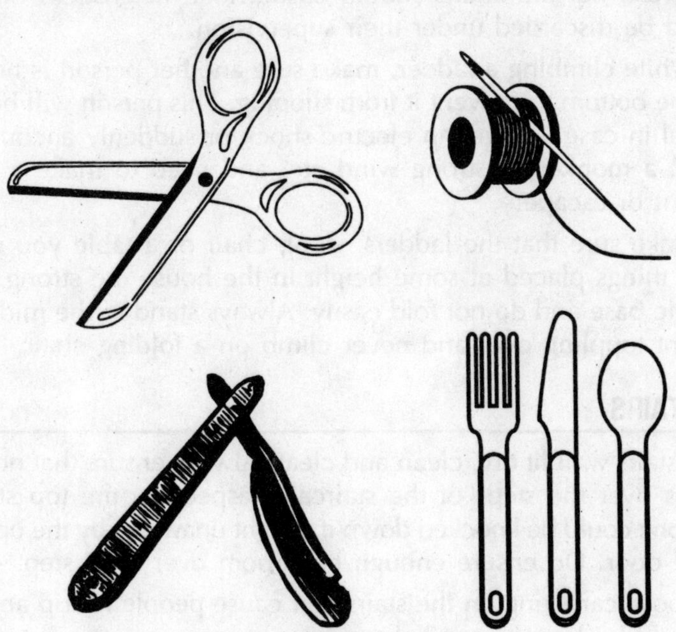

Common domestic items which may cause injury.

Walk Carefully

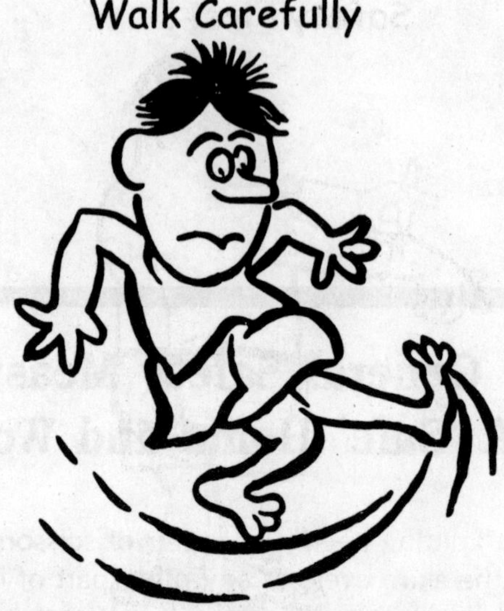

and emotions. Even matchboxes, cooking gas lighters, cigarette lighters etc. need same precautions. Some children have this hobby of collecting matchboxes of different types from different countries, hotels etc. but the adults should ensure that matchsticks of these should be discarded under their supervision.

While climbing a ladder, make sure another person is holding it at the bottom to prevent it from slipping. This person will be very helpful in case you get an electric shock or suddenly encounter a lizard, a monkey, a strong wind etc. and need to make a quick descent or escape.

Make sure that the ladders, stool, chair or a table you use to reach things placed at some height in the house are strong, have a stable base and do not fold easily. Always stand in the middle to prevent toppling over and never climb on a folding chair.

❐ STAIRS

Keep stairs well lit dry, clean and clear. Always ensure that no door swings over the steps of the staircase, especially the top stop as someone could be knocked down if caught unawares by the opening of the door. Do ensure enough headroom over each step.

Loose carpeting on the stairs can cause people to trip and fall. It should be kept in good shape.

Safety First . . . . .

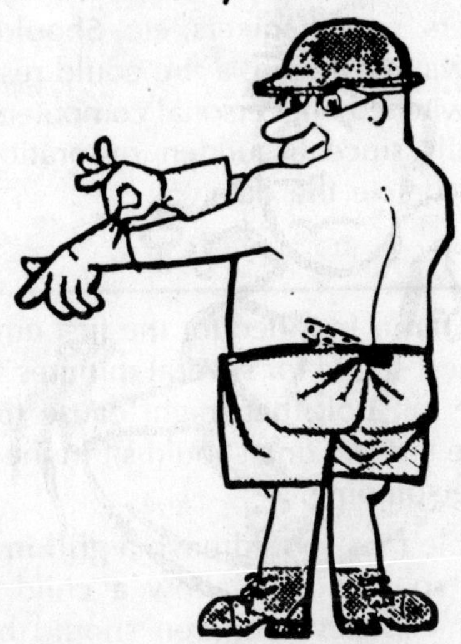

There should be railings or handrests on both sides of the stairs, even if there is a wall on one side. The railings give support to children as well as to the old and infirm.

Everyone in the house should make it a point to wipe a staircase dry if a wet patch is found. If this cannot be done, then post a sign to warn users that the stairs are wet, or block entry to the stairs.

Do not slide down the bannisters of a staircase. A fall may result in severe head injuries.

Children can fall from trees, and from roofs which are unprotected by a high parapet wall. They should not be allowed to climb or fool around them.

No one should sit or stand on a window sill, balcony railings, terrace parapet, etc. as even slightest distraction may result in a fall.

Provide enough natural or artificial light in corridors, hallways and passageways between rooms and upon the stairs so that it is safe to walk and no obstacle remains hidden from view. Night lights should be provided in the bedrooms and corridors.

❐ POWER CUTS

If power failures are frequent, one should keep a torch in each room, and keep candles and matchboxes handy but out of the reach of young children.

In case of power failure, turn off power appliances such as electric irons, toasters, ovens, mixers, etc. Should the power come on when you are away or asleep, a fire could result if any of these appliances are left switched on. Personal computers should be turned off when power fails since a sudden restoration of power may damage the disc or delete the data.

❒ CEILING FANS

Whenever a ceiling fan is installed for the first time or after repairs, let it run at the highest speed for several minutes. Any defect in the roof hook or in the fan bolt that might cause the fan to fall will show up. During the test, no one should sit in the region where the fan might fall while spinning.

Pedestal and table fans should have a grill in the front and the rear, small enough so as not to allow a child to put his finger through to touch the blades. Children should be warned of the dangers of the rotating blades of a fan.

❒ REMEMBER PRACTICAL SILLY JOKES ARE DANGEROUS ?

Never pull a chair from underneath a person trying to sit on it. The unexpected fall from even about half a metre (18 inches) could

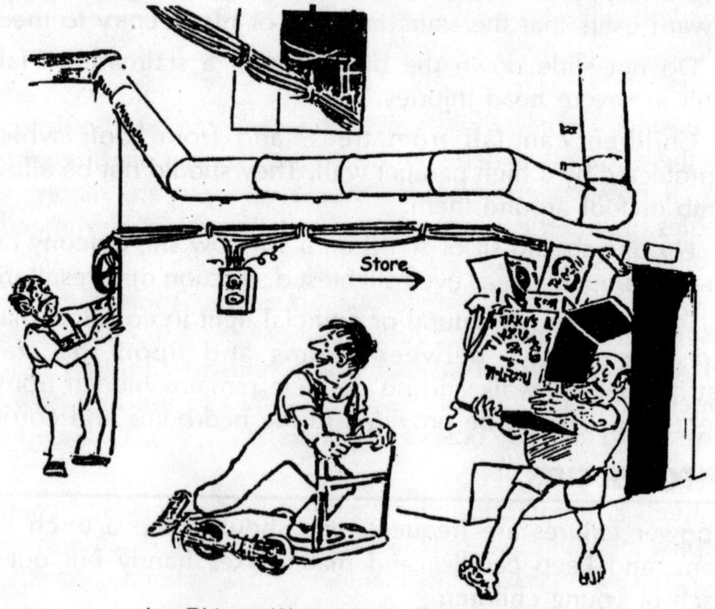

Joy Ride at Workplace is Dangerous

fracture his thigh bone and also injure the spine, neck or head if he hits a piece of furniture or a wall nearby.

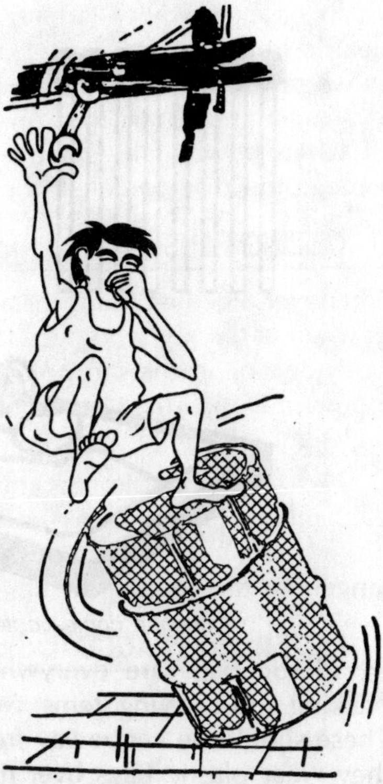

Never put a pencil or anything sharp underneath a person trying to sit on a chair. It can lead to serious bleeding and may require an emergency operation.

Another item of personal safety concerns the clipping of nails. While pressing the nail-cutter, one should close the eyes momentarily till the nail is clipped and lands on the ground. Sheared nails act as very sharp, tiny missiles which can badly injure the eyes. They travel very fast and do not generally give the eyes a chance to close.

After using a needle, keep it threaded. Such a needle is easy to handle and, should it fall down, it will be easy to retrieve and locate.

Besides kitchen forks, knives, scissors, can and bottle openers, etc. there are other items in the household that are sharp and can hurt, if not properly handled. Some of these are razors, sewing needles, geometrical instruments, and dissection instruments used by biology students.

Other potentially dangerous household tools are hammers, chisels, screwdrivers, etc. Add some of your gardening equipment and one has a virtual arsenal in the house ! Children should be properly taught which of the above things to use and how to use them. Sharp toys like bows and arrows, darts, etc. also need special attention

Keep all toxic consumer products in their original containers. Keeping them in cups, milk bottles, mineral water, soft drink bottles, etc. can result in their accidental ingestion which may prove harmful.

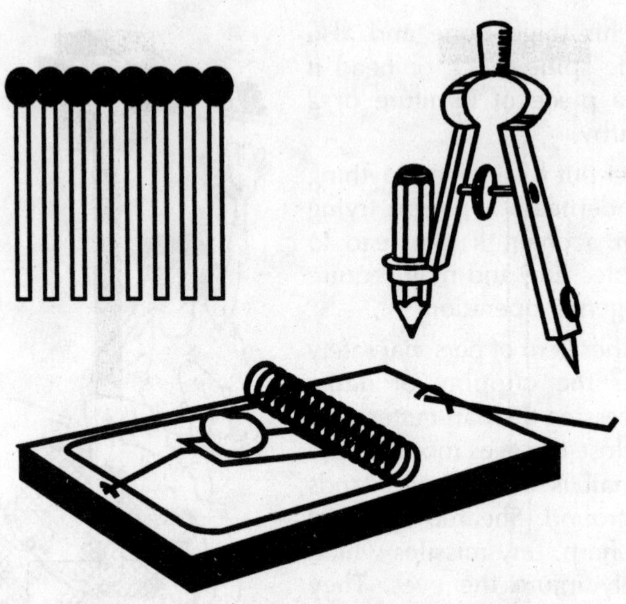

Common domestic items which may cause injury.

Plastic bags are everywhere nowadays. These are used for packing and carrying items, waste bags, etc. and come in all sizes. These should be kept away from children as they can suffocate, if they wear plastic bags over their heads and faces as hoods. Tiny tots may even put them in their mouth and choke.

Close all cupboard doors and table drawers after the job is done; otherwise children running around, and elderly persons with impaired vision, can get severely hurt.

Keep walkways approaching the house, and the steps outside the house, as well as all open courtyards, free of slippery areas caused by wetness or algae growth.

If there is a full length clear glass door in the house, put some decoration on it so that people know that it is a door and not an open passage to walk through.

Repair any frayed or worn out edges of rugs/carpets and other floor coverings so that no one trips over them.

If you serve alcoholic drinks at a party, do not leave bottles outside. Empty all partly consumed glasses immediately after the party so that children cannot get to them. Even a small amount of alcoholic drink can cause brain damage and may also prove fatal to a small child.

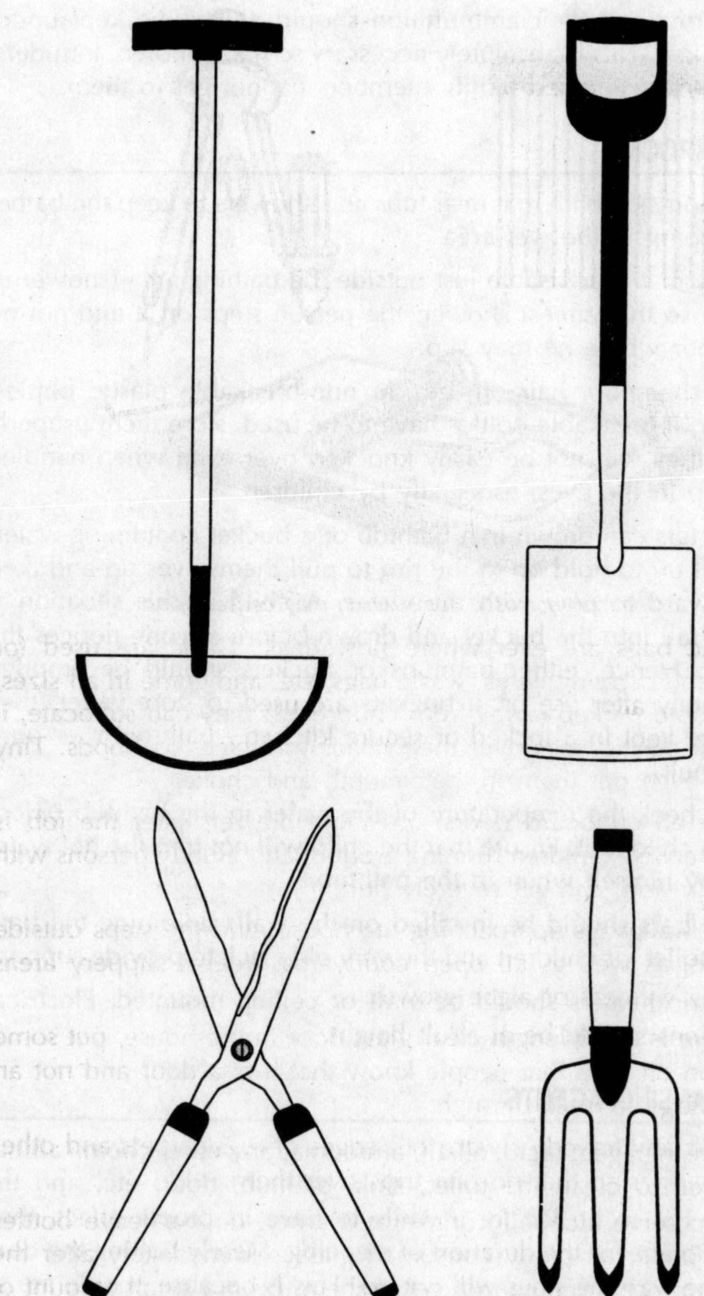

Gardening equipment which can cause injury.

Firearms and their ammunition should always be kept under lock and key. This is absolutely necessary so that children, intruders, and irate, impassioned family members cannot get to them.

❐ BATHROOMS

Place a non-skid bath mat near tubs and showers to keep the bather from slipping in the wet area.

A dry mat is advisable just outside the bathing area (shower or bathtub), so that after a shower, the person steps on it and not on a wet floor where he may slip.

Buy shampoo, hair oil, etc. in non-breakable plastic bottles. However, if breakable bottles have to be used, store them properly so that they will not be easily knocked over even when handled with soap in the eyes, especially by children.

Tiny tots can drown in a bathtub or a bucket containing water. They will try to hold on to the rim to pull themselves up and then lean forward to play with the water. A child in this situation is likely to fall into the bucket and drown before anyone notices the accident. Hence, either bathtubs or buckets should be emptied immediately after use or, if buckets are used to store water, they should be kept in a locked or secure kitchen / bathroom, or on a higher shelf.

Do check the temperature of the water in the bathtub before putting a child in it. Ensure that the child will not turn the hot water tap on by himself when in the bathtub.

Handbars should be installed on the walls adjoining the bath tub and toilet for children and the very old / sick to provide support.

Electric heaters should be wall or ceiling mounted. Electrical connections should be at adult height.

❐ CLEANSING AGENTS

If a cleansing agent (acid, alkali, ammonia, any other chemical) has been used to clean the toilet, sink, bathtub, floor, etc. and the cleanser has to be left for a while to have its proper effect, then lock the place for the duration of cleaning. Merely bolting the door or putting warning sings will not do. This is because people are so used to their bathrooms that they will simply not look at notices but will enter them blindly from sheer habit. Children are more likely to think that they will stay clear of cleansing agent and yet may touch it inadverently or slip in the treated zone on a wet floor.

Most cleansers have a corrosive and harmful effect on the body and even prompt medical treatment does not always remove all the scars caused by these chemicals. Appropriate safety items like gloves, safety goggles, shoes etc. should be worn at the time of their handling. Fresh water and a clean cloth should be kept handy to wipe off any spills on your body.

Many times drain cleansers suddenly erupt out of badly clogged drains probably due to the gas generated by the action of the cleanser on the material clogging the drains, taking the person cleaning the drains by surprise and can seriously injure his face, eyes, hands etc. So keep away from drain opening to ward off such a mishaps when cleansers are used. You must have read in the newspapers that people have died while cleaning manholes or gutters.

Wash several times thoroughly to get rid of even the last traces of cleansers, after finishing your job. Shoes or bathroom slippers worn during washing must also be washed thoroughly to avoid cleanser being carried into other rooms of house. Acid or chemicals used for cleaning the toilet or bathroom must be kept in a locked cabinet, properly labelled.

Children should be strictly kept away from the vicinity of area where strong chemicals are in use or are accessible as the child can spill it over himself or taste it and cause himself serious injury, while you go to answer a phone or a door bell or nature call.

Avoid smelling as the mode of identification of a chemical because several chemicals could smell alike or your sense of smell could be numbed by a cold or other illness.

❐ SAFE HANDLING OF TELEPHONES

—Avoid using the telephone in the bathtub, shower, swimming pool or in the rain as any contact with water could give an electric shock.

—Do not use the phone during any thunder or lightening storms, as far as possible because any electrical surge through the phone wires could cause a shock.

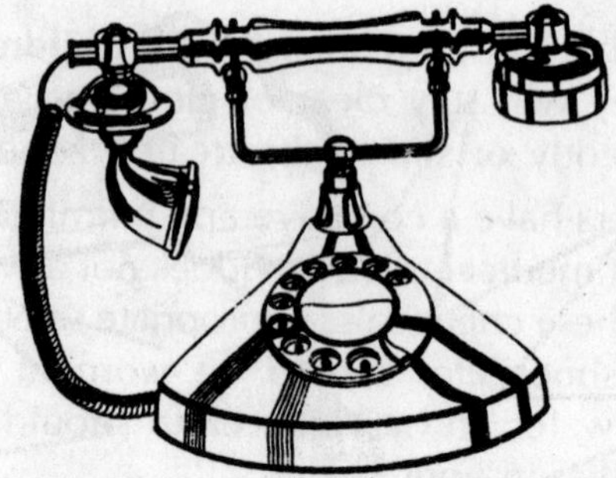

— Avoid using telephones near a running computer as it may malfunction due to electrical signals from telephone.

— Use a phone located away from a gas leak area, as the telephone's electrical contacts could create a tiny spark when you dial which might ignite the gas and cause fire.

❐ KITCHEN SAFETY PRECAUTIONS

A kitchen commonly has sharp knives that can hurt, boiling water or hot food that can scald, and water spills or fruit peels upon which an unsuspecting person can slip or fall. Inflammable materials such as gas, kerosene, matchboxes, cooking oil etc. are also stored in kitchen making it potentially the most danger prone area in a house.

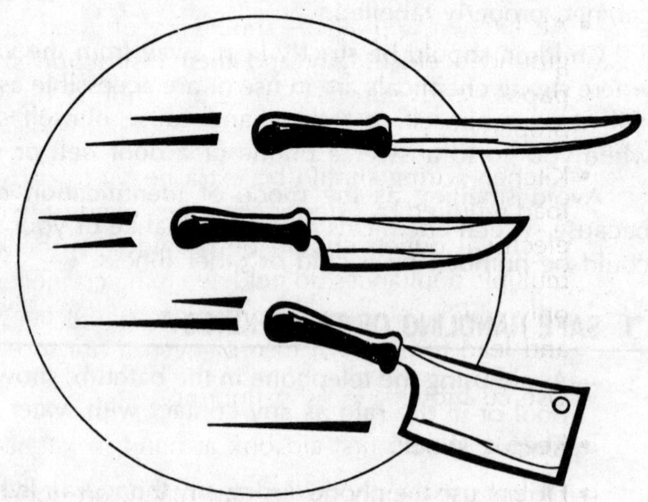

Playing with kitchen knives can cause injury to kids

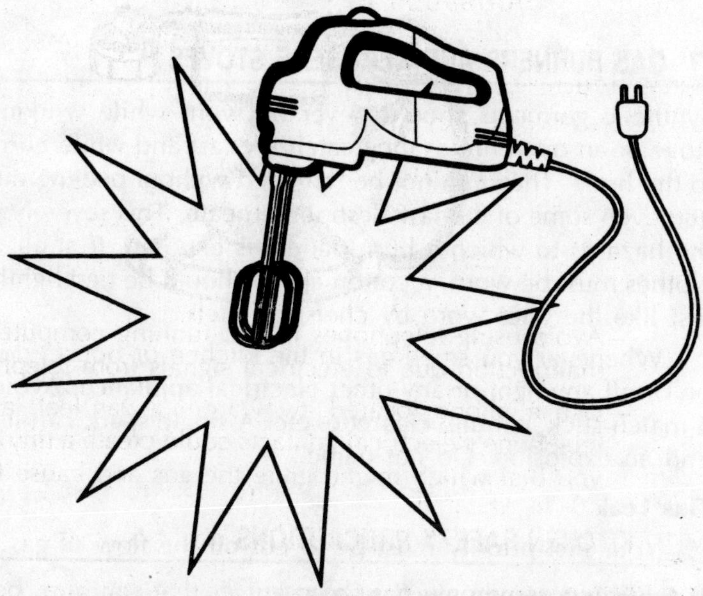

Carelessness can cause injury while using electrical appliances

- Do not allow young children to use the kitchen as a play area even when no cooking is being done.
- Kitchen should be well lit.
- All kitchen appliances should be of good quality, properly grounded electrically and their instruction sheets, warranty papers and purchase receipts should be kept in a file properly.
- Kitchen wiring should be extra heavy to carry the excessive load required by grinders, toasters, ovens, mixers etc. Enough electrical outlets should be provided in the kitchen so that multiple appliances do not have to be connected to one outlet only which can cause overdrawing of current from that outlet and lead to a blown fuse or even a fire too.
- Use cushioned non-slip flooring.
- Keep a locked first-aid box at hand in kitchen.
- Fit bolts that only adults can reach, on doors.

❐ GAS BURNERS AND KEROSENE STOVES

Synthetic garments should never be worn while working near a stove or an open fire as they catch fire fast and while burning stick to the body. They can not be removed without peeling off the skin and even some of the raw flesh underneath. This severely increases the hazards to which a burn patient is exposed. If at all, synthetic clothes must be worn, a cotton apron should be tied tightly on top, just like the ones worn by chefs in hotels.

Whenever you smell gas in the kitchen or house, do not turn on or off any light or any other electrical appliance. Avoid lighting a match-stick, candle, cigarette, etc. A single spark can lead to fire and an explosion. Do not panic.

Gas Leak

Your first priority must be to cut off the flow of gas.

If there is a strong smell of gas

(1) Turn off the main gas tap next to the meter / cylinder.

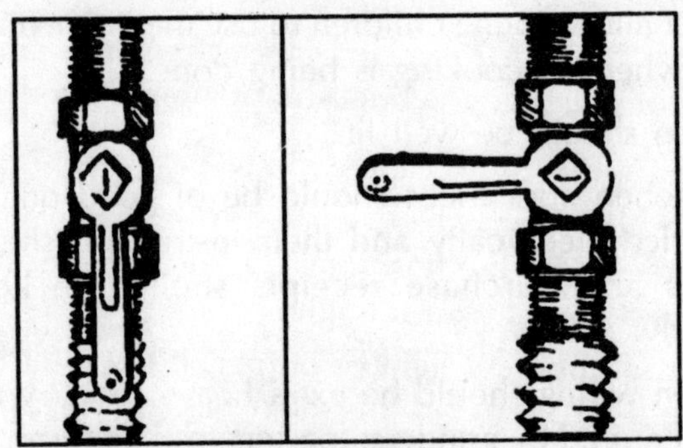

(2) Open doors and windows.

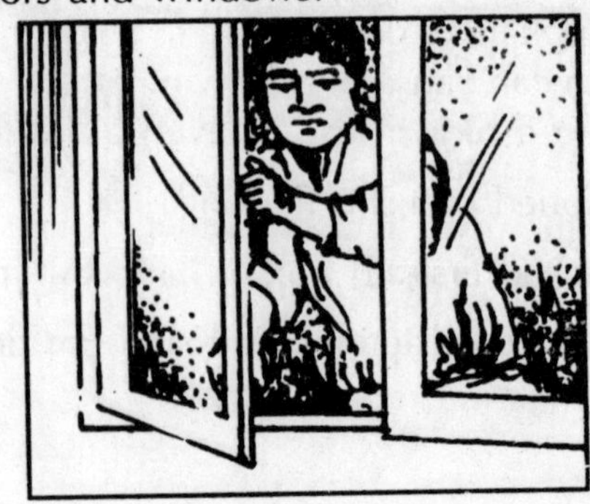

(3) Put out cigarettes or naked flames and switch off electric appliances.

(4) Get the unconscious person into the open air and put him in the recovery position.

(5) Telephone your local area gas office immediately – day or night. Find it under 'Gas' in the phone book.

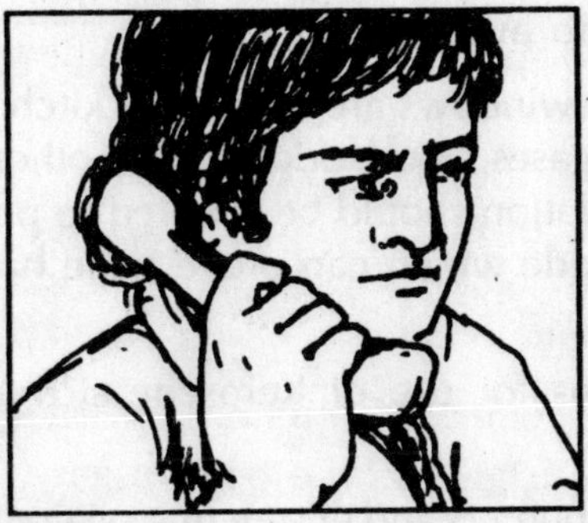

GAS OFFICE

Tel ....

....

....

....

....

- Do not try to trace the leak with a naked flame (Match or lighter).
- Do not enter a room or area where the smell of gas is especially strong. The build-up of fumes may overpower you.

If there is a slight smell of gas

(1) Trace the source immediately. Often the pilot light on a cooker or gas fire has gone out, or a burner on the cooker has blown out in a draught.

(2) Turn off the pilot light or burner. If the pilot light does not have a tap, turn off the main gas tap next to the meter / cylinder.

(3) Put out cigarettes, extinguish naked flames; switch off any electric equipment in the room.

(4) Open doors and windows to let the gas disperse. Wait for the smell to go.

(5) Relight the pilot light or burner.

(6) If the smell persists or returns, telephone your local area gas office immediately — day or night.

(7) Do not attempt repairs yourself.

Gas companies and manufacturers of gas burners give very detailed and informative brochures on the safe use of gas cylinders. These should be followed for installation, testing, use and storage of gas cylinders in the house. The rubber pipe should be visually examined atleast once a week to see that it does not have any crack or that it has not been chewed up by cockroaches etc. It should be replaced frequently to avoid a major leak.

A good vent, exhaust fan or windows are a must for kitchen for the easy dispersal of smoke, gases, food odours and other bad smells. Sufficient fresh air circulation should be ensured to prevent accumulation of carbon monoxide which can prove quite harmful for health.

Following safety precautions for use of Kerosene stoves can prove to be quite beneficial :

(*i*) Avoid using re-soldered burners and ensure that oil container is made of a seamless metal sheet, without any manufacturing defects.

(*ii*) Do not overpump the stoves, lest it bursts and burns people nearby. Preferably operate stoves at medium pressure.

(*iii*) Avoid overheating stoves by long and continuous use.

(*iv*) Do not try to refill them with kerosene while they are ignited or still hot.

(*v*) Avoid placing them on the floor since they can easily get knocked over, especially by children.

(*vi*) Check the joints regularly for leaks.

(*vii*) Avoid using a cooking stove as a room heater because it can be very dangerous and fatal too.

(*viii*) Store kerosene away from stove and other sources of heat.

The handles of pots and pans used during cooking should be turned inwards towards the walls, as hot pans may be knocked down by a child or a cook in hurry, if their handles are jutting out of cooking platform.

Keep matchboxes away from stove and burners. They could catch fire spontaneously.

❐ BLAST INJURY

Explosion in the industries or due to bombs can cause many causalties. The possible injuries will be extensive burns, fractures, damages to ear drums, shock and wounds due to flying glass or other debris.

Management

- Reassure the causalty.
- Move the victim with as little disturbance as possible to a safer place.
- If the casualty's general condition and injuries allow, raise him into a half sitting position with support to his head and shoulders.

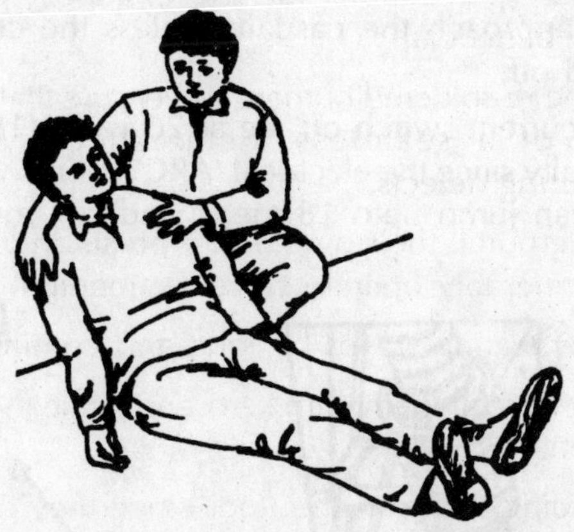

- Loosen any constricting clothing around neck, chest and waist.

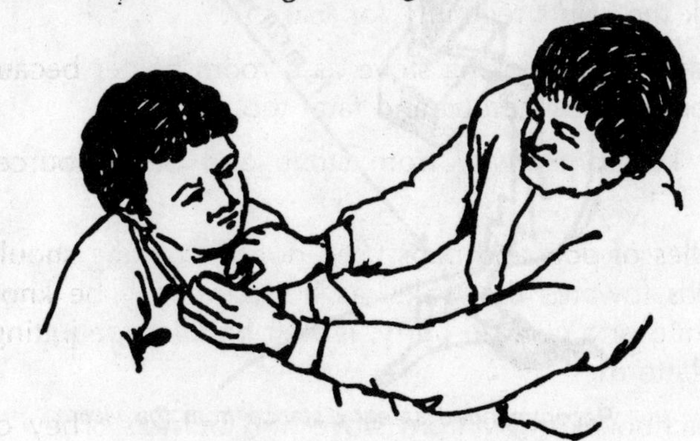

- Control bleeding, wound or burns.
- Immobilize fracture, if any.
- Check breathing and pulse at 10 minutes interval.
- If unconscious open his airway and complete ABC resuscitation.
- Remove to hospital on a stretcher.

❒ ELECTRICAL BURNS

Electrical burns occur due to high voltage industrial machinery and lightening. Much damage occurs at or close to the points of entry and exit.

Management

- Do not approach the casualty unless the current has been switched off.
- Till the current switch-off, be at 20 yards (18 m) away from the casualty since the electrical 'ARC' in high voltage industrial cables can jump upto 18 meter and kill you.

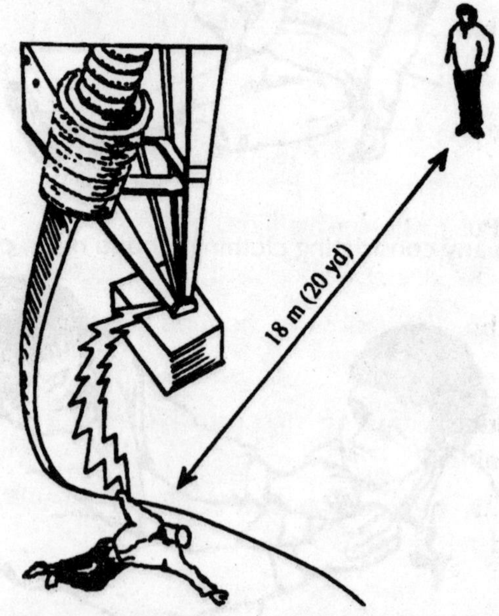

Recommended safety distance from the victim

- Treat as per general burn.
- If breathing and heart actions are affected treat accordingly with complete ABC resuscitation.
- Arrange urgent removal to hospital as a stretcher case.

❒ POISONING

A house contains many substances, such as bleach, insecticides and paint stripper, that are highly dangerous to children. If a child or anybody swallows one, get medical help quickly.

Routes

- Swallowing
- Breathing
- Injection

First-Aid Mangement

(A) **If unconscious** :

- Do not induce vomiting.
- Lie him on his back on hard and flat bed.
- No pillow.
- Turn the head to one side.
- If excessive vomitting :
  - Put to lie on his side.
  - One leg stretched and other leg bent at knee on thigh.
- If breathing slow or stopped : Artificial respiration.

(B) **If conscious:**

- Induce vomiting (If corrosive poisons – do not induce vomiting).
- Plenty of cold water to drink, which will delay absorption and replace fluid loss.
- Milk is good for the purpose.

COMMON POISONS

1. **Aspirin**

   First -Aid : – Induce vomiting
   – Sodium bicarbonate : drink (One table spoonful to a tumbler of water)
   – Strong coffee / tea

2. **Arsenic (Rat poisons)**

   First -Aid : – Induce vomiting

3. **Carbon Monoxide**

   First -Aid : – Artificial respiration.
   – Oxygen inhalation

4. **Sleeping tablets**

   First -Aid : – Induce vomiting (Give Mag. Sulph. 2 tea spoonfuls in a glass of water)
   – Hot Coffee / tea
   – Keep him awake

5. **Mercury** (From teething powder of mercury itself)

   First -Aid : – White of egg in water
   – Then milk
   – Then induce vomiting

6. **Lead** (From hair dyes)

   First -Aid : – Induce vomiting then Mag. Sulph. in water.

7. **Opium and Morphia**

   First -Aid : – Potassium permangante with water : drinking
   – Hot Coffee / tea.
   – Keep the patient awake.

8. **Phosphorus** (match stick head and rat poisons)

   First -Aid : – Induce vomiting.
   – Large quantity of water.
   – Tender coconut.
   – Do not give oils as they dissolve phosphorus.

9. Prussic Acid (used in photography and tender bamboo seeds)

First -Aid : – An emergency
– Start artificial respiration.
– Induce vomiting.

10. Follidol

First -Aid : – Induce vomiting.
– Water or tender coconut drink.
– Artificial respiration.

11. Insecticides

First -Aid : – Vomiting.
– Artificial respiration.

12. Acid

First -Aid : – Do not induce vomiting.
– Water or sodi. bicarb. to drink.

13. Alkalies

First -Aid : – No vomiting
– Water or tender coconut drinks or orange juice.

14. Dettol & Phenol and other disinfectants

First -Aid : – Do not induce vomiting.
– Mag. sulph. : 4 tsf in a litre of water.

If a Child Swallows a Household Chemical

Household substances contain many harmful substances such as bleach, insecticides, paints, etc. Sometimes children out of curiosity swallow, if those substances are within their reach. In such cases :

- Get medical help quickly.
- Try to discover what the substance swallowed is (But remember, the child may become unconscious at any time, so do not waste time unncessarily).
- If conscious, induce vomiting (not in case of corrosives).
- If corrosive and burns, give water or milk to drink.

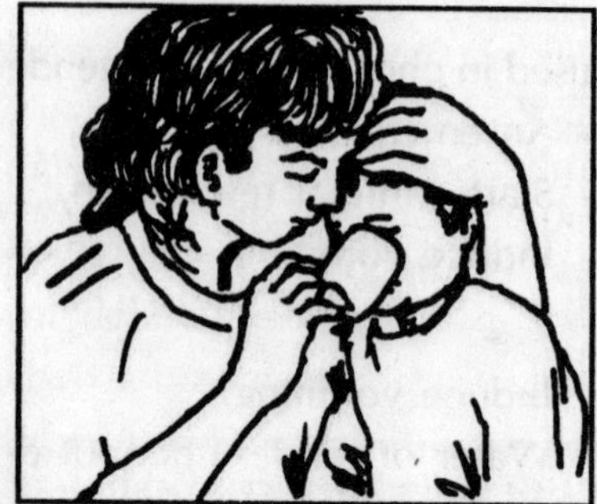

- If unconscious (apply ABC rule if required) place him in recovery position.

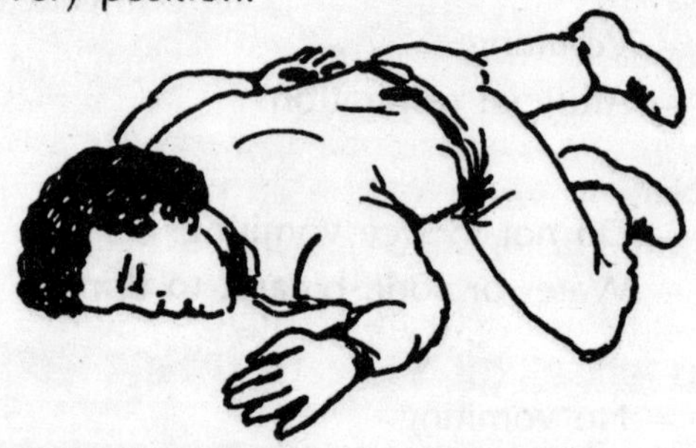

- Remove to hospital as a stretcher case.

Alcohol poisoning

In alcohol posioning the casualty will have the following warning signs.

- Breath will smell alcohol.
- Vomiting.
- Partly conscious or already unconscious.
- Pulse rapid and weak.
- Breathing will be shallow.
- Eyes blood red.
- Pupils may be dilated.

Management

- Maintain an open airway.
- If the casualty becomes unconscious or having vomiting, place in the recovery position so that he does not choke on his vomit. Complete ABC resuscitation if necessary.
- Remove to hospital as a stretcher case.

Industrial Poisoning

In industry, some people may be in contact with dangerous chemicals or gases at their workplaces. Those are grouped as :

(a) *Irritants* e.g., Ammonia, Nitrous fumes etc.

(b) *Asphyxiants* e.g., Carbon dioxide

(c) *Toxic gases* e.g., Carbon monoxide, hydrogen cyanide.

(d) *Toxic vapours* e.g., those given off by volatile chemicals such as carbon-tetrachloride or trichloroethylene.

If the casualty is trapped in an enclosed space, never attempt to rescue, unless you are fully equipped with, and practised in the use of breathing apparatus and life-lines.

Management

- Take the patient to open air
- If required start ABC resuscitation.
- Transport to hospital/medical centre.

Drug Overdose

An overdose of any drug (either an addicative drug or an ordinary medicine) is serious and requires urgent medical treatment. Symptoms of drug overdose include abnormal dilation or contraction of the pupils of the eyes, vomitting, difficulty in breathing, unconsciousness, sweating and hallucinations.

If a person takes a deliberate or accidental overdose

(1) Ask the casulty what has happened. Obtain any information about the drug that you can as soon as possible. The casualty may become unconscious at any time.

- Do not try to induce vomiting. It wastes time and may be harmful.

(2) If the person is unconscious, put him in the recovery position.

(3) Telephone and ask for an ambulance.

(4) Collect a sample of vomit and any bottles or pill containers that are near the casualty. Send them to hospital with the patient, as evidence to assist treatment.

❐ SHOCK

This is a manifestation of changes in which the circulation fails, because either the pressure or volume of circulating blood has fallen to a dangerous level.

This is because the blood flowing to the vital organs is insufficient to keep them supplied with oxygen and functioning. It is a serious condition, which can prove fatal. The body reacts to shock, by diverting available blood to the vital organs (e.g. brain, heart and kidneys) away from less important tissues.

What is Shock ?

Prostration of body arising from sudden exhaustion of vital activities.

❐ CAUSES AND MANAGEMENT

Cause of Shock

- Injury
- Emotion
- Medical emergency (colic, perforation, appendicitis).

Types of shock

(a) Nerve shock

(b) Haemorrhagic shock

(c) Toxic shock

(A) Nerve Shock

Definition. Faintness to complete unconsciousness.

Warning sign

- Pallor
- Beads of sweating
- Over-breathing
- Sensation of heat

Other signs and symptoms

- Cold, pale and clammy skin
- Pulse : feeble
- Breathing : irregular

- Pupils : dilated
- Muscle : Loss of muscle tone

(B) Haemorrhagic Shock

Signs and symptoms

- Face and skin : Pale, cold and clammy
- Blueness : Lips and finger tips
- Pulse : Rapid and feeble
- Respiration : Shallower air hunger
- Pupils : Normal or dilated
- Patient may be (i) apprehensive or restless, or (ii) talkative and abnormally cheerful. In either case unconsciousness may supervene.
- Pain : May not be there.
- Vomiting
- Intense thrist
- If fluid taken in, vomiting may result.

(C) Toxic shock

What causes ?

Poisonous substances formed, which gain entrance to the blood stream and loss of fluid from the blood into the tissues.

❒ SPOILED FOOD

Most cases of food poisoning occur because the food is not suspected to be spoiled as it does not taste or smell bad. So be sure about your food quality.

❒ CHOPPING AND CUTTING

Knives, forks, scissors etc. should be properly kept in the storage tray only and one should be careful while cleaning them. The cutting and sharp edges should be on the inside and their handles on the outside in the storage tray or on the storage shelf so that they can be easily picked up by their handles.

❒ FREEZER FOOD

If the power goes off for a long time, the frozen food will thaw in the freezer. Avoid refreezing this food since harmful bacteria might germinate. If the food has thawed, cook it straightway or dispose it or get some ice to keep the food frozen continuously.

❒ IF BURNT, POUR WATER

Do not ever try to run if your clothes catch fire since it will only fan the fire. Immediately drop to the floor and roll or cover yourself with a blanket to put out the fire.

If burnt, pour water over the affected area till the pain subsides. Tap water can be used, to cool the skin surface and reduce damage done by heat. Contact a doctor or a hospital soon.

❒ PLASTIC AND GLASS CONTAINERS

Plastic contains numerous chemicals, solvents, plasticizers etc. and in order to cut corners, some dubious manufactures use cheaper, harmful ingredients in disproportionate amounts which can later badly affect the food and contaminate it. They are generally good for dry food and wrapped food but not necessarily for liquids, juices, syrups etc. unless they are certified by a government body, for such usage. Whenever a new utensil is used for the first time, do remove all the labels and wash the new utensil in soap and plenty of hot water to remove any temporary polish on it or any traces of chemicals last used on them in the factory. Utensils with enamel coating inside should not be used for cooking since it may contain harmful chemicals and lead which will continue to leach out i.e. get into food in small traces over the life span of utensil because of the high temperature needed for cooking and their reaction with spices, lime and other ingredients used in cooking.

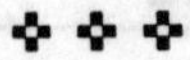

CHAPTER

2

Safety of 'DEAR' Children

Children are generally unaware of the dangers posed by different items and situations. They need special protection and extra guidance in all their activities during their initial years.

Children tend to go to kitchen frequently as the mother is mostly there and the father and older children are out of the house. The child needs attention and the mother is the best source, so the continuous attempts to enter kitchen. Kitchen, as we all know, has a lot of hazardous activities going an like boiling, frying, cutting, grinding, crushing, scrubbing etc. and an innocent child can grab the knife, sweets jar, steaming kettle, the fork, cups etc. He may try

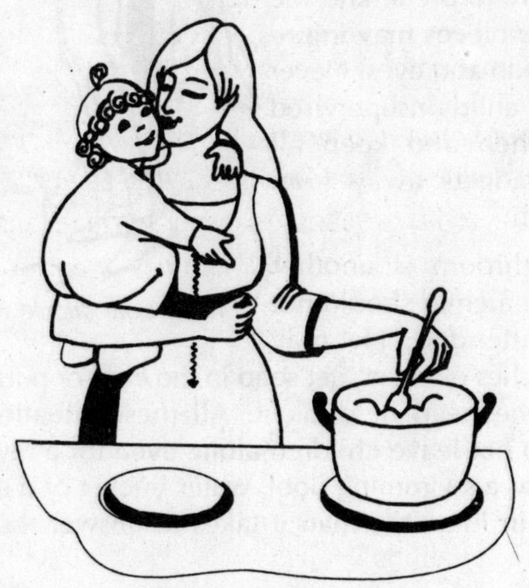

Avoid preparing food while holding a baby in your arms.

to open boxes or containers and would like to taste what they contain (even pepper, red hot chilies, spices etc).

The child enjoys emptying the containers an floor, mixing their contents, playing with them and may even put harmful things in his eyes or mouth or rub on his body.

Avoid any cooking while holding a baby in your arms as the child may try to jump on to the stove or may feel giddy with all the pungent smells and the fumes.

Avoid holding a hot drink in your hand, with a child in your hand as the child can in a fraction of a second try to grab the item, which may scald the child and even yourself.

The table cloth should not be left hanging too low as the child may hold and pull it down, bringing all the dishes down and also hurting himself. Do avoid allowing a child move around freely with a glass milk bottle is his hand because should the child fall, the bottle is most likely to break and the broken glass pieces may injure the child's skin and eyes. Never ever leave a child unsupervised in the kitchen and keep all electrical gadgets away from child's reach.

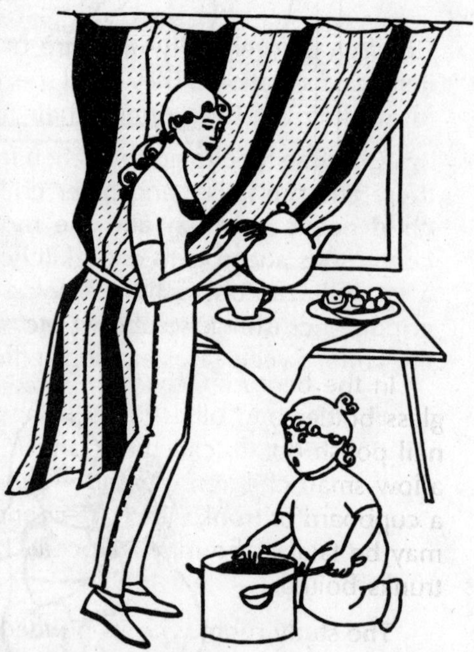

Table cloth should not hang too low.

The bathroom is another place where a child should not be left unattended. He may drown in inches of water, get soap in the eyes or pour toilet cleansing fluid over the head or drink it. All these situations can be very harmful. Do not leave children alone even for a few seconds in the bathtub, near a swimming pool, water bucket or a toilet bowl. They can drown in less time than it takes to answer the telephone or a door bell.

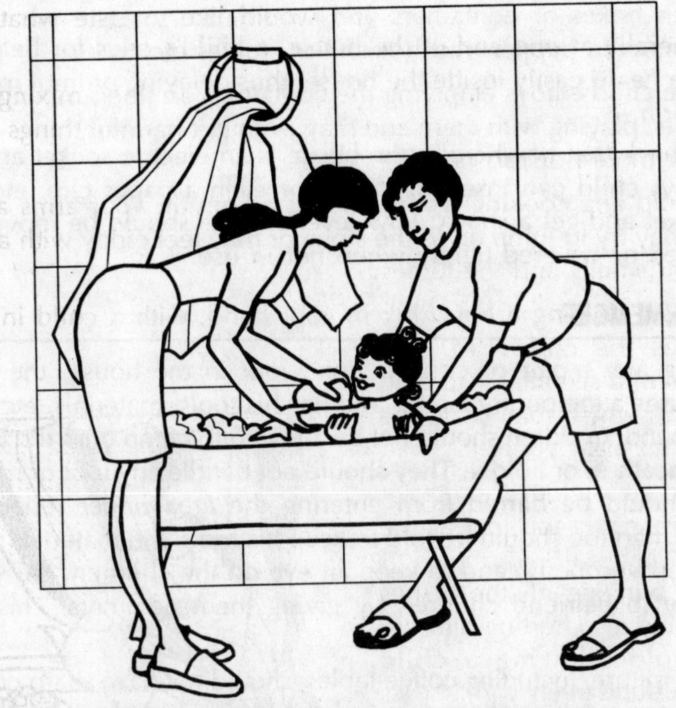

Don't leave children unattended in a bathroom.

In the bedroom, the dressing table is very inviting with all its glass bottles and other fancy things. Anything made of glass, e.g. nail polish bottle, can break and injure a child. Therefore, do not allow small children there alone. A child can also lock himself in a cupboard or trunk which he cannot open easily from inside. This may be fatal as he may suffocate. Hence, keep all cupboards and trunks bolted.

The study room with its pointed pencils, pens, ball-point pens, ink bottles, pins, paper clips, and other such items can also be quite inviting to a child. Yet, all of these items can hurt a curious child. So do not leave these items on the table when you are not using them. Keep them in a drawer.

Do not let the child stay alone in storeroom, workshop or a garage. These places are generally full of a variety of potentially dangerous items, tools and gardening equipment. He can get badly hurt in numerous ways. Furthermore, as the workshop or the garage is generally at one end of the house, a child's cries for help may not be heard easily inside the house, thus delaying prompt medical attention.

Check that nowhere in the house is an electric socket at a low level. A child can insert his finger or even a paper clip, etc. into a socket and get a shock. Low level sockets should be moved up, plugged or covered tightly when not in use.

❐ REMEMBER

During any repair or construction work in the house, the repair man uses a temporary ladder and has his tools, materials, etc. lying all around. Children should not be allowed to climb onto the ladder, sit beneath it, or hold it. They should not handle any tool or material and should be barred from entering the area under repair. The repair man too should be told to keep his tools and materials within sight and properly, and to keep an eye on the children. He should not try to befriend children by giving them hammers, chisels or nails, etc.

Furniture, including coffee-tables, should not have sharp corners. Their corners as well as edges should be rounded since children are likely to fall upon them while running around. For the same reason, do not use a glass-top table if a child can reach it.

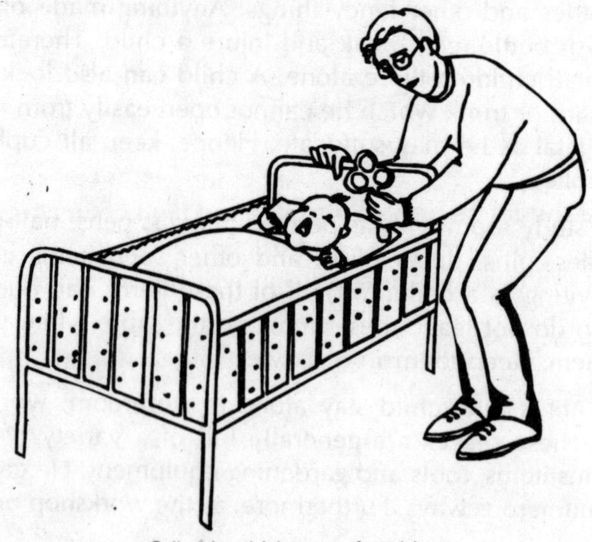

Crib should be comfortable.

There should be no locks or bolts on the inside of the doors to children's rooms. If a small child bolts or locks himself in, he may not be able to unlock the door and may get hysterical or frightened.

Nowadays most parents use cribs, playpens, strollers, walkers, and high chairs for their young children. Ensure these are made safe for them.

Check that there is no space in a crib around the mattress for a child to insert his head and suffocate. If a child can stand up, see that he will not fall out of the crib. In a crib there should be no toys with strings as strings can strangulate a child.

In a playpen, no side should be down when the child is in it. The sides should be at least 50 cm high. The playpen should be stable and not fold accidentally or collapse on any side.

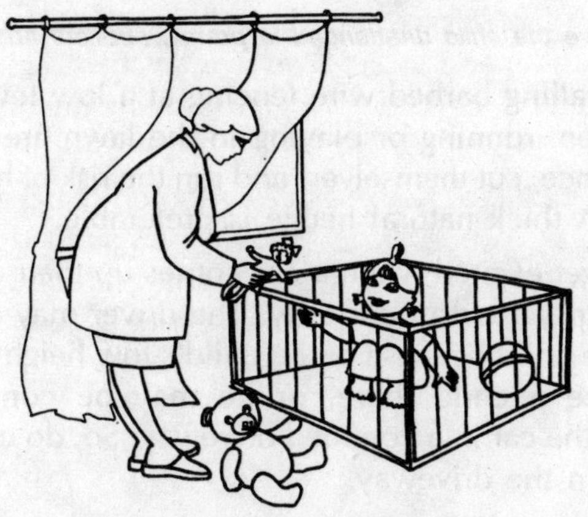

Playpen should be safe.

There should be belts in strollers and high chairs to prevent the child from falling over. The construction of these items should be such that the child's clothes or skin will not be pinched, sheared, or cut.

Walkers, carriages and strollers should have brakes that cannot be released by the child.

Do not leave infants unattended in prams, strollers and walkers as they may slide down a ramp, or the child, if able to walk, may wander off and get lost.

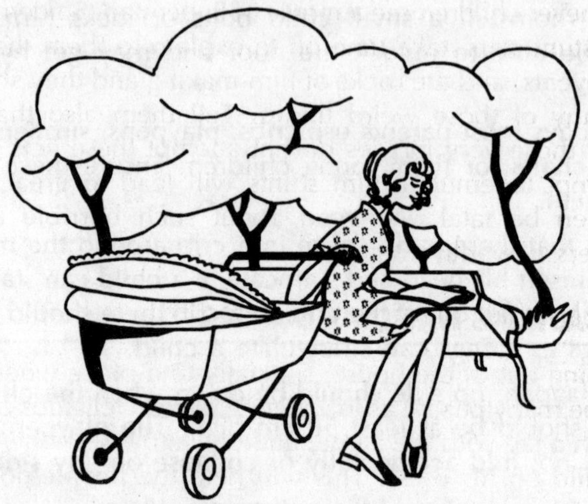

Don't leave the child unattended in prams, strollers and walkers.

Avoid installing barbed wire fencing at a low level around the house. Children, running or playing in the lawn are very likely to run into the fence, cut themselves, and run the risk of heavy bleeding and tetanus. A thick natural hedge is preferable.

Children get excited when a car comes up their driveway, and they run towards it out of curiosity. The driver may not always be able to see the child because of the child's low height, also he least excepts to see a child there, or he may be concentrating on manoeuvring the car in a confined driveway. So, do not let children play near or in the driveway.

Do not let small children handle marbles. airgun bullets, beads, small stones, gravel, knives, forks, scissors, toothpicks, sewing or injection needles, pins, drawing pins, etc. These can cause serious injuries. A round object could also get lodged in the throat, nose, or ear. A child should not put a spoon handle, pencil, or even a plastic straw used to sip cold drinks in his mouth and run around the house. If he hits a wall or falls down, the item can damage the back of the palate. There is no easy cure for this and the recovery is slow and rather painful.

Small children should not handle an umbrella, either open or closed. Umbrellas have been known to cause injuries to the eye. Therefore, always put them on an upper shelf, or hang them high, out of the reach of young children.

Whenever children see a movie of Superman, Spiderman, WWF, or other stunt stars, take time off to explain to them that these are not real events, and are tricks of film-making and they should never attempt any of those weird things. Tell them also that even the heroes of those very movies do not attempt these acts in real life. Any attempt to emulate film stunts will lead to great harm, and could even be fatal. We read about such horrible attempts in newspapers nowadays regularly.

❐ PRECAUTIONS IN CROWDED AREAS

When going out of the house, specially to a place where there are likely to be many people as in wedding parties, religious celebrations, etc. attach a tag with the name, address, and telephone/fax number of the child on his dress. This will help the people/police restore your child to you should he get separated/lost.

Label the child's clothes and school bag with the name on the inside where it is not visible to strangers. A stranger could, after reading the name, strike a conversation with the child convincing him that the stranger is a family friend and may mislead the gullible child.

Instruct children not to accept gifts from anyone, nor invitations to parties from mere acquaintances.

If the child expresses any fear about particular persons or a place, listen to him carefully and draw out the entire story. Take necessary steps to improve the situation. Do not underestimate or brush aside a child's fears. He has no one else to go to and talk about them.

Keep a list of names and phone numbers of your child's friends and their parents. It would also help to keep a list of the teachers' names and phone numbers, and the school office phone number.

Children should be trained not to hitch-hike or accept a ride with anyone they do not know, even if told that the child's parents are hurt and want to meet the child. The child should tell the person to contact the school principal.

Children should not listen to any adult who wants them to keep a secret from their parents. They should inform their parents if any adult wants to take their picture, give them a gift or money, even if the adult is known to them. They should seek their parents' permission.

Girls should not wear a *chunni* wrapped around the neck. It can choke them during play, or it may get accidentally caught in the wheels while riding on a scooter, motor cycle, escalator, or a bicycle.

The above instructions should be augmented by one's own experiences and the advice of elders. Sharing information with neighbours also proves mutually beneficial.

❐ TOYS

Children need toys as much as they need parental love. However, before buying a toy, some thought should be given to the kind of toy to buy, depending upon the age of the child, so that the toy to buy, depending upon the age of the child, so that the toy will not only be fun but also safe. Toy industry sources agree that making toys safe will not increase the cost to the consumer. What are needed are toy safety laws as well as a consumer movement to ensure their enforcement.

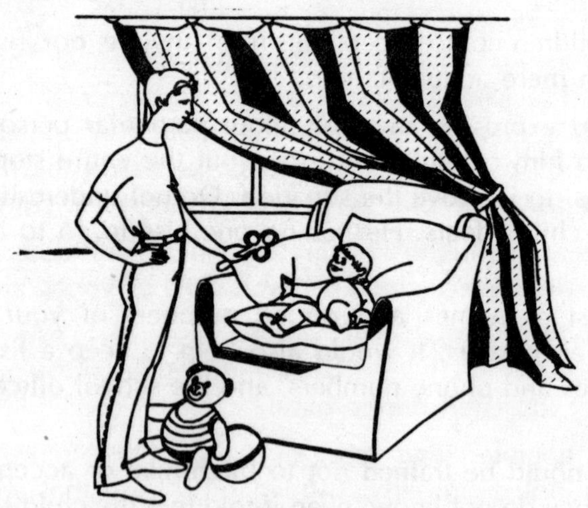

Toys should be safe and comfortable.

All toys and play equipment must be of good quality, installed correctly and maintained properly. Children must be taught how to use them safely.

Toy packaging should not have any staples since in the excitement of opening the packet, a child can be hurt by it. Further, a loose staple lying on the floor can injure someone's foot. Even worse, an infant may try to eat it or may put it into the eyes.

Adults should read the directions for use on all the toys they buy and explain them to children.

Toy should not have any sharp edges or corners lest they hurt, cut or pierce the skin, eyes, nose, ears, etc. Parents should check the toy cupboard periodically for broken toys which should be discarded right away.

A rusty toy should be discarded because it can cause tetanus if it cuts the skin.

No arrows, rubber or plastic balls, or sparks should come out of toy-guns and pistols since they have the potential to cause grave injury, sometimes irreversible or sometimes fatal. Do not permit bows and arrows for the same reasons.

Tops having sharp pointed spikes or nails can hurt a child's eye or skin. Do not let small children play with them.

Toys should not be very small, nor have tiny removable parts that can get into the nose or ear, or be swallowed.

Do not buy toys which make a noise when shaken. They may contain small pebbles or lead shots. Should the toy break open, an infant or a toddler may try to gobble the pebbles and lead shots, and may even choke on them. For the same reason the tiny tots should not be allowed to play with pebbles, marbles, coins, etc.

Make sure that the button eyes on teddy bears and dolls are not loose. If they come off, they could be swallowed by young children.

Be careful with toys that require home assembly. Ensure that a child cannot disassemble them. Check frequently that the nuts and screws have not loosened during play.

Electrically operated toys may give a shock if immersed in water or not handled properly. Instead buy those that work on batteries.

Small children love to wrap things around their necks. Toys with long strings may thus cause strangulation of a child in some unexpected situations.

The paint or coating on toys should not contain any dangerous chemicals. Some of the chemicals to be avoided are : ammonium nitrate, asbestos, lithium hydroxide, copper sulphate, selenium, chromium, barium, mercury, and all lead-based chemicals.

If a toy is such that a child will be tempted to stand on it, whether or not the toy is meant for this purpose, rest assured that he will try to stand on it! If it is an unstable toy, the child will fall and hurt himself badly. This includes toys such as tricycles, stools, etc. Sometimes, if a toy, a table or a chair is close to a window, it might entice a child to step on it to see the view outside. This may lead to a fall from the window. Such items should not be left near windows, or the windows should be kept locked or have grills/panes.

Teach older children to keep toys meant for them away from the younger ones. Encourage children to check and correct each other when unsafe measures are adopted at play. They can exchange their experiences and help each other.

Buy only those toys that are not hazardous for even the youngest member of the family.

Do not let your children use low profile riding toys such as plastic tricycles outside the house since these are too low to be seen by approaching cars. The plastic design also makes for poor traction, thus making the tricycle hard to manoeuvre or stop.

Skateboards excite a lot of youngsters but they generally do not know how to use them safety. A lot of accidents are caused by these. Proper protective equipment (non-slip shoes, hip, elbow and knee padding, helmet, special gloves, padded jackets) should be used.

All outdoor play equipment should be kept in good shape. This applies to swings, slides, see-saws, merry-go-rounds, etc. These should not be rusted, nor should they have sharp edges or corners, etc. The safe use of such equipment should be taught to children.

Games and toys should be stored safely. Ideally, the storage chest should have no lid. If it must have one, a sliding lid that will not cover a child if he falls into the chest, or one whose cover will remain open in any position, is preferable. The chest should have ventilation holes that will not be blocked if it is placed next to a wall. These holes can provide life-saving air should a child be trapped inside.

If a truck or other container is being used as a toy chest, remove the lid altogether to avoid the danger of a child falling in and the lid closing on him.

It is likely that with more sophisticated toys coming into the market, some specific precautions need to be taken. For this, it is essential that the instructions accompanying the toy be read and understood thoroughly.

Nowadays markets are flooded with imported toys especially Chinese make which are dirt cheap and attractively packaged but they are highly hazardous, unsafe, non-standard apart from most of them being of very inferior quality. We should avoid buying them.

Do not leave your child unattended at the beach. He can drown.

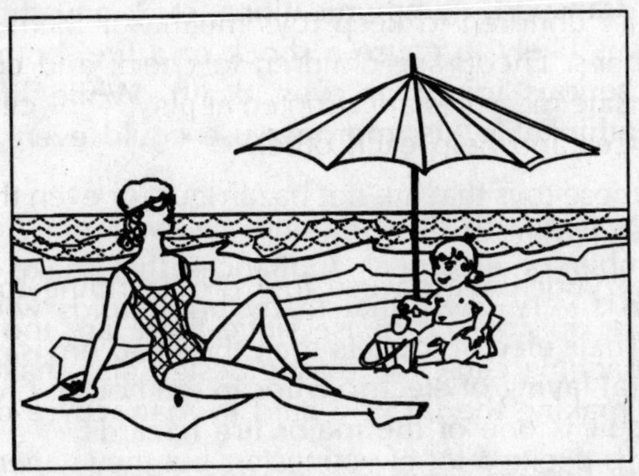

Keep your tiny tot away from pets and stray animals. They may bite or may even be carrying some infection.

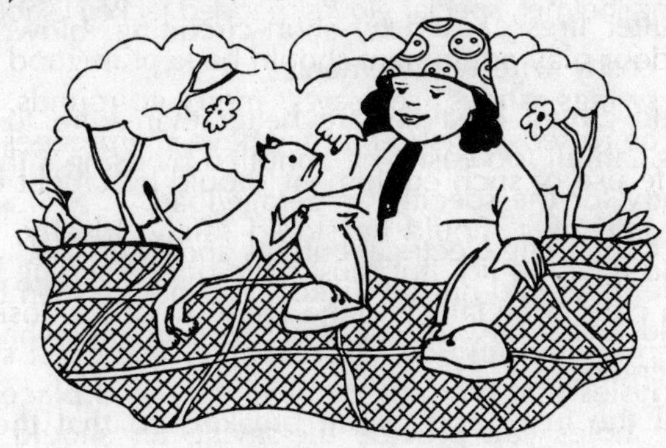

❖ ❖ ❖

CHAPTER 3

Electricity and Fire : Friends or Foes?

As we all know, electricity is a good servant but a real bad master. While it can be used to provide comfort in various ways (light, heat, cooking, transport, communications, etc.), any slight misuse or carelessness is likely to cause a shock or a fire, both of which can result in serious injury or even death. While life without electricity is unthinkable, its improper use could even make you loose your life.

With higher standards of living and the availability of an ever increasing number of electrical appliances that make life more comfortable, it is very likely that many households will connect more items to their electric outlets than they had envisaged at the time of the initial laying of electric wires in the house. Overloading an electric circuit is one of the major fire hazards.

Poor quality fixtures, improper maintenance and repairs can lead to electric shocks. Hence, it is prudent to put in extra-thick wire for the anticipated loads right at the beginning instead of having to suffer fires caused by short-circuiting, blown fuses, or undertaking costly wire replacements.

Automatic circuit breakers are better than wire fuses whose effectiveness can all too easily be annulled by using a thicker wire than necessary for the specific amperage/load.

The box containing electrical cutouts and fuses should be easily approachable. It should not be locked. All mature members of the family should know how to use the fuse-box and what to do in times of emergency.

Label all the fuses and circuit breakers so that the room or appliance to which each is connected is easily identifiable.

This comes in handy during an emergency. Do not rely on your memory.

There should be a main switch for each room so that it can be used in case of an emergency. Having to run to the main switch for the entire house, which may be located on a floor other than the one where the emergency has arisen, could be difficult. This could have a fatal effect because in electrical emergencies even seconds count.

Do not play with electric switches. Some of the poorer quality ones may become loose or get broken, and when used give a shock. Any cracked, broken, or exposed switch, plug, or socket must be replaced right away.

On all electric appliances, 3-wire plugs should be used. The electrical ground or earth should be a definite one and not a superfluous one. With sophisticated and costly electronic items and personal computers, etc. being used these days, the need for proper earthing has become more important.

❒ EXTENSION CORDS

Any extension cord used should be quite capable of taking the current it is supposed to carry. It should not dangle or be left to run on the ground. Wires left like this can be hazardous to small children, elderly people, or those with poor sight. They may trip and fall. Therefore, the choice of an electric cord, and its proper installation are very important.

Do not use an extension cord permanently. Get a regular line laid, or change the location of the fixture, so that an extension cord is not necessary.

The cord should not lie over wet or hot surface. Nor should electrical wires lie under mats, carpets, or in the doorways where they are likely to get crushed and their insulation cracked, leading to short-circuit fires and electrical shock.

Sometimes, at public and family functions, there are several electric cords connected to microphones, video cameras, audio cassette recorders, projectors, lights, etc. that trail on the floor. The users of these equipment generally move around with the cords in tow. This can cause an unexpected nasty fall.

Temporary lighting is used for marriages, religious functions, large meetings, etc. One should not string bare wires or wires with cracked insulation on tree tops as live wires can cause fires and electrical breakdowns, short circuits, electrocution, etc. Ensure use of properly insulated and standard wire and hang it very carefully.

❐ ELECTRICAL APPLIANCES : A MODERN BOON ?

The instruction booklets for operation and maintenance of electrical as well as other appliances should be readily available in case the need arises, or if spare parts have to be ordered. The following precautions are a must too.

Every time you clean or empty a blender, mixer, grinder, toaster, power-lawn mower, etc. switch it off and pull the cord out of the power socket so that it is no longer connected to the power supply. This is to ensure that no one knowingly or unknowingly turns the power on while you are cleaning it.

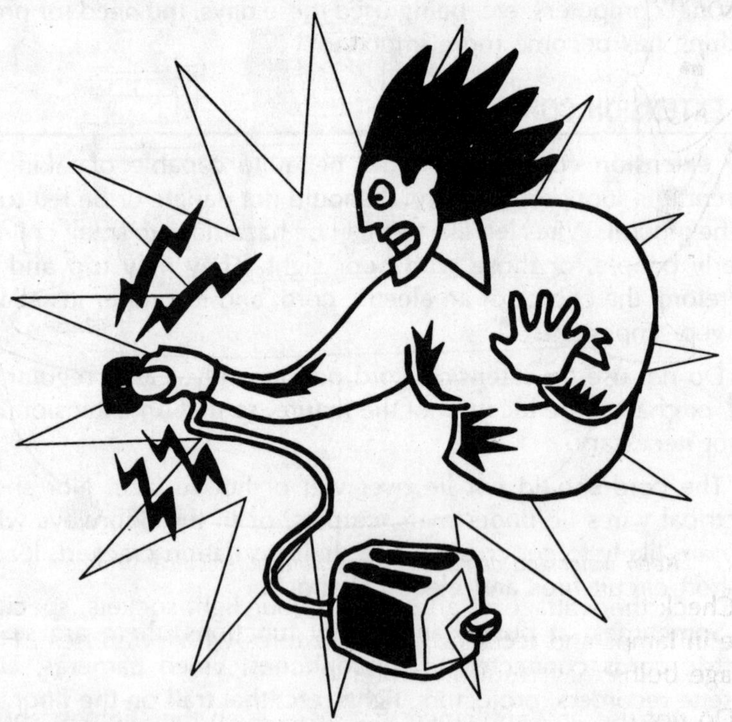

Ensure your hands are dry before using electrical appliances.

Before using any electrical appliance, or turning the switches on and off, make sure that your hands are dry. Remember, water is an excellent conductor of electricity.

Connect only one appliance to one socket. This will ensure that when one appliance is switched on, another does not get switched on at the same time. Also the current drawn will be within limits and no excessive heat will be produced which could melt the wire insulation or cause a fire.

Always use a plug, and not bare wire ends in a socket. The bare wire could become loose and give a shock, or it could cause sparking and fire.

Keep water (and any dampness) away from all electrical fixtures. Do not use any appliance with wet hands or while standing on a wet floor.

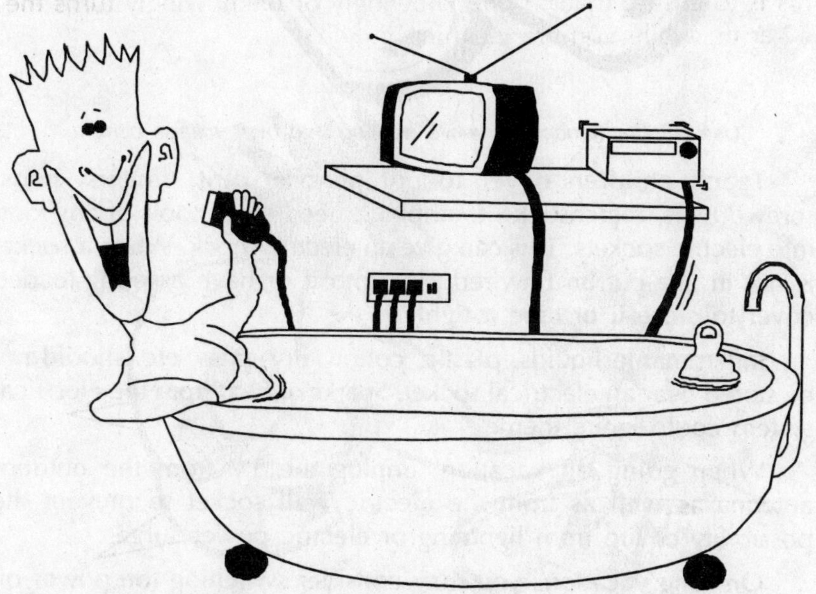

Keep water and dampness away from all electrical fixtures

Check the wattage of all bulbs in your light sockets, specially those in lamps and recessed ceiling fixtures which trap heat. High wattage bulbs may result in a fire.

Do not use any appliance that gives even the slightest shock. Get it repaired and tested by a professional. It is advisable to have an electric leak detector at home and test appliances and plugs periodically, or whenever leakage is suspected.

To prevent electrical shocks, always use insulated tools with plastic or non-metallic castings and handles.

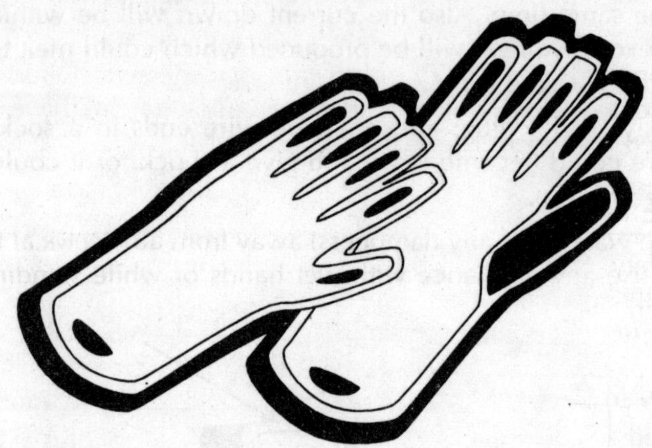

Use Rubber handgloves while working with high voltage current.

Teach children never to put pencils, pins, fingers, pens, screwdrivers, matchsticks, toothpicks, needles, or tools of any kind into electric sockets. This can give an electric shock. When a socket is not in use put an unwired plug into it or have a spring-loaded cover to close it or tape it tighly.

Inflammable liquids, plastic, cotton, dry grass, etc. should not be stored near an electrical socket. Sparks or heat from the electrical system could ignite them.

When going on vacation, unplug the TV from the outdoor antenna as well as from the electric wall socket to prevent the possibility of fire from lightning or electric power surges.

On long vacations you may consider switching the power off from the mains itself, specially if the wiring is old. However, this may not be possible if refrigerators, electric alarms, etc. are to be left operating.

Do not place the TV or any other major electrical appliance close to a wall or near furniture. Allow sufficient space for air circulation so that the heat generated by the appliance can be dissipated.

For the same reason, do not cover the air vents in these appliances with cloth or paper or plastic when they are in use. The covering material as well as the appliance can catch fire.

Do not put any liquid or any food item on the TV. Spills can seep through the vents and cause a fire or shock as well as damage the TV.

Do not expose the TV set to rain or excessive humidity. This can lead to shock or a fire. If water does get in, have the TV examined by a repair person before using it.

❐ FIRE HAZARDS

Fire safety features have to be strictly designed into buildings especially high-rise ones. Hence, architects, structural engineers, construction people, interior designers, city authorities, and the owners of buildings should all be interested in precautions against fire. They should follow all the applicable building codes and approved practices.

The ever-increasing incidences of fires in multi-storeyed buildings are a dangerous trend.

A house has a lot of inflammable items in the form of gas, liquids and solids. Some of these are cooking gas, matchboxes, gasoline or petrol, kerosene, nail polish remover, paints and thinners, furniture polish and wax, cigarette lighter fuel, oil, any kind of plastic, clothes, specially synthetic ones, rugs, upholstered furniture, wood panelling etc.

A single match is enough to start a fire

The above list is not an exhaustive one but it should give an idea that, except for concrete and metal, the rest can catch fire easily. One should, therefore, take all the necessary steps to avoid fires, detect them, fight them, and escape from them safely should the need arise.

The safety nuggets given below will help reduce the chances of fire and also in fighting a fire should one break out.

Fire in the kitchen

Do not store cookies, candy, etc. above the cooking range or stove. Children will try to get to them even if the stove is hot and in use. They are likely to get burnt.

Do not use the oven for storing pans containing oil leftover after being used for frying or for storing of utensils. It is very likely that someone will turn the oven on to warm it without first looking inside to check for the stored items. This may cause a fire.

Inflammable items

Inflammable liquids, cardboard boxes, rags, etc., should be stored away from heaters, furnaces, cooking ranges, stoves, and even from direct sunlight.

Do not use or store aerosol cans near open flames or near a source of heat, including sunlight. The increased pressure in the can due to the heat-induced expansion of the gas inside will result in an explosive rupture, throwing pieces all around. This could hurt people and property, and the contents of the ruptured can, if inflammable, could ignite causing a fire. For the same reasons, do not puncture or incinerate an aerosol container even when empty since some amount of gas will always be there.

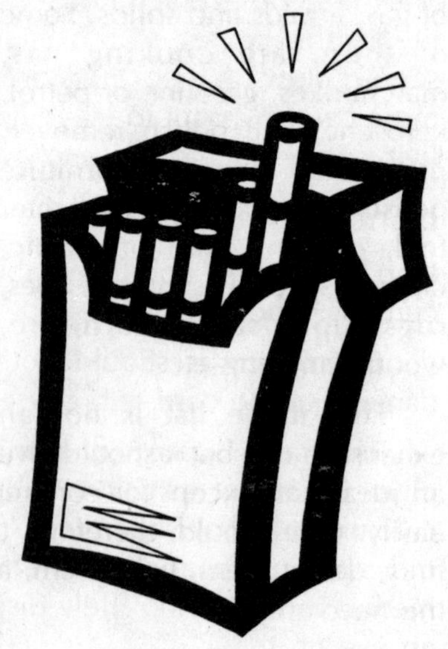

Do not let drapes, furniture, newspapers, other reading material that are combustible near the stove or near an electric room heater. Ensure that even a breeze cannot bring any of these near an open fire or a very hot surface.

Cigarettes

Do you know that the temperature in a cigarette can be over 900°C and when a puff is drawn (which brings in the air), it

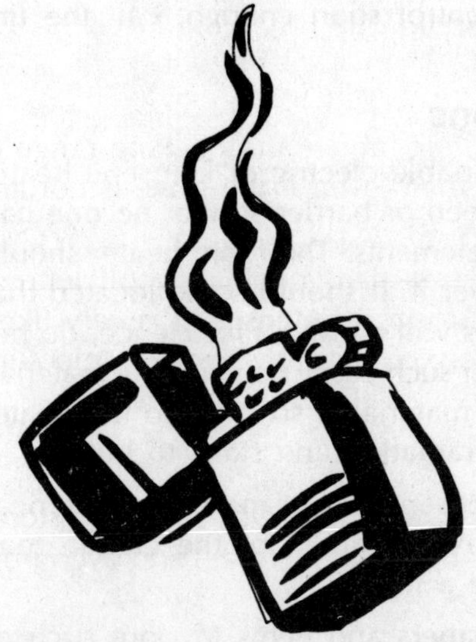

Items like a lighter should not be given to children as they can start a fire while playig with it

can shoot upto 1200°C. Such a high temperature can ignite most of the materials and hence, one should be extremely careful about the disposal of cigarette butts. Even guests should be requested not to smoke in bed.

Keep cigarette lighters and matchboxes out of reach of children. They may be tempted to try to use them. This may cause a serious fire in the house, or the child's clothes may catch fire causing serious burns. If there are smokers in the family, then one has to be more careful as not to leave lighters and matches in the bathroom, living room, bedrooms, etc. within the easy reach of children.

Upholstered Furniture

If possible, select non-flammable fabric for upholstered furniture and curtains. Place the upholstered furniture away from sources of heat.

Electric cords should not go underneath furniture since any damage to the cord can cause a short-circuit fire or give a shock.

The major cause of furniture catching fire is a smoldering cigarette or hot ash. It usually happens when the smoker is not careful, feels drowsy, or keeps an ashtray on the furniture itself. The old, the infirm and people under the influence of alcohol or medication may not safely dispose of a cigarette butt or ash. Keep an eye on them.

Toxic gases from a furniture fire can cause suffocation. If the fire cannot be brought under control soon enough, call the fire brigade and rush outdoors.

Common Useful Precautions

If there is a fireplace or a portable electric or kerosene heater in a room, there should be a screen or barrier so that no one can directly touch the fire or the hot elements. The room heater should be so placed that no one trips over it. It should be so located that it does not get knocked over. This will cause a fire. Hence, do not place it over rugs, carpets and other such easily combustible material. Also ensure that no combustible material is so close to the heater that the material gets heated by radiation and starts to burn.

Never place oil lamps, incense sticks, candles, on or near combustible materials. These may fall down or the candle may burn down to its base and cause a fire.

Every house has important papers and items to store such as house plans, house deeds, insurance policies, passports, cash, jewellery, adoption papers, wills, property transaction papers, bank papers, important medical documents, horoscopes, school certificates, college degrees, etc. These should be kept in a fire-proof filing cabinet which can withstand heat from a fire for several hours. Such cabinets should also be strong enough to withstand a fall of several metres if the floor gives in. Such papers are irreplaceable and hence the extra cost of such a filing cabinet is well-justified. Duplicates of all the papers should be maintained at other premises for safety's sake e.g. in your office, at a friend's or relative's house.

Fire poses a severe threat in high-rise buildings since smoke rises up and the fire spreads rather fast to the upper floors. Hence, install smoke detectors and fire alarms on each floor.

Escape Plans

There should be an escape plan from the house in case of a fire. It should take various scenarios into account in the sense that a fire could be in any one or more sections of the house simultaneously. Hence, one may need several alternate plans. Practise the plans frequently to keep everyone aware, and paste an escape plan in the guest-room as well.

Children are likely to hide under a bed, inside a closet, or in a bathroom in case of fire. They should be told that these are not safe places in such situations.

All windows and doors that have security bars should open easily from inside to provide a means of escape in case of a fire.

Fire Extinguishers

Fire extinguishers are very handy for putting out small fires. Each house should have at least one. It should be recharged as recommended by the manufacturer. No one should try to save on the cost of such recharging since a false sense of security in an antiquated fire extinguisher is worse than not having one at all.

The use of the fire extinguisher should be taught and demonstrated to household personnel capable of handling such a unit which may weigh a couple of kilograms. However, if mishandled, the carbon dioxide or other gases released from a fire extinguisher can choke a person and cause significant harm.

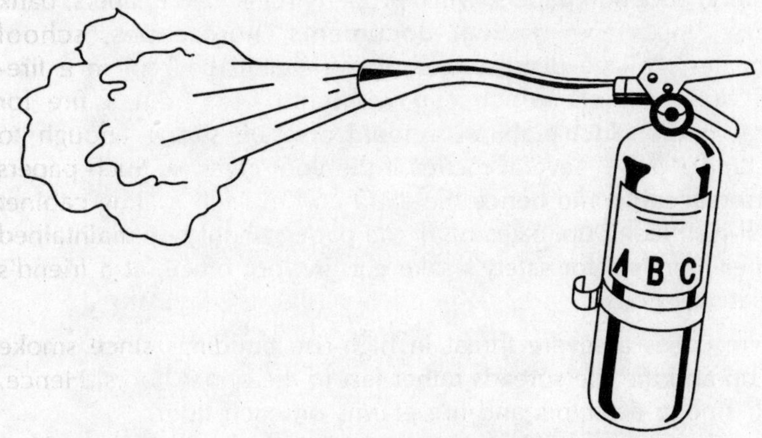

Fire extinguisher

In case of fire due to oil, grease or *ghee,* do not use water to put it out. Oil being lighter than water, will float over it and will continue to burn, thus spreading the fire all around. Use sand over such fires. One can also try smothering the fire with a blanket, jute bag, etc. If it is in a pan, cover the pan, thus effectively cutting out the air supply to the fire.

In case of an electric fire, cut the power supply. Then throw sand on it or use an appropriate fire extinguisher. Do not use water, it being a conductor of electricity and may electrocute people fighting the fire.

In case of a big fire, do not try to fight it regardless of its origin. Get out of the building as quickly as possible and raise the alarm. Do not try to collect your belongings. You may get trapped inside in the process as even seconds count in such a situation.

It has already been said that fire is a good servant but a bad master. Do not let it ever get out of control, even momentarily.

Remember. A minor lapse can cause loss of valuable lives, property, time and give lifelong suffering.

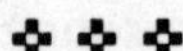

CHAPTER

4

Medical Safety : You Just Can't Ignore

Medicines are playing an increasingly important role in maintaining the health of individuals, in today's jet age.

❒ HANDLING EMERGENCIES

It is a must that every house has a first-aid box. It is imperative that this box is not kept locked in a cupboard. Keys are the worst things to find in an emergency. It is also important that all the people in the house be given a basic training in first-aid.

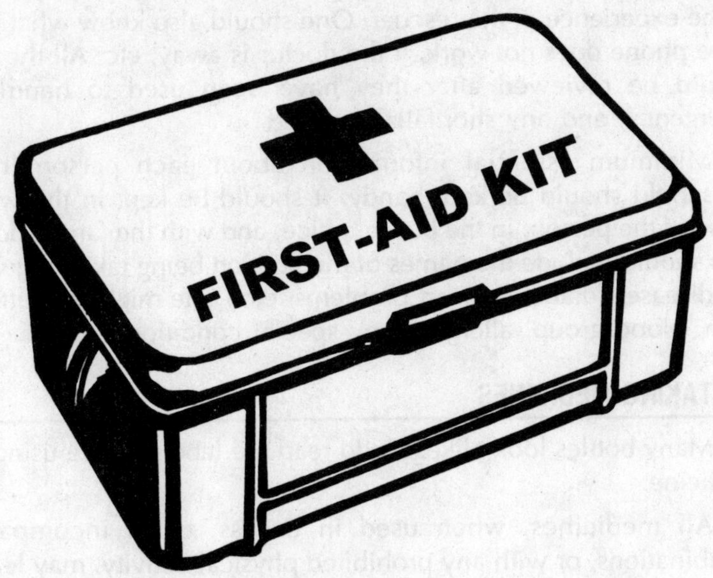

First-Aid Box

Important phone numbers of all members of the household, police, doctor, hospital, ambulance, fire-brigade, relatives and friends, and immediate neighbours should be readily available.

When people from one state or country move to another, it is likely that the family members may not know the language of the adopted place. If this is the case, they will not be able to talk to the neighbours or the police. In such cases, they should rehearse a few phrases to use in an emergency so as to be able to give the person at the other end of the telephone line some idea of the emergency situation, the location of the house, and also say that the caller cannot answer any questions since he does not know the language. It would be ideal if some mock exercises are conducted as to how to make an emergency phone call during a hypothetical emergency situation.

Everyone in the house should know what to do should someone get hurt. The injuries can be of several types : burns, electric shock, accidental poisoning, drug overdose, cuts by sharp-edged items, fall resulting in a fracture, heart attack, epileptic attack, etc.

One should know who to contact (doctor, hospital, etc.) in case of an emergency, and other preliminary steps to be taken. These steps would of course depend upon the extent of the injury as well as the experience of the rescuer. One should also know what to do if the phone does not work, if the doctor is away, etc. All the steps should be reviewed after they have been used to handle an emergency, and any shortfalls removed.

Minimum essential information about each person in the household should be kept handy. It should be kept in the wallet/ purse of the person, in the house, office, and with the family doctor. This should include the names of medication being taken regularly, the diseases (diabetes, heart problems, etc.) one might be suffering from, blood group, allergies, any special conditions, etc.

❐ TAKING MEDICINES

Many bottles look alike. So do read the labels before using any medicine.

All medicines, when used in excess, or in incompatible combinations, or with any prohibited physical activity, may lead to life-threatening situations. Sometimes an out-of-date medicine may do harm rather than good. This applies to all medicines including vitamins, sleeping pills, even herbal and folk medicines, etc.

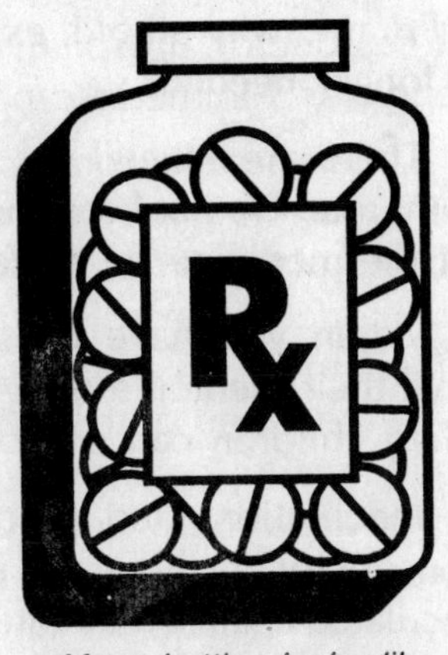

Many bottles look alike.

Vitamins for children are often sugar-coated. Children may take a large dose assuming them to be candy. This can be very dangerous. Keep all medicines away from the reach of children.

Fancy coloured pills and medicine containers attract children right from the time they begin to crawl. Keep all such items out of their reach.

Do not drink medicine directly from the bottle since you may ingest more than required.

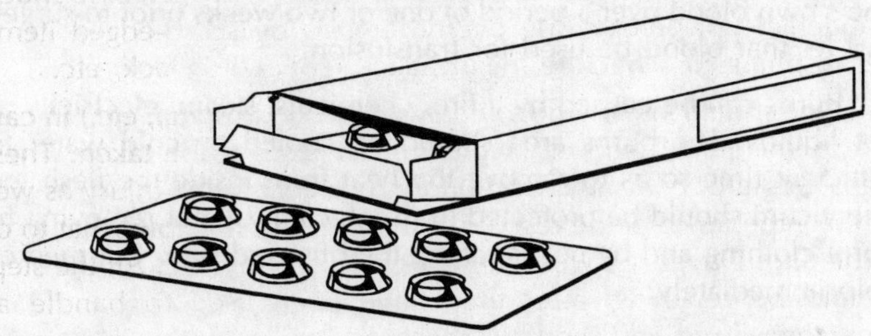
Keep all medicines, specially fancy coloured pills away from children

A thermometer is a useful aid in the diagnosis of fever and to follow its course of treatment. It can, however, be catastrophic if it breaks in the mouth and the patient swallows some of the mercury. Hence, when using it with children or with a patient who is sleepy or prone to epileptic attacks or violent temper, one should be very careful and vigilant. In case of accidental swallowing of the mercury, the patient needs an emergency stomach wash in a hospital and no time should be lost in contacting a doctor.

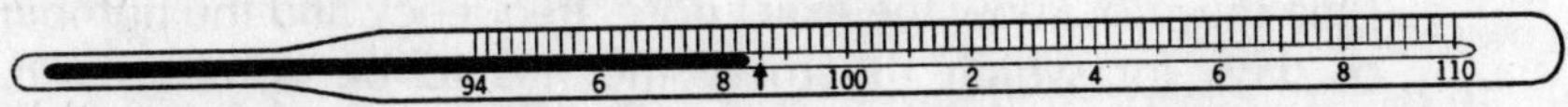

Thermometer

The medicine cabinet should be cleaned once a year. Destroy and drain away all old, expired medicines as well as those that are no longer needed.

There are several medicines that come in squeeze tubes like toothpaste. Do not keep medicine and toothpaste in the same place, lest the medicine be mistaken for the paste or vice-versa.

When you have guests visiting, be extra careful. They may leave their medicine on a table or in an easily accessible handbag where children can get to them.

Inoculations and vaccinations should be done as advised by your doctor. If there are pets in the house, every one should be inoculated against their bites and scratches. Tetanus shot on a regular basis is very helpful. Blood transfusion is a life-saving measure. With the spread of diseases like hepatitis and AIDS, thorough testing of blood to be transfused is necessary. Alternatively, one may donate one's own blood over a period of one or two weeks prior to surgery and let that blood be used for transfusion.

Burns can be caused by a fire, chemicals, steam, electricity, or hot liquids. The burns area should be cooled by cold water for sufficient time so as to remove the heat from inside the flesh too. The victim should be protected from infection by not removing his burnt clothing and by not touching the blistered skin. Get medical help immediately.

❒ MEDICAL ADVICE IS ESSENTIAL

- Do not take any medicine without the advice of a physician, even if the same medicine has been used before. There are several reasons for this.
  - It may not be a correct medicine for the current ailment. It may be outdated.
  - Some medicines need testing before being administered, even if these have been used earlier.
  - One may not know the exact dose, frequency and the number of days for which the medicine has to be administered. Sometimes, the dose has to be changed from the one previously given.

- Sometimes, a few tests may be required during the course of the treatment.
- One may require another medicine to control the side effects of the first, or may need a supplementary medicine and/or vitamins.
- Some medicines may have to be taken on an empty stomach while others may only be taken after some food has been ingested.
- If the person is already on some other medication, then the possibility exists of adverse interaction with the new medicine.
- Whether or not one may have fried and spicy food or milk, etc. with the medicine needs to be known too.
- Special or specific signs or reactions may need to be observed during the course of the treatment. At the onset of these, the physician may need to be consulted. Only a physician can advise on all the above points.

❐ VITAL INFORMATION ABOUT MEDICINE

The doctor, the pharmacist, and all the literature that comes with the drugs provide a lot of information about the medicines one is taking. Some of the things that one should know are :

The reason for which the drug has been prescribed. In case this medicine is not available in the market, the alternative to be used.

What specifically is it supposed to do and how quickly ? The recommended dosage — the number of pills or teaspoons to be taken at a time and how often in a day, plus the number of days the medicine has to be taken.

In case more than one medicine has been prescribed, how should they be spaced during the day and whether these should be taken together or with some time gap between them ?

Whether the medicine should be taken before or after the meals and how long before or after the meal ? Should the tablet or powder be taken with water, or milk or fruit juice or honey ? What are the side effects, if any ?

The other questions to be kept in mind are :

What other medicine, vitamins, etc. should be taken, or precautions exercised to minimize the side effects ? What are the interactions with other medicines, vitamins, specialized foods that one might be taking ?

The dietary restrictions to be observed in terms of eating sugar, fats, spicy foods, etc. What specific items should be taken, e.g. water, fruit, fruit juice, soup, etc.?

What activities should one avoid such as driving, reading for long periods of time, sitting straight for a long time, etc. ? Are short naps recommended ?

Is there a tapering of medicine intake with time or a sudden stoppage at the end of the recommended period ?

How should the medicine be stored — in a refrigerator, or in a cool dark place ? Are there any special precautions that need to be taken for pregnant women, small children, very old people, or people with some other diseases ?

Is there any testing to be done prior to giving the medicine : sensitivity test for penicillin or sulfa drugs, for example ? What steps should be taken if the tests prove that the medicine is not suitable ? What alternative medicine should be taken in that case ? What tests, if any, should be done during the course of the treatment ? Where should they be done ?

Under what conditions should the patient stop taking the medicine altogether and call the doctor ? Should any other step be taken immediately to ward off any harmful effect of the discontinued medicine ?

The patient and at least one more adult in the family should understand all these points and accordingly carry out the regimen of administering the medication.

If you are on a life support system at home, do have an alternate power supply (battery or generator) available.

With medical and health care systems becoming more sophisticated, it is imperative that users understand each new equipment or medicine very thoroughly before starting to use it. A constant dialogue between the patient (his family members) and the doctor on the one hand, and the doctor and drug company/ equipment manufacturer(s) on the other, will prove beneficial to all the parties concerned.

❐ CARING FOR THE AGED

With increasing life expectancy, breakage of joint family system, and higher living standards, the safety of the growing number of the aged is a major concern. They have special needs due to :

1. Changes in the ability to smell a leaking gas or a burning item, increase in reaction time to any event, and lack of alertness in the morning if sleeping pills has been taken at night. Most accidents involving the aged are found to occur during the morning hours.
2. Arthritis or other physical problems which decrease or slow down the movement of various muscles and joints.
3. Lapses in memory which may contribute to inattention to important things like food on the stove and inability to notice wet floors. This increases the probability of slipping over a wet surface.
4. General decline in strength which makes it difficult to lift loads including grocery bags.
5. General decline in vision may result in inability to see danger in many situations, specially when the light is low or the contrast in the scenery is not sharp. Adjustment from light to darkness or vice versa also takes longer. The angle of vision too decreases; thus, the field of vision is reduced.
6. Hearing sensitivity also decreases with age.

Hence, in a household with elderly members, a number of precautions need to be taken. Many of these can be taken care of at the time of construction of the house.

1. Fire alarms should be installed in rooms and hallways and tested periodically.
2. Grip bars should be installed in the bathrooms and bathtubs to prevent falls.
3. Hand rests or banisters should be used on all the stairs.
4. Bright lights must be used in rooms including bathrooms. There should be a lamp or light switch and a telephone within the reach of the bed for use at night.
5. The base of a walking stick, if used, should be at least as wide as the top. If the stick is used at an angle, a narrow

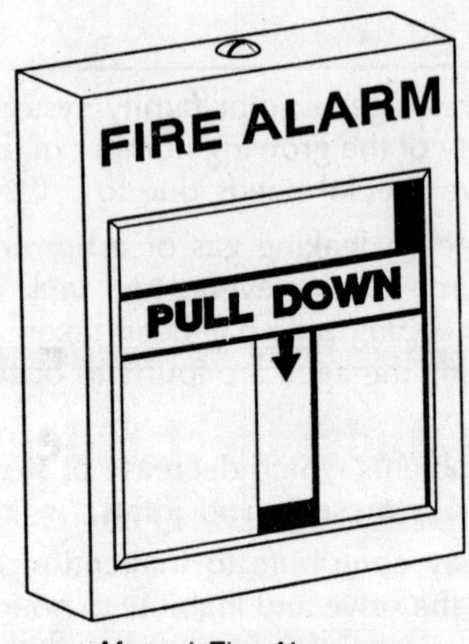

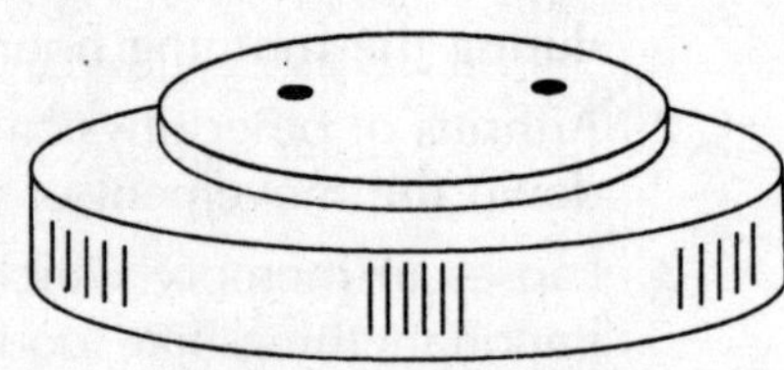

Manual Fire Alarm *Automatic Fire Alarm*

base results in slipping, specially while rising from a chair or a bed.

The elderly should be extra careful about smoking in bed, using a step stool, using sharp implements or power tools, having too much furniture crowding the house, lifting heavy loads, etc. They should be especially careful in the kitchen, the bathroom, roadside and while driving.

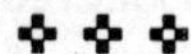

CHAPTER

5

Tools and Insecticides : Danger in Disguise

With increasing technological progress, the services of mechanics are becoming more costly and also difficult to get. Hence, many people prefer to do their own household repairs. This requires the use of tools some of which are sharp and heavy, and some of which are electrically operated. Adequate precautions need to be taken for the safe and proper use of these tools.

It is important to read the instructions that come with any tool before using it.

Do not wear a tie, scarf, dangling jewellery, ring or loose clothing while working with any kind of tool or repairing any machinery.

Use safety goggles, hand gloves, etc. as the situation requires. The regular prescribed glasses may shatter and hurt the eye if hit by a flying piece of wood or metal unless these are safety glasses.

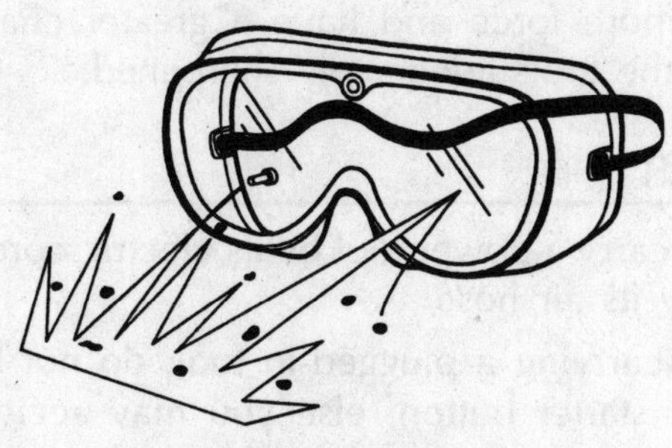

Safety Goggles

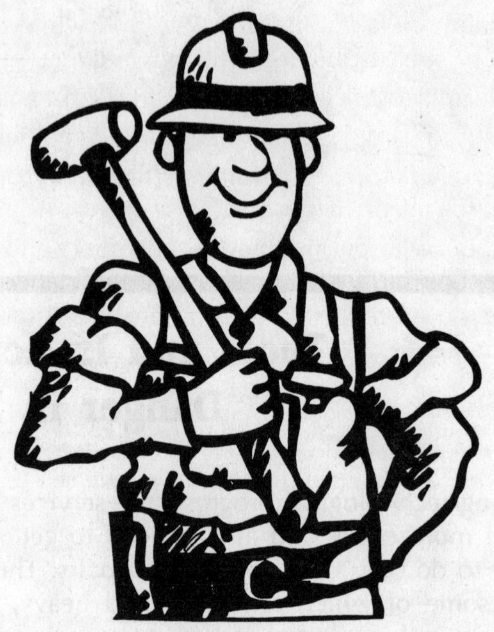

Use of head gear

Use spark resistant tools made of aluminium, brass, plastic or wood in places where inflammable substances or gases may exist.

The work area should be dry, clean, and well-lit.

Maintain tools with care and commonsense as recommended by the manufacturers.

Check for cracks in the wooden handle of a hammer or an axe. It may result in the metal part of the tool flying off and hitting someone hard. Replace cracked handles.

Blunt tools can be more hazardous than sharp ones because they require more force and have a greater chance of slipping. Hence, keep the tools adequately sharpened.

❐ REMEMBER

1. Never carry a power tool by its electric cord or a pneumatic tool by its air hose.
2. When carrying a plugged-in tool, do not keep your finger on the starter button, else you may accidentally start the tool.

3. Disconnect tools during servicing, and while changing any accessory such as blades, drill bits, cutters, etc.
4. Keep electric cords clean and away from heat and sharp edges.
5. Use proper guard, face shield, etc. and keep observers away.
6. Use a 3-pin, properly grounded plug. Do not use electric tools in a wet or damp area.
7. Hand tools with plastic handles like pliers and screwdrivers are not necessarily electric-shock proof. Hence, always stop the electric current before using any hand tool on electric wires or electrical appliances.

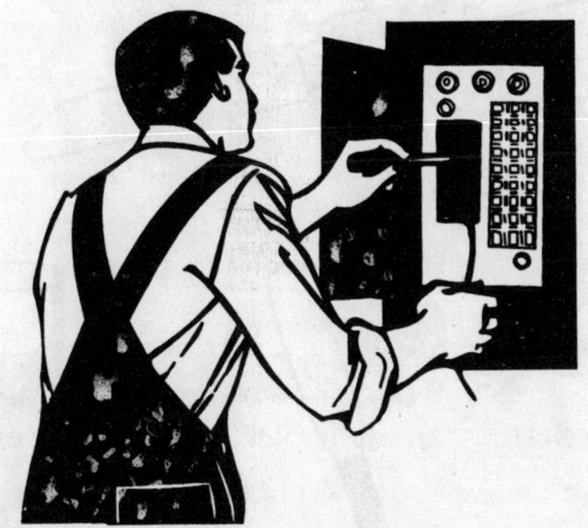

It is very important not to let children handle any tool nor have access to the tool box. Serious accidents may occur.

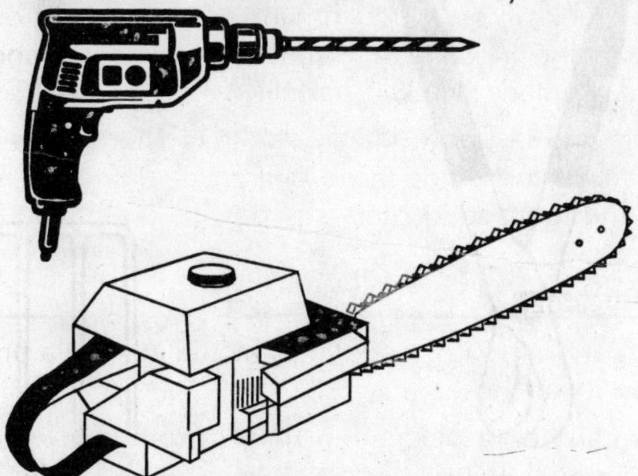

Tools of any kind should be kept out of reach of children for their safety

❐ USE OF GARDENING TOOLS

Gardening involves the use of sharp tools and chemicals in the form of fertilizers and insecticides. To keep this hobby free from any mishap some important precautions need to be taken.

1. A gardener should have tetanus shots regularly. Some bacteria from the soil, or cuts caused by a rusty tool, can cause tetanus.

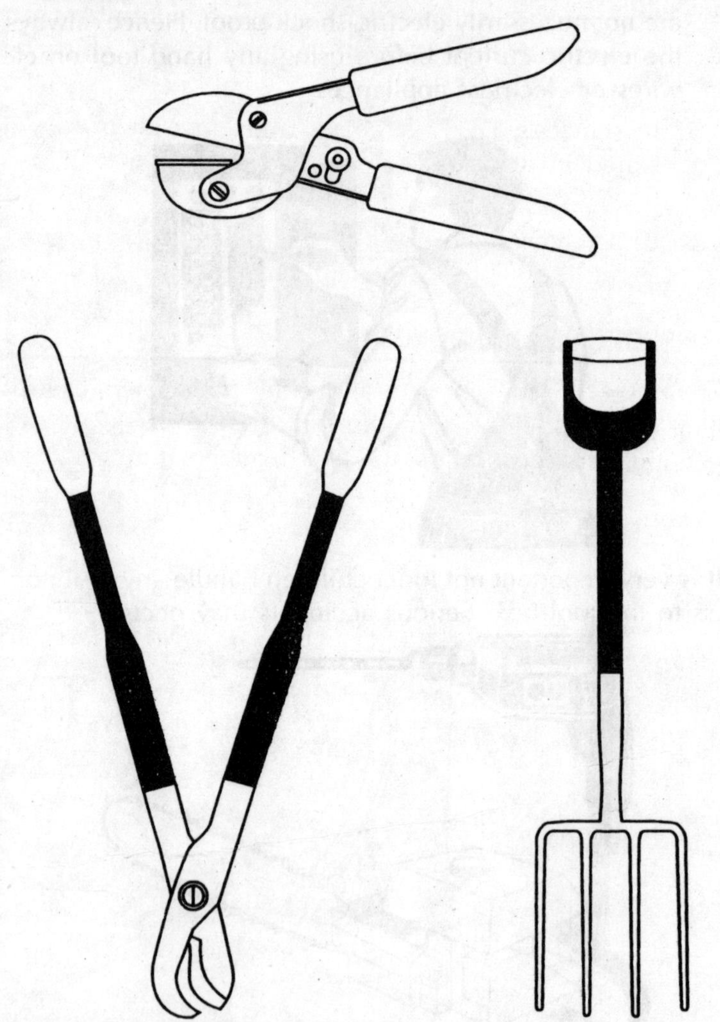

Gardening tools being sharp, care should be taken while handling them.

2. A gardener should wear full-length trousers so that no insecticide spray can harm, or pieces of stone churned over by the lawn-mower can hit his legs directly.
3. It would be ideal if good eye-safety glasses are used. Do not spray while wearing contact lenses since the chemical in the spray can damage them.
4. Shoes that cover the whole foot should be worn to protect from insect bites, insecticide sprays, and from any gardening equipment which may fall on one's foot or which one may step on accidentally.
5. Insecticides, DDT, gamexine and other chemicals must be stored in a locked cabinet and each container or packet properly marked.
6. Children should not be allowed to handle these items, which should be kept well out of their reach.

❐ INSECTICIDES HANDLING

Insecticides, DDT, gamexine and other toxic chemicals used for killing pests and insects should be used properly. All necessary precautions like covering of the face, accidental inhaling, exposure

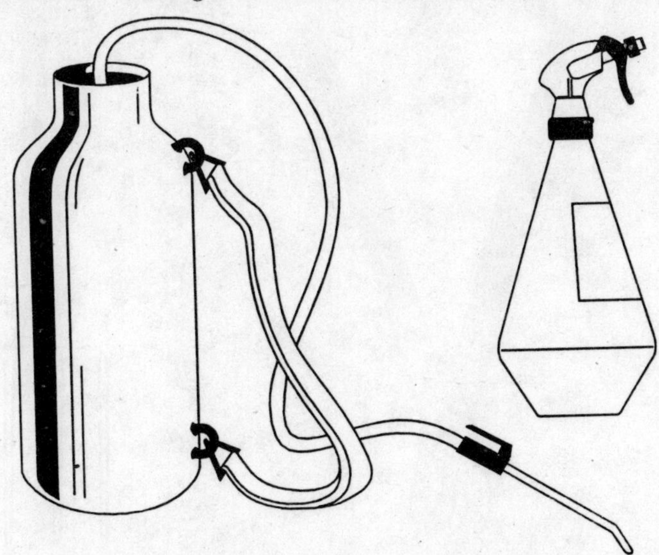

Equipment used for spraying insecticides on plants

to the skin, etc. should be taken into consideration. Any accidental spray on a person can be very harmful.

Since insecticides, when used, are likely to remain on the surface for a couple of days, warning signs must be put on the lawn, kitchen gardens, and flower pots so that no one touches them or walks on the sprayed grass.

Do not let a pet chew the grass of a freshly sprayed lawn. It can prove to be lethal. The person who has sprayed insecticide in the lawn or farm should bathe thoroughly afterwards, paying special attention to the hands, hair and any other parts that could have been exposed to the spray. If you have any breathing problem like asthma, or if you are on a strong medication of any kind, or have had any major medical treatment or operation, you should consult a doctor before taking up gardening.

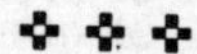

CHAPTER

6

Enjoy Safe Swimming

As everyone knows, swimming is lot of fun and a very good exercise too. Yet it must be remembered that accidents during swimming are common and often fatal.

Children between the ages of one and three are the primary victims of drowning in swimming pools at home. Some parents put their wards through early swimming training and think that the child can then be left alone in a pool without fear of drowning. But, it must be remembered that while drowning young children seldom splash or cry for help loud enough to alert people nearby.

❒ VITAL CHECKLIST TO PREVENT CHILDREN FROM DROWNING

1. Never evr leave a child unsupervised near a pool. Do not let fences and barriers around a pool give a false sense of security. Children usually find a way to get around them.
2. Do not rely on the floatation device being used by a child as completely safe. Always keep the child in sight when he is in the pool. Beginners should also be under constant supervision.
3. Children under three should not be trained in a group, but on a one-to-one basis by a trained swimming instructor. Drowning accidents can occur during a group training of small children because several children may need attention at the same time which cannot be provided by one instructor.
4. Do not keep toys near the pool. A child playing with them could fall into the pool. This is specially true with tricycles, balls, etc.

5. No one should push playmates, jump on another person, or do any other kind of potentially dangerous activity in the pool.
6. In any social gathering around a pool, someone should keep a vigilant eye on the pool, specially if children are present or if people are drinking alcohol.
7. There is a myth that a drowning person comes up thrice before he finally goes down. This is simply not true.

Remember. Safe behaviour by adults will serve as s guide for the young.

❒ BARRIERS

Effective barriers against unauthorised entry into the pool should be erected. All doors and windows to the pool should be the self-closing and self-latching type. The latches should be at such a height that these cannot be reached by a youngster who wishes to enter the pool area.

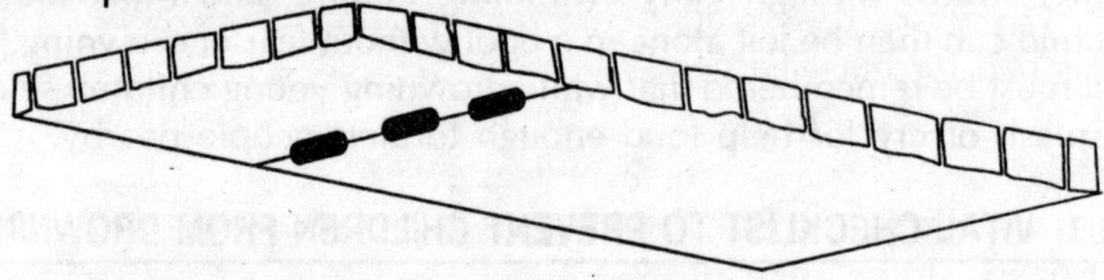

Float line in swimming pool

A float line should be stretched across the pool to indicate where the deep part begins. This will forewarn all swimmers.

❒ DIVING

No one should dive into a shallow pool. First, determine the depth of the pool or river bed and ensure that there are no submerged objects such as rocks, stones, or trees. Before diving, ensure that there are no other swimmers or divers in the area.

Anyone who has taken alcohol or drugs that produce drowsiness should not be allowed to swim or dive. Diving means keeping an eye for obstacles, judging distances and depths, as well as monitoring speed and direction so as not to collide with any one or anything. For all these functions, mental and physical alertness is necessary.

Anyone with a history of epilepsy or heart attack should get his doctor's permission before attempting t o swim. Such a person should never swim alone.

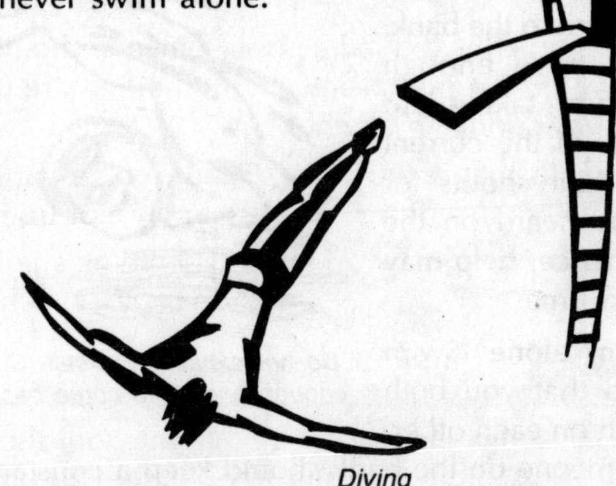

Diving

Never dive in an above-ground swimming pool. These are rather shallow. A dive in them might result in a grievous injury.

Physicians do not advise swimming immediately after a meal. It is bad for the digestive system.

It is wise not to go for a swim during a thunderstorm. One may be momentarily blinded by lightning and may collide with someone or hit a wall. In rivers, storms may result in a sudden surge of water which can prove dangerous.

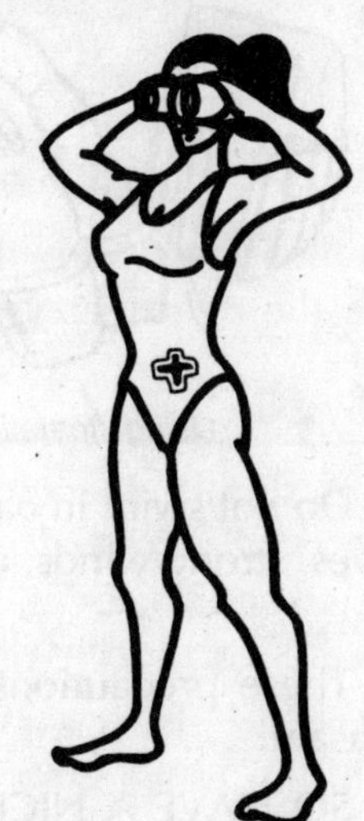

Ensure presence of life-guard before venturing to swim in a river or sea

❒ SAFE SWIMMING IN RIVERS

In a river, one should swim at a distance from the bank since a river is generally shallow at the banks and may have submerged steps for bathers or rocks hidden from view.

Keep a distance from boats of all types. Do not hold on to them. The boat can turn upside down. Similarly, keep away from any floating object and be careful about water creatures.

Do not exhaust yourself. It is possible to wander quite far off from the river bank in your initial enthusiasm. You may then lack the stamina to return to the bank. Make sure you have enough energy left to return, taking into account the flow of the current in the stream. Your shouts for help may not be heard on the river bank and hence, help may not reach you in time.

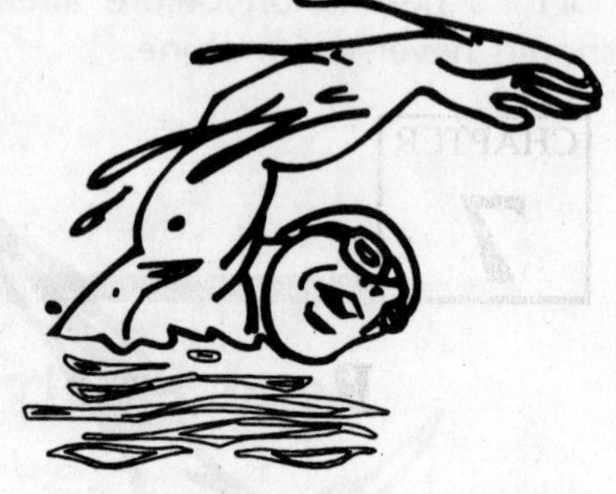

Do not exhaust yourself. Conserve enough energy to come back safely

Do not swim alone. Swim with a friend so that you both can keep a watch on each other. Alternatively, someone on the bank should keep a constant watch and arrange for rescue in case of an emergency.

Do not swim anywhere near a bridge or dam gates regulating the river flow. There are lots of circular currents or whirlpools which can entangle even a good swimmer.

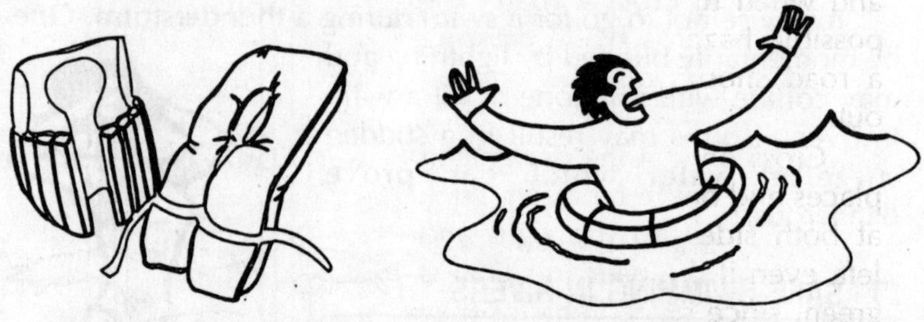

Using floatation devices is recommended for novices.

Do not swim in case of floods, heavy rains, thunderstorms, high waves, strong winds, chilly weather, or too many boats in the river, etc.

These precautions will help make swimming safer and more pleasant.

SO HAVE A NICE AND COOL DIP !!

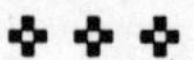

CHAPTER

7

Road Safety : Save Precious Life

The rapid technological advances in the last few decades has made transportation very fast but at the same time the results of mishaps are becoming quite horrible and hair raising. Hence, it is really important to take adequate precautions and also to teach young children about road safety.

❐ ROAD CROSSING

The young must be taught how and when to cross a road. The possible hazards while crossing a road should also be pointed out.

Cross only at the designated places and not in between. Look at both sides, to the right and left, even if the pelican signal is green, since some vehicles may not be able to stop in time and may hit the pedestrian.

While waiting to cross the road near an intersection, stand at least half a metre away from the kerb. This is to save your feet from buses or trucks which, while turning, often get their rear wheels on the pavement.

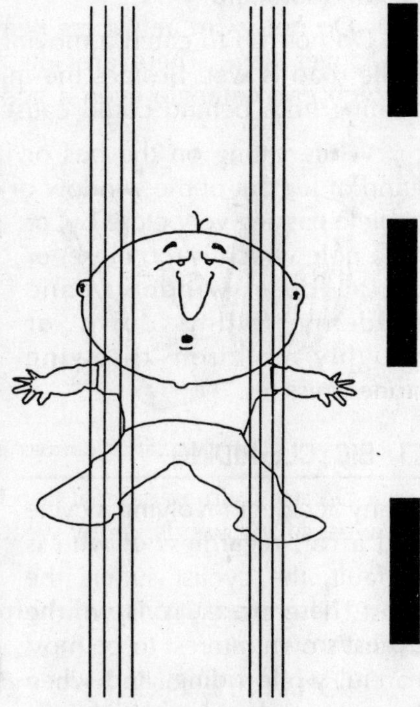

Possible hazards while crossing a road should be pointed out to the young regularly

Cycle rickshaws are very common and at some places

especially small towns, the only available mode of transport. However, even after many years of use, their basic design has more or less remained unchanged. Passengers can fall down when a vehicle hits from the rear, or the driver has to apply the brakes suddenly. Severe injuries, fractures and even deaths have resulted from a sudden, unexpected fall from a height of just over one metre onto a hard road with other traffic moving up too close for comfort and sometimes adding to the injury. Hence, passengers should sit firmly holding the side bars or the frame. It is important that the rickshaw is not loaded over its carrying capacity of two persons. Rickshaws carrying lots of young school children need special attention.

❐ TRAVELLING BY BUS

While riding a bus, do not hang on the outside of the bus or stand on the footboard.

Do not run to catch a moving bus. You may fall down, or slip if the road is wet. Besides the injury caused by the fall, a vehicle coming from behind could cause further injury.

While sitting on the bus or in a train, do not put your head, hand or leg out of the window or door. You may get hit by another vehicle passing very close by, or by a pole which is too close, or by a loose window pane suddenly falling down or naughty children throwing stones/missiles.

❐ BICYCLE RIDING

In any accident involving a cycle and a car, regardless of who is at fault, the cyclist suffers the most. Therefore, it is in the cyclist's own interest to be most careful while riding, and when being overtaken by vehicles.

Be careful on roads under repair and pieces of stones or

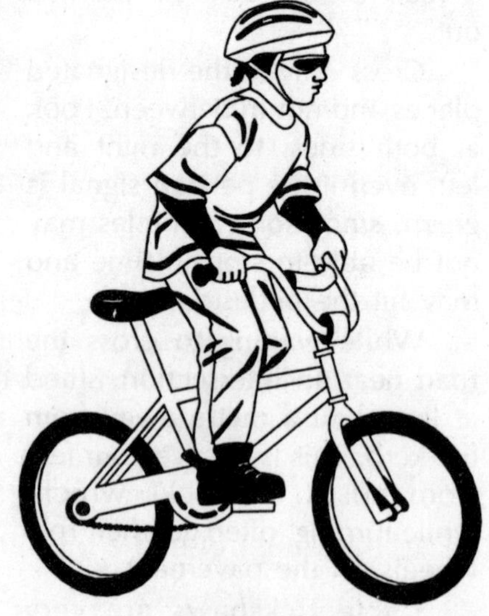

Riding a bicycle

other items lying on the road. Be watchful of pedestrians, pets or stray animals suddenly coming onto the road to cross it. Be careful of motorists trying to jump a traffic signal, and a bus or truck making a wide turn, etc. Keep an eye on the traffic around you, and adopt all the safety measures, some of which are listed below.

1. Children and learners should not ride on the main road until sufficiently experienced.
2. Since over two-thirds of the accidents occur at intersections, turns, etc. signalling your intentions at least 30 meters before turning and carefully observing the traffic signals and signals of other vehicles are very important for safe riding.
3. The cycle should be of the right size, neither too small nor too big. A wrong size can cause discomfort and may not be easy to handle and control efficiently.
4. For riding comfort, safety and longevity of the bicycle, it should be properly maintained. This basically means :
   (*a*) Keeping the tyres inflated to the correct pressure;
   (*b*) Adjusting the brake shoes to be within 3 mm of the rim and ensuring that they are in good shape;
   (*c*) Oiling and greasing the components as recommended;
   (*d*) Checking the tension in the cycle chain.
5. If you ride the bike a lot, and specially over long stretches of roads where there are no repair shops, learn how to do simple repairs such as mending a puncture etc. Carry essential repair tools in a bag, including a small air pump.
6. A bicycle should have the following accessories for safety : headlight, rear light, horn or bell, rear-view mirror, front and rear reflectors, pedal reflectors, spoke reflectors. Wearing reflector armbands and legbands makes a cyclist more visible to other vehicle drivers on the road at night. Even if the law does not require it, one should always wear a helmet, especially if there is a lot of traffic on the road. Reflector strips on the helmet make for better visibility
7. Be careful of traffic on blind curves.
8. On a road, a bicycle is a vehicle and not a toy. Therefore, do not ride it in a reckless fashion nor race with others.

9. Do not cycle holding it with one hand, or without holding the handle bar, even on a road with light traffic. You may be thrown off the cycle and you can get hurt badly.
10. Do not wear any ear plugs or headsets in your ears. This would hinder your hearing traffic noise and horn sounded by another vehicle.
11. Whilst cycling, do not carry load, or a small child in your lap or on your shoulder. This would be unsafe for you, the child, as well as other road users.
12. If an extra person is to ride, there should be a carrier at the back. Ensure that the passenger's foot does not get caught in the moving spokes. Install a barrier between the rear wheel and the child's legs.
13. For small articles, books, etc. have a basket or a carrier or both so that your hands are free.
14. Watch out for items and clothes that dangle. They may get into the spokes. This includes purses, bags, sarees, lower ends of wide trousers or pajama legs.
15. Use less-travelled roads and plan your itinerary thoughtfully. Do not cycle on highways where the traffic moves fast. It is very unsafe, unless bicycle lanes exist separately.
16. Do not hold on to another vehicle playing on the road. 'Hitching' a ride like this can lead to a catastrophe.
17. It may be unlawful to cycle on pavements and pedestrian pathways. You may hit someone and both may be injured.
18. While riding in a cycle lane be on the lookout for cars backing out, children rushing out of houses, etc. Take extra precautions when coming onto the main road from the cycle lane.
19. On the road, ride as close to the sidewalk as is possible, not in the middle of the road where the traffic moves at a higher speed.
20. Do not ride very close to parked cars. You could be pushed off your cycle by a car door suddenly opening.
21. Motorists have blind spots in the rear corners where other vehicles are often not visible in the rear-view mirror. Do not ride in these blind spots.

22. Fast moving buses and trucks cause air turbulence which can unsettle a cyclist. Stay at a safe distance from such vehicles.
23. If several people are cycling together, form a single file so as not to obstruct the traffic. This will also minimize the chances of any accident.
24. At night, do not look directly at the headlights of the vehicles approaching you. This could interfere with your vision and blind you temporarily, and you may not be able to spot pot-holes, pedestrians crossing the road, etc.
25. If the road is covered with loose gravel, sand, or fallen leaves then get down and walk with your bike since riding is not easy under such conditions.
26. Avoid pot-holes and broken manholes. These can cause damage to the bike and may also result in the rider falling down.
27. Since dogs have a habit of chasing cyclists and it is often difficult to pedal fast enough to move out of the harm's way due to the traffic, it is best to get down and walk slowly past a dog. If possible, walk with the bike between yourself and the dog.
28. Never ride a bicycle in the wrong lane or on the wrong side of the road.
29. It is very important to control speed when going downhill.
30. If you are tired or/and caught in heavy traffic, or when the road is uphill, walk with your bike rather than ride on it.
31. In rain, take care that your raincoat does not get stuck in a wheel or pedal.
32. During or after rainfall or snowfall, the road is likely to be slippery. Ride slowly and watch out for oil patches, water puddles, icy patches, etc. Do not brake hard lest you skid and fall. Keep good distance from other traffic since cycles as well as other vehicles need longer distances to come to a stop on a wet road. Be cautious and turn slowly on such roads.
33. In cold weather, protect your hands with appropriate gloves but ensure that hand movement or grip is not restricted.

34. Ride slowly during bad weather.
35. If you have to stop in a hurry, do not completely slam on the front brakes. This could result in skidding of the bike. Apply both the brakes cautiously and gradually.

❐ RIDING ON TWO-WHEELERS

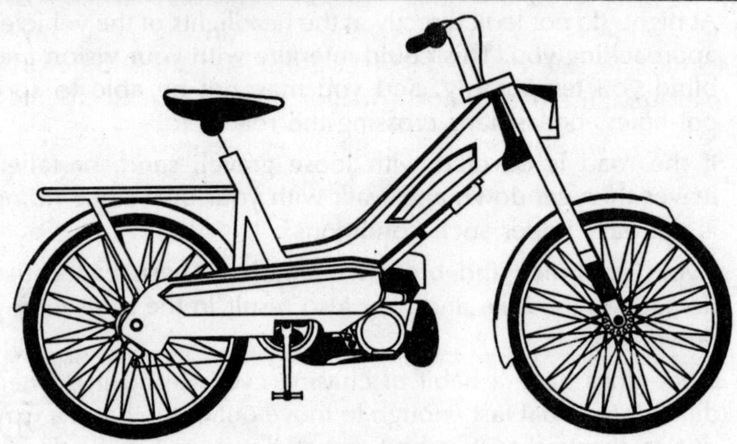

Riding on two wheelers

Though motorized two-wheelers provide speed at a low cost, they do not provide safety. A two-wheeler accident usually proves more damaging and more expensive than one on a bike or in a car. To reduce the frequency and severity of accidents, one should follow all the defensive and safety procedures.

1. Keep the vehicle properly maintained. Check the conditions of clutch, brakes, light, horn, tyres and fuel gauge, orientation of rear view mirror etc.
2. Not more than two persons should ride on it. Each one should wear a helmet securely fastened.
3. Keep an eye on the traffic behind, using the rear-view mirror to see if someone is trying to overtake. Give him way as soon as it is safe to do so.
4. Keep an eye out for pedestrians, cyclists, school-children, animals, slippery roads, pot-holes, etc.
5. Follow all the road safety rules, overtake with extreme caution if you must, and maintain a safe distance from the vehicle ahead of you.

6. Be extra careful at night and during bad weather such as rain, dust-storm, etc.
7. Carry a first-aid box for emergency use.

❒ DEFENSIVE DRIVING

Defensive driving is anticipating situations or factors that can possibly lead to accidents, and manoeuvring your driving in a way that enables you to stay out of accident-prone situations. Safe driving has to be practised. It is not a matter of luck that accidents are avoided.

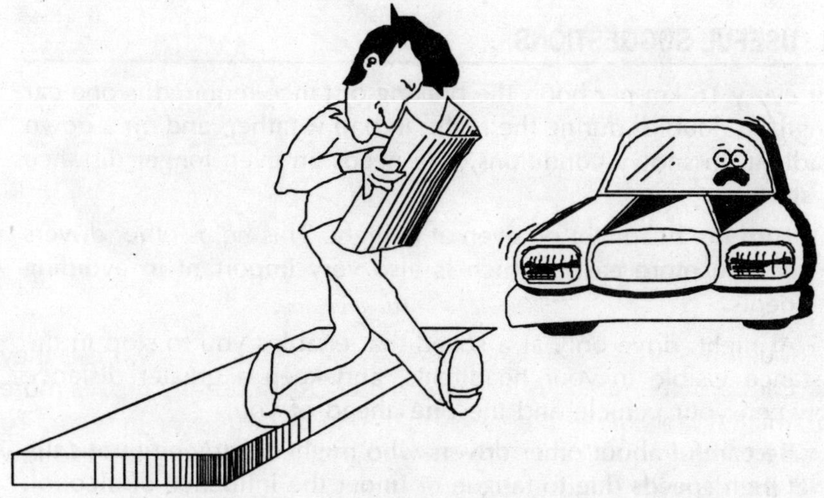

Defensive Driving : Be alert for errors on the part of other road users while driving

Following guidelines can be very useful.

1. Show care, courtesy, and consideration for other road users.
2. Have a complete knowledge of traffic rules and regulations.
3. Be alert for illegal moves and errors on the part of other road users whilst driving.
4. Show concern for accident prevention.
5. Always expect the unexpected. Give right of way, do not claim it. Observe lane discipline.
6. When being overtaken, do not increase your speed or try to prevent the other vehicle from overtaking you.

7. While riding in a car, lock the doors from inside and do not lean against them when the car is in motion. They may open and throw the passenger out.
8. Do not disturb the driver or ask questions, specially in heavy traffic, in unfamiliar areas, and when the driver is in a hurry.
9. Do not drive after drinking alcoholic beverages, even if it is only beer. Alcohol impairs one's driving abilities.
10. Do not smoke while driving at night since the nicotine and carbon monoxide in cigarette smoke can hamper night vision.

❒ USEFUL SUGGESTIONS

For every 16 km per hour, the braking distance required is one car length. It doubles during the night, in bad weather, and on a down gradient. In snowy conditions, one needs an even longer distance to stop.

Turn the headlight on even at twilight. This helps other drivers to see you more easily which is also very important in avoiding accidents.

At night, drive only at a speed that enables you to stop in the distance visible in your headlights, and keep a greater distance between your vehicle and the one ahead of you.

Be careful about other drivers who might be driving erratically or at high speeds due to fatigue or under the influence of alcohol. Keep sufficient distance around your vehicle to take a defensive measure should the need arise. For this, keep a constant watch on the traffic behind and around you by looking frequently in the rear-view and side mirrors.

If you see the police chasing a car, get out of the way and pull up at the earliest. Major accidents can occur during a high speed chase. Give way to all emergency vehicles, such as ambulances and fire-brigades.

Be extra careful on an undivided two-way road, specially on turns.

Don't use the high beam when there are other vehicles, cyclists, or pedestrians on the road. Your high beam may temporarily blind them.

When passing a road repair zone or a procession, slow down.

If you are tired, let another person drive. If no other driver is with you, then take a rest, eat a light snack, and, if possible, wash your face and eyes before resuming driving. If none of this is possible, take a taxi.

While driving, keep anger from building up due to traffic or red traffic lights over which you have little control.

If a problem in the car forces you to stop, pull off the road, turn the emergency lights on and warn the oncoming traffic with a white cloth or flares. Wait for a police vehicle to come by. If you are working on the car, be careful of the approaching traffic.

If you spot someone in trouble on the road, report it to the police. They are better trained to help and can call for additional assistance as necessary. Of course, there may be instances involving human life where you may yourself have to help out because time is important. In that case, try to get several people to help and someone should also contact the police or hospital right away.

Your car should be checked for winter worthiness and for icy road conditions if these are likely to exist in your driving region.

A small child should always be carried in a safety seat placed in the middle of the rear car seat and securely fastened. He is not safe in your lap. In an accident he could be thrown against the dashboard or your own body could crush him.

On slippery roads, pedestrians and cyclists may slip and fall; therefore, be cautious in your driving and give them extra space. Give old people some more time to react.

❐ OLD AGE DRIVERS

As the average age and the living standards increase, there is an increasing number of old age drivers for beyond the age of retirement.

With age, reflexes become slow, muscular strength is reduced and some joints may become arthritic. Vision changes occur as well. Peripheral vision decreases, glaucoma and cataracts cloud vision, lens hardening makes close focusing difficult; pupil size decreases cutting down the amount of light reaching the retina thus affecting vision, specially at night, and the ability to adjust from light to darkness decreases as well.

These vision problems affect judgements regarding distances, cars pulling out of driveways, quick interpretation of the road signs, turning signals, etc. The ability to distinguish objects with slight differences in shades decreases, so they may not see in time a pedestrian wearing dark clothes crossing the road at night. While it is true that the total number and severity of accidents in which older drivers are involved is less than those is which young drivers are involved, the number of accidents per kilometre driven by older drivers is quite significant. Of course, they are law-abiding, courteous, non-competitive, and cautious drivers.

When older people are involved in an accident, they receive more injuries and their recovery is slower because of their fragile bones and advanced age.

Some older drivers find busy intersections difficult to cross and may make wrong turns.

Some are on medication and hence, should consult their doctor about the advisability of driving.

Diabetes can cause fluctuating vision, dizziness, and even unconsciousness, if care is not taken. Strokes, epilepsy, Alzheimer's and Parkinson's diseases cause dizziness and tremors, and impair memory and concentration. If an older driver suffers from any of these ailments, heart disease and deteriorating vision and hearing, it is essential that a doctor be consulted regarding the advisability of driving.

Do not let driving a car become an issue of personal pride. Your safety and that of others may be at stake. Road skills and safety depend less on your age than on your overall health.

Older people should avoid heavily tinted glass windows since they require more light to see clearly than do the young.

In order to reduce the number of accidents, older drivers may be required to take driving tests at periodic intervals to assess their driving capability. They may be restricted to day-time driving, if need be.

Road signs should use larger letters, shiny material and contrasting colours. The signs should be well-maintained, clear, and not broken. Sadly, all these things are missing very much in most of the countries.

❐ SAFETY OF CHILDREN

Children, being small, cannot see beyond parked cars from the pavement and hence, do not know the status of the traffic on the road. They also have less knowledge about road safety. So, they are likely to run out from behind parked cars onto the road while chasing a ball, a kite, or a friend.

Children cannot correctly judge the speed, the distance of a car, and gaps between the traffic. They often cannot quickly determine the direction from where a car, or the sound of a horn is coming. They cannot always tell whether something is moving or is stationary.

Children sometimes cannot separate fantasy from reality. They think they can stop a car by signalling with their hands, or that they can bounce back at the last moment as they see in cartoons. They can, therefore, act carelessly with regard to traffic.

Children may misunderstand traffic signs. A sign post for drivers to warn them that 'children might be crossing' may be interpreted by a child to mean that it is safe to cross the road without bothering to watch out for traffic. They think that drivers will always slow down on seeing the sign.

Children believe that when they see a vehicle, the driver of the vehicle sees them too. This, however, is often not the case. The short height of children makes it difficult for drivers to see them.

Car horns should be used with discretion. The sound may startle a child. He may run backwards into the path of oncoming traffic. He may, on the other hand, take it to mean that the driver has seen him and is asking him to move faster and may get into the next traffic lane in a hurry and be run over by the oncoming traffic. Either way, he faces a situation that could be injurious and even fatal too.

❐ DRIVING IN THE RAIN IS A PLEASURE ?

The risks on the road increase during the rains, therefore, the driver should be very alert. Road conditions change from one stretch to another due to fallen branches of trees, oil leakage, pot-holes, etc.

Pedestrians tend to concentrate more on protecting themselves from the rain rather than from the traffic.

Cyclists, two-wheeler riders, hand-cart pullers, rickshaw pullers, etc. cannot use umbrellas; so rain water splashes onto their eyes and reduces their ability to see clearly.

You need more time to see and be seen, to react and to stop, since braking distance increases on wet roads. Hence, drive slowly and leave more distance between you and the vehicle in front.

The car may skid if you speed, brake, or steer suddenly on a wet road. Hence, be careful. Test the brakes after driving through water.

In extreme conditions, avoid driving altogether.

Civic authorities should use pavement reflectors to guide drivers, specially at turns, in bad weather and at night.

Larger rear-view mirrors give a better idea about the rear traffic and compensate to some extent for the decrease in peripheral vision in older drivers.

The headlights should be such that they increase the length of the road that is visible, but do not increase the glare onto the approaching traffic.

Carry a flashlight, warning flares or reflectors, necessary tools, water, some food, first-aid box and a fire extinguisher in the car. Also carry a spare fan belt, engine hoses, car registration and insurance papers, etc.

If brakes fail, try pumping them to see if they can be reactivated. If this does not work, use the hand brake slowly or shift to a lower gear.

If a tyre blows out, hold the steering wheel tightly since it will vibrate intensely. Try to keep the car under control. Then slowly pull onto the side of the road.

If the engine overheats or the oil pressure gauge lights up, pull off the road and check for the source of trouble, oil levels, etc. If the alternator light comes on, do not stop till you reach a service station, else you may not be able to start the car again. Get the system checked.

It is essential that vehicle drivers observe all the traffic laws of the city.

Remember someone is waiting for you as well as for the others at HOME.

CHAPTER

8

Picnics and Kite-Flying : 'Play' Safe

Everyone loves picnics in the stressful 'Modern' life.

A picnic is a wonderful way to relax and spend time in natural surroundings. It involves delicious food, fun-filled games and sometimes, a campfire. If you keep in mind a few precautions, the fun and joy will not be spoiled by an accident.

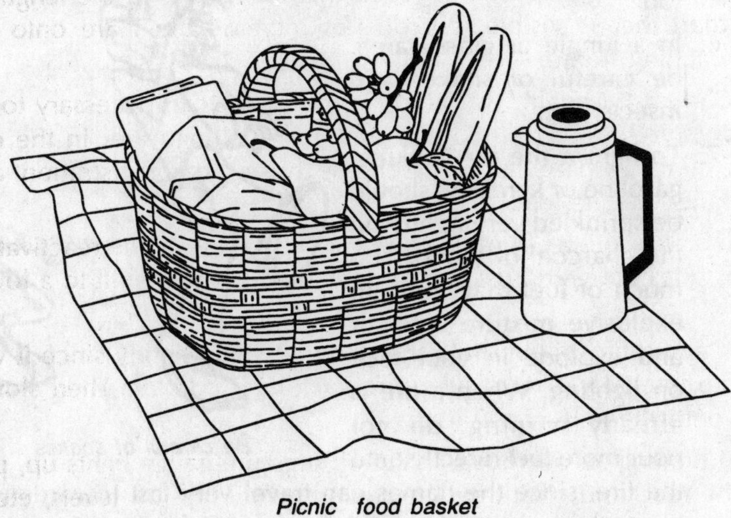

Picnic food basket

❒ PICNIC FOOD

1. Keep each sandwich in a separate plastic wrapper and keep them all in an icebox so that they remain fresh.
2. Use small containers for pre-cooked food so that the core of the container can also get cold in the icebox, otherwise, the food in the middle will remain warm and may get spoiled.

3. Cook the food well. Bacterial poisoning is a real danger.
4. Do not leave salad, etc. in the closed trunk of a car for long. The high temperature inside may spoil it. Milk, meat, fish, custard, etc. should be finished quickly or they are likely to get spoiled.

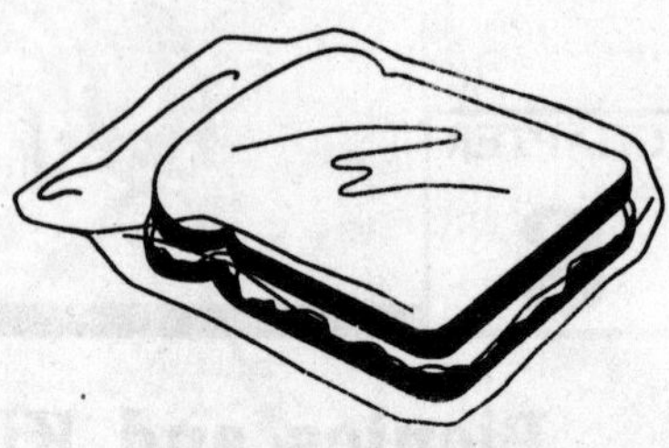

Keep each sandwich in separate plastic wrapper

5. Wash hands very thoroughly. Do not decide they are clean by just looking at them because you cannot see the bacteria crawling about. They are there for sure even though they are not visible. Wash knives, picnic tables, cutting boards, etc. too.
6. In a jungle or grassy area, be careful of snakes and insects, etc.

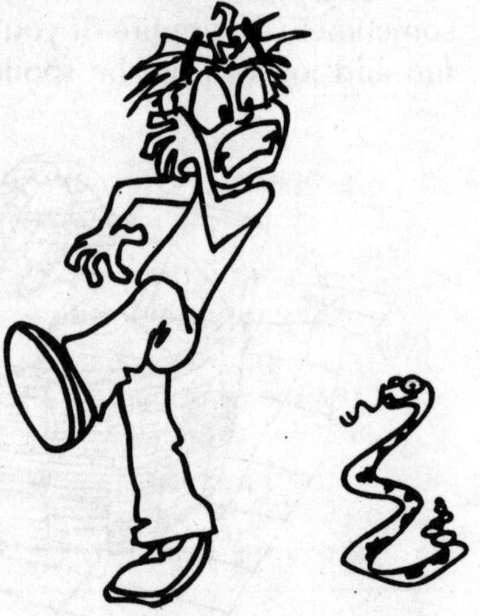

Be careful of snakes

7. To light a fire for cooking, gasoline or kerosene should be sprinkled very lightly on the charcoal or wood. Too much of fuel may form an explosive mixture with air and explode in your face on lighting. When a fire is already burning, do not pour more fuel directly onto the fire, since the flames can travel very fast towards you. Use a ladle instead to add the fuel to the fire.
8. Do not touch a hot cooking grill nor let any loose clothing come into contact with it.

❐ CAMP 'BON' FIRES

1. Always go for the camp fire away from combustibles such as tent, plastic materials, bed sheets, electrical wires, waste paper etc.

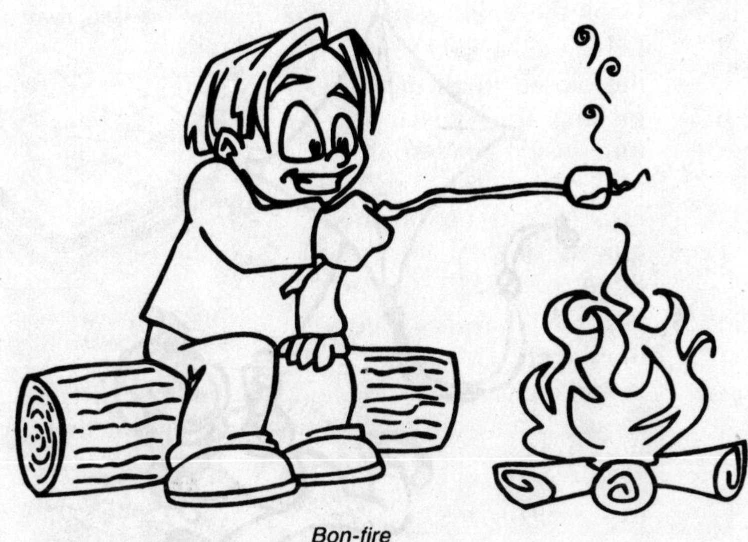

Bon-fire

2. Preferably keep the fire small and do put it out completely before leaving the place. A few buckets of water or sand should be kept ready for use in case of emergency.
3. If children are going on a picnic with friends (or with school or club), find out the names, addresses and phone numbers of their friends, the places being visited, mode of transport, time of departure and return and children should be strictly instructed to inform their parents or guardians if they will be returning later than expected.

❐ ENJOYING KITE FLYING

Many people love to fly kites, especially children but a few precautions will make it safe and more enjoyable.

1. Fly the kites from a ground level lawn, garden, park or open space but if it must be done from a roof-top, then the roof should have at least one metre high wall all around. Entry to the roof must be locked or blocked to prevent children from falling through it, while moving back and forth engrossed in flying his kite or observing other kites. There should be atleast two persons on the roof to help out in an emergency.

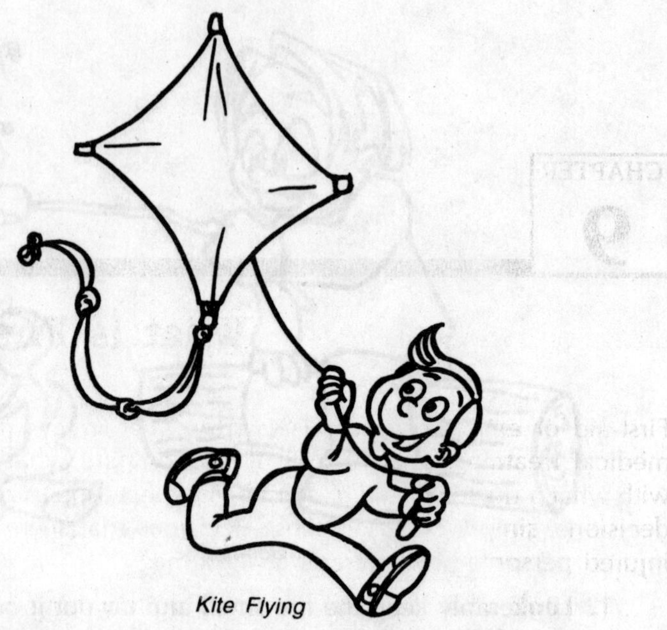

Kite Flying

2. Children should be clearly instructed to avoid climbing onto the boundary walls, rush up and down the stairs while looking at kites in the sky or while trying to catch a 'cut' kite, as they may loose their balance and tumble down the stairs or off the walls.
3. Loose poles or wooden staff should be removed from the roof to prevent children from using them to catch other kites as they may fall over the side walls onto the street or the ground below.
4. Avoid entangling kites in TV antennae, as they may be damaged.
5. Do not fly a kite if the sun in above your head since long exposure to hot sunlight can be very harmful to skin and eyes.
6. Do not fly kites from a roof which has an electric pole or wires in close vicinity as children may be tempted to untangle kites caught in them using a stick or metal rod and hence may get an electric shock, which can be fatal. We have read so many reports of such unfortunate incidents in daily newspapers.

CHAPTER

9

What is First-Aid ?

First-aid or emergency care is exactly what it says it is. It is not medical treatment and you shouldn't compare what you can do with what a doctor would do. Nobody expects you to make medical decisions, simply common sense decisions that seem to be in the injured person's best interests at the time.

1. **Look after yourself** — don't do anything hazardous or thoughtless that puts you in danger or there could be twice the problem for someone else to cope with. Get the casualty and yourself away from hazards as soon as possible. Don't get trapped by collapsing buildings, gas, smoke or fire.
2. Look first for essential problems.

   Check for : breathing, choking, bleeding, consciousness.

   Action on these can save life — anything else is a frill and can be done while awaiting professional help.
3. Get help as soon as the life-saving is under way. Don't try to do without professional aid — it's their job, they have the equipment and knowledge and are used to taking the responsibility when things go wrong. Tell the professionals over the phone how many casualties there are, what happened, exactly where you are, your telephone number and whether special equipment is needed.
4. Reassure the injured person and keep him as happy as possible under the circumstances. Combine confidence (which you may not feel) with kindliness.
5. Organise bystanders — don't let them stand around making remarks that could upset the casualty. 'Give him air' is a

common cry that goes up in such situations. This is nonsense, of course, because the casualty will have plenty of air. What he does need is emotional 'air', *i.e.*, calm, reassuring care and not a crowd of fussing people standing around him.

6. If there are several casualties, decide quickly which most needs urgent attention and if necessary quickly show a bystander how to do artificial respiration or heart massage.
7. Don't worry yourself into doing nothing for fear of doing the wrong thing. You are, after all, not expected to know about all the conceivable complications that might arise from your actions. It's better to turn an unconscious person carefully into the recovery position and clear the airway every time, because 99 times out of 100 you'll be doing exactly the right thing. The other case in 100 will have a broken neck and you could possibly injure him further but this is the price we have to pay. Take the calculated risk — you'll wish someone would do so for you or for a member of your family.
8. Once you have carried out life-saving procedures, do nothing, unless you are absolutely sure of what you're doing. **Inactivity is the most difficult activity.** Harm can be done by piling blankets on injured people (which overheats them); giving drinks of tea to everyone in sight (dangerous as injured people vomit easily and may drown themselves in the tea you've just given) sitting people up (who should be kept flat because they may have a back injury); and taking people off into cosy front rooms 'in the warm' where they are overlooked by the emergency services or simply can't be found at all.
9. Take charge and organise. If you've read this book you'll be in a much better position to cope with problems than the average bystander, so protect the casualty from ill-informed actions. Ask others to help in other ways while you do the first aid. Of course, should there be a doctor or nurse in the crowd, they can take over.
10. Always stop when you see an accident unless professionals are already on the scene. The simple actions described in

this book will enable you to save life and prevent further injury.

Knowing what to do puts you in a privileged position but it also carries responsibilities. Don't pass by — one day it could be you or your family lying there.

❒ FIRST-AID PRIORITIES

1. *Assessment of the situation* : Observe what has happened quickly and calmly. Look for dangers to yourself and the victim. Never put yourself at risk.
2. *Make the area safe* : Protect the victim from danger. Be aware of your limitations.
3. *Assess all victims and give first aid* : Treat those with life-threatening conditions first.
4. *Get help* : Quickly ensure that all specialists help summoned is on the way.

The general principles of first-aid are as follows :

1. One should be in control, both of oneself and the problem.
2. One should be gentle but firm, calm and logical.
3. One should speak to the victim kindly but purposefully and reassuringly.
4. One should build up rapport while handling to the victim.
5. One should explain fully what one plans to do.
6. One should give honest answers rather than give misinformation.
7. One should not let the victim be alone and unattended at any time.
8. One should not separate a child from its parents or guardian.
9. One should send the victim to a doctor or hospital by quickest means.
10. One should inform the relatives of the seriousness of the problem.
11. One should inform police about serious accidents.

❐ QUALITIES OF A PERSON GIVING FIRST AID

1. One should be a good observer, able to note the cause and effects of the injury.
2. He should be able to act quickly.
3. He should not panic or get excited at a critical time.
4. One should be resourceful, able to use whatever things are available.
5. One should be able to reassure the apprehensive victim and his relatives. One should be clear in his instructions to the victim, his relatives, and the onlookers.
6. One should be able to control the crowd.
7. One should be able to obtain help from onlookers as required, e.g. for directing traffic, making phone calls, turning off electricity or gas etc.
8. In case there are multiple injuries, one should have the ability to judge injuries to be managed first.

❐ RESPONSIBILITIES OF A FIRST AIDER

1. Gaining access to the patient in safest and easiest way.
2. Assessment of the situation quickly, such as finding out whether casualty is unconscious, conscious, alive or dead.
3. Identification of the injury or the nature of illness affecting the victim.
4. Giving early and adequate treatment in a sensible order of priority.
5. Arranging for the removal of the casualty to hospital or the clinic of a doctor.
6. Remaining with a casualty until handing him over to the care of a doctor.

Things to be avoided by the first aider

1. Forgetting that he is not a doctor.
2. Handling the victim unnecessarily.
3. Moving a patient unnecessarily.

4. Removing clothing unnecessarily.
5. Examining wounds by opening which have already been bandaged by someone else.
6. Moving a patient with a fracture or suspected fracture until splints have been applied.
7. Neglecting shock.
8. Failing to give artificial respiration when needed.
9. Reducing dislocations, except of the finger.
10. Burning a patient with a hot water bottle or other heated object.
11. Failing to remove false teeth, tobacco or any other eatable from the mouth of an unconscious patient.
12. Permitting air to reach a burned surface.
13. Leaving a tourniquet on over 20 minutes without loosening.
14. Putting oneself at risk by attempting heroic measures in difficult situations.
15. Acquiring communicable diseases from the victim.
16. Declaring the victim to be dead.

❒ FIRST AID KIT

The materials necessary for first aid are kept together in a first aid kit or some other suitable container. These kits should be kept in the work place, in home, sports and leisure facilities and vehicles.

The contents of the kit at workplace and leisure center must conform to the legal requirements. You may add things to your kit at home depending on your requirements. The kit should be clearly marked and easily accessible. It should be kept in a cool and dry place. It should be checked and replenished regularly, so that all required items are always ready to use.

Contents of a first aid kit are shown in the following table. These may vary according to the duties performed, rules of the organisation and special needs for the occasion.

❐ FIRST AID KIT

Item	Quantity (Number)
For assessment purposes	
Flashlight	1
Thermometer	1
Tongue spatula	1
Blood pressure instrument	1
Gloves, rubber	1
Writing pad and pen	1
For treatment purposes	
Bandage, triangular	2
Bandages, assorted sizes	6
Gauze pads, sterile	6
Sticking plaster roll	1
Cotton wool packet	1
Swab sticks	6
Eye pads	2
Safety pins	12
Eye pads	2
Light plywood splints	2
Screw capped bottles, wide mouthed	2
Urethral catheter	6
Gastric lavage tube	2
Intravenous drip set	2
Hypodermic syringe, 2 ml	1
Hypodermic syringe, 5 ml	1
Injection needles No. 22, 24	2
File for cutting ampoules	2
Scalpel	2
Pocket knife	1
Scissors, blunt and sharp tipped	1 each
Artery forceps	1
Toothed forceps	1

Dextrose 5% solution for intravenous use	2
Oral rehydration therapy pack	1
Tetanus toxoid ampoule	2
Adrenalin injection 1 : 1000 ampoule	1
Atropine injection ampoule	1
Antihistaminic tablets packet	2
Antispasmodic tablets packet	2
Paracetamol tablets packet	1
Antiasthma tablets packet	1
Antacid tablets packet	1

Medications for external use

Methylated spirit bottle	1
Tincture of iodine bottle	1
Tincture of benzoin bottle	1
Lignocaine 2% tube	1
Eye drops bottle	1

❒ POISONING

What is a poison ?

Anything which when taken into the body affects if adversely. Poisons can be tables taken in excess (of which the commonest are painkillers, sleeping tablets and iron tablets); fruits and plants (e.g., mushrooms and berries); chemicals (e.g., weed killers, domestic cleaning fluids and turpentine substitute (turps); bites (such as those

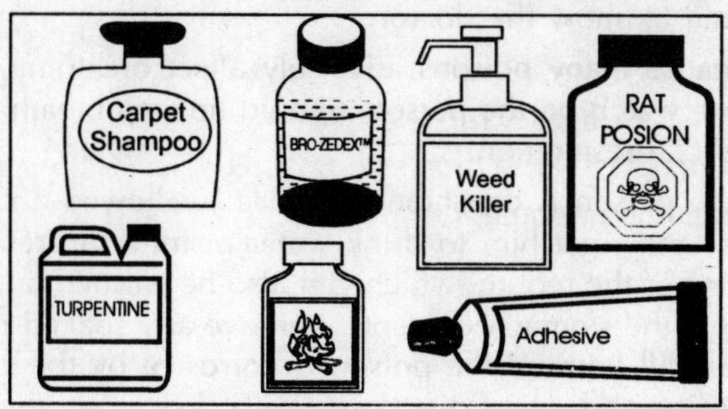

Household poisonous chemicals

from a snake); gases (like coal gas or industrial gases that are absorbed through the lungs); and agricultural pesticides that are absorbed through the skin.

It is usually obvious what sort of poisoning is involved, so we will look at them group by group.

Swallowed poisons

Usually a child. It is difficult to know how much was swallowed unless you know how full the container was in the first place.

1. Any swallowed poison must be treated seriously. Get medical help as soon as possible. Ask someone to telephone a doctor/ambulance or take the person to hospital by car or other means at once.
2. Always take the container along with you so that the doctor can identify the poison and so possibly remedy it quicker. Tell the ambulance people what has happened and ask their advice (where applicable).
3. Do not delay because children can go downhill very quickly even though they seem all right at first.

While awaiting medical help

1. Remove excess poison from the mouth, keeping pills, berries or containers for the doctor to see.
2. If the person is conscious, ask what he took. Do this quickly in case he lapses into unconsciousness rapidly.
3. If the person is unconscious, turn him into the recovery position so that he will not suffocate or vomit. Keep any vomit to show the doctor.
4. Because many poisons adversely affect breathing, keep a close watch on the person. Should he stop breathing, give artificial respiration.
5. If the person is conscious and has swallowed a corrosive substance, get him to drink water or milk to preserve the lining of the mouth (which can also be washed out) and to dilute the stomach contents. Remove any soaked clothing. You will know if the poison is corrosive by the chemical burning and white discolouration it leaves on the mouth, lips and clothes.

6. Never give anything by mouth to an unconscious person no matter what you think he has taken.
7. Never make a person vomit if he has taken anything containing petrol, turpentine substitute or anything corrosive such as strong acids and alkalies. The substance will already have done plenty of damage going down and can only do more on its way up. Give these people milk or water to drink as this helps protect the stomach lining and to some extent prevents absorption of the chemical.
8. Never give salt water to make the person vomit. If the person has taken poisons other than corrosives, thrust three fingers well down the back of his throat to make him vomit. Little children can be held upside down as this is done. The person may even be able to make himself sick like this.
9. Never try to make anyone vomit if he is unconscious.
10. Keep a close watch on the person until help arrives.

Some commonly swallowed poisons

All of these should be kept away from children. Although they rarely kill, they can cause many unpleasant effects and worry both child and parent.

After shave lotion
Alcohol
Ammonia
Animal medicines
Antifreeze
Bleach
Brake fluid
Carpet cleaning fluids
Caustic soda
Detergents (including bubble bath and washing-up liquid)
Disinfectants
Dyes
Fertilisers
Fire lighters
Garden chemicals
Glues
Insecticides
Lavatory cleaners
Lighter fuel
Medicines
Metal polishes
Methylated spirit
Mothballs
Nail varnish
Paint and paint strippers
Paraffin
Perfumes
Petrol
Rat poisons
Shampoos
Turpentine substitute (turps)
Weedkillers

Drugs are among the commonest causes of accidental poisoning in children. Aspirin, other painkillers, iron tablets, anti-depressants and sleeping pills are drugs which if taken in excess lead to serious illness or even death in children. Always keep medicines locked away out of the reach of children, preferably in a proper medicine cabinet. Many medicines come in foil strips with each tablet sealed safely away from children. If you have loose tablets, buy child-resistant containers with screw tops that can be undone by adults but not by children.

Some poisonous plants

There are surprisingly large numbers of poisonous plants. The best rule is to each your children never to such or eat anything unless given to them by their parents or by other adults whom they know. Most of the poisonous plants listed below are unpleasant to eat and so are difficult to consume in large enough quantities to be harmful but even so — play safe with children.

Older children can be taught which plants are dangerous but even they should be taught not to eat anything.

Should your child swallow anything but the smallest amount of any of these plants, get medical help but do not panic.

Some common examples :

Aconite (all of the plant)
Broom (seeds and pods)
Bryony (berries)
Daffodil and narcissus bulbs
Daphne (berries)
Deadly nightshade (berries)
Hemlock (young leaves and unripe fruit)
Honeysuckle (berries)
Laburnum (seeds and pods)
Laurel (leaves and berries)
Lupin (seeds and ponds)
Potato (fruits and green tubers)
Pyracantha (berries)
Rhubarb (leaves)
Yew (berries)

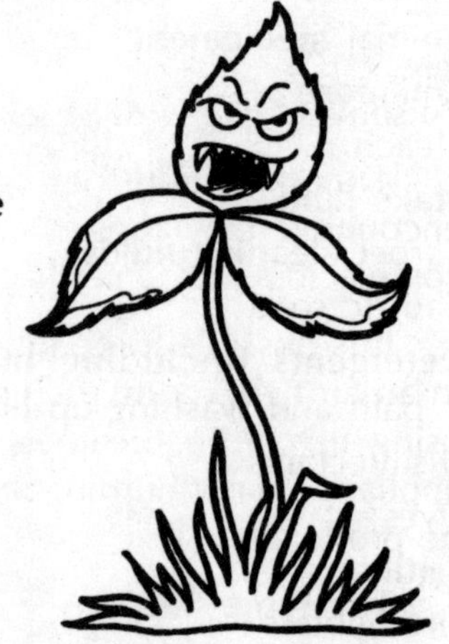

Agricultural poisons absorbed through the skin

There are so many chemicals used today in agriculture that it is difficult to generalise about them. The disturbing thing is that many of them are now available for the domestic market and so can present as a hazard even if you live in a city. As the symptoms are so variable it makes sense to say :

If you ever get any strange feelings after using pesticides, weed-killers or fertilisers, do not neglect them. Early, vague symptoms can quickly change into serious ones, so do not delay.

Some of these poisons affect breathing, some others nerve conduction and many are absorbed through the skin or the lungs.

What to do

1. Stop the person using the chemical.
2. Remove him gently from the area.
3. Remove contaminated clothing.
4. Wash exposed areas of the skin (preferably using rubber gloves yourself).
5. Give artificial respiration if breathing has stopped.
6. Look at the container for suggested remedies. As a precaution, wear gloves when handling chemical container and send it to the hospital with the person.
7. If the victim is sweating a lot and is hot, fan him and sponge with tepid water.

Poisoning by gas or smoke (fumes)

Although industrial gases and vapours of various kinds are encountered by those working with them, the gases most of us come across are domestic gas, carbon monoxide and carbon dioxide.

It is possible to be killed by gas because if a person is trapped in an air-tight room, the gas displaces the oxygen (which he is also using up as he breathes) and the person suffocates. Also, if an appliance is not burning properly, poisonous carbon monoxide may be produced.

The same happens with smoke but smoke has the additional disadvantage of actually damaging the lungs.

If you find someone in a gas or smoke-filled room :

1. Take a few deep breaths before entering.
2. Go in quickly, holding your breath and lift the victim to safety.
3. If you cannot remove him for any reason, throw open all the doors and windows, turn off the gas, leave and go back in as soon as the gas has dispersed. Do not do this if the place is on fire as it could draw the fire to the victim.
4. If the room is filled with smoke, a wet cloth or towel wrapped across your mouth and nose may help to keep a little of the smoke out of your lungs. Keep low and if you cannot lift or drag the person clear, get help.
5. Ask someone else to go for help.
6. Give artificial respiration if necessary.
7. If the person is overcome by exhaust fumes in a closed garage, open doors, switch off the engine and proceed as above.

Prevention note

1. Have all gas appliances serviced regularly (at least once a year)
2. Never meddle with appliances yourself.
3. Never block up ventilators — natural gas burns safely with plenty of air but produces poisonous carbon monoxide if it has too little air.
4. Never leave the car engine running in a closed garage — the poisonous carbon monoxide in the exhaust can overcome you quicker than you think.

Some common do nots

- Do not use a tourniquet to stop bleeding — the chances are you will do more harm than good by cutting off the blood supply for too long.
- Do not throw the head back for a nosebleed — this makes the blood trickle to the back of the throat from where it is swallowed. Subsequent vomiting can make the nosebleed worse.

- Do not give people salt water to make them sick when they swallow tablets. Do not give any water because rather than diluting the poison, water speeds up its absorption in the stomach.
- Do not use antiseptics undiluted — they are no more effective than in the correct dilution and can damage the body.
- Do not force a damaged elbow into a sling — you may do serious damage to the nerves and blood vessels nearby.
- Do not force a zip fastener open if the foreskin is caught. Cut the bottom of the zip open and peel open the teeth of the zip from below.
- Do not try to remove beads or other foreign bodies from children's ears and nose — leave them to the experts.
- Do not leave hand injuries hanging down — keep them up to stop swelling. Pin the cuff to the person's lapel or dress high up on the chest.
- Do not cover wounds or infections of the fingers with nylon fingerstalls for more than an hour or so. The warm, moist conditions favour the breeding of germs.
- Do not use other people's medicines.
- Do not give anything by mouth to someone you suspect has broken a bone — he may need an anaesthetic later.
- Do not make an emergency pillow for someone who has collapsed in the street — you may endanger his breathing by bending the neck forwards.
- Do not leave an unconscious person for longer than it takes to summon help.
- Do not move anyone you think has damaged his back unless he is threatened by danger.
- Do not give unconscious people anything to drink or eat. Wait until the person is alert enough to hold a cup for himself.
- Do not remove people from the scene of the crash because the ambulance crew may never find them.
- Do not take people to hospital by private car after a serious accident or illness because you deprive them of the treatment they would receive in the ambulance.

- Do not try lifting a vehicle off someone — you will probably hurt yourself or fail and let it drop back on the person, so inflicting even more damage.
- Do not touch anything until the mains supply has been switched off when you arrive at the scene of an electric shock.
- Do not cover people up more when they have a fever.

❐ SELF-HELP SECTION

This section is not meant to be a medical encyclopaedia, nor a way of making the reader into a professor of medicine overnight! The subjects covered are basically those which, whilst not life-threatening, can be distressing, painful or simply worrying until you can get medical help. If you suffer from longstanding arthritis or bad breath, the chances are that you will have to come to terms with it, find a satisfactory treatment or at least be prepared to seek 'non urgent' medical advice. All the conditions covered here are sufficiently worrying in the short term to constitute an emergency — but not in the usually accepted sense of the word. If an epileptic friend has a simple fit, for example, it would be reassuring to know what to do (and what not to do), then you would not panic.

As with the rest of the book, this section is not meant to replace medical advice from your doctor but should enable you to do something useful while you are waiting for the doctor to visit or for an appointment at the hospital and may even prevent you going to the local casualty department with something you could treat yourself.

If you are in any serious doubt about any condition — call your doctor. Do not use this section to outwit, out-diagnose or replace him. Having said this though, it is the responsibility of each of us to do what we can to help ourselves and our families. If we all insisted on medical care for all of the things in this section, every time we had them, doctors would be completely overwhelmed. Drawing the line is always difficult but the following gives you guidance on this too.

Abscess

A bad spot or boil containing pus anywhere on the body. The treatment for any collection of pus is to let it out. Nature will do this eventually but in the meantime it can be painful and inconvenient to wait. If the abscess is on the face or hands it can be dangerous as well as painful. Always get medical help early for abscesses in these areas and never interfere with them.

For other abscesses, draw the pus out by applying a hot water bottle to the area over a simple dressing and keep it covered afterwards with a fresh, dry dressing. Doctors always say you should not squeeze a pimple but people do it everyday and come to no harm. When there is a definite white or yellow 'head' to an abscess or boil you can squeeze it after washing your hands thoroughly. Never squeeze so hard as to damage the surrounding skin and if the head does not come out easily, stop, wait another day and try again if necessary.

Never dig around with a needle, penknife or similar instrument. If the pus would not come out on its own, see a doctor.

Never use waterproof dressings such as nylon fingerstalls or occlusive adhesive dressings because the bacteria in the abscess grow especially well under such wet, warm conditions and can spread to cause a wider and more serious infection of the tissues around the boil.

If you think the boil is spreading or if you notice any thin red lines in the skin surrounding an abscess, get medical help.

Always seek medical help for any abscess that is interfering with the use of a joint.

Never take the odd couple of antibiotic capsules or tablets that you happen to have in the medicine chest as this can lead to half-treated infections that never properly clear up. If you need antibiotics, your doctor will prescribe a proper course. Badly and half-treated abscesses can readily be troublesome for a very long time. If you take a few left-over tablets or stop a proper course early, you may permit the infection to flare up again and it may not respond to that medicine the second time around.

Alcoholism

This is a complex disease that is almost impossible to treat at home. If a member of your family is an alcoholic you will need help in order to lead a normal family life. Because alcoholism is a 'family disease', it has insidious effects which can be damaging to any or all of the family.

Angina

A severe pain in the chest, arms or neck caused by starvation of blood to the heart muscle. Treating angina is often easy because the person who suffers from it has usually been told what to do his doctor when the diagnosis was first made.

The problem with treating angina at home is that it is difficult (if not impossible) to distinguish between a really bad angina pain and a heart attack. Even doctors cannot always tell the difference without doing an electrocardiograph test. It someone has angina, sit him in a reclining position or lie him down; loosen any tight clothes; keep calm and help him to take one of his heart tablets. If the pain does not go within half an hour, or if he becomes ill, call a doctor.

The person who has the angina is usually the best judge of how he feels. If he is really ill with an episode, you will have to take over. Get an ambulance or a doctor if (1) he stops breathing or his pulse stops; (2) he goes very pale, sweaty or even blue; (3) he loses consciousness; (4) the pain goes on for more than half an hour after taking the angina tablets; or (5) he becomes very distressed.

Should it be necessary to call for an ambulance, tell the ambulance officer as much as you can about the person's angina because in some areas there are specialised cardiac ambulances which they can send out. Simply saying "Dad's collapsed on the sofa" tells them nothing.

Arthritis

Pain in a joint or joints. What you are to do depends on whether the pain has come on suddenly 'out of the blue' or has been with you for some time. Long term pain in the joints does not call for emergency action, but a painful, swollen joint of sudden onset can be very distressing.

Rest the part involved, take painkillers, apply heat to the area and see your doctor as early as you can.

Blisters

These are produced by burns or by repeated rubbing and chafing of an area of skin. Under normal conditions, do not *burst* blisters because doing so increases the risk of infection. Simply cover them with sterile, dry dressings and leave them. However, should the blister be so awkward because of its position that it causes a restriction of movement and function, prick it carefully as follows. Wash the blister itself with antiseptic solution, sterilise a large needle by boiling it or passing it through a flame until red hot, keep the needle away from anything else while it cools, pierce the blister in two places at the base and absorb the fluid that emerges on clean, new, cotton wool or gauze. Cover the whole area with a dry dressing until healed.

Breast abscess

Nearly ten per cent of breast feeding mothers suffer from a breast abscess in the weeks following childbirth. These abscesses are almost entirely preventable in the first place and arise only because the 'modern' mothers feed their babies in such a strange way. Because they breast feed by the clock (if indeed they breast feed at all), the breasts become engorged (swollen) and the pressure within the breasts can block a milk duct. The blocked duct shows as a red, hot, tender lump in the breast and this often makes the woman feel shivery or 'flu-like'.

First-aid measures include feeding the baby much more frequently (to empty the breast); not limiting the length of feeds; massaging the lump gently but firmly towards the nipple; ensuring that your bra does not press on any particular area of the breast; varying the position in which the baby feeds at each feed and even during a feed; and using hot or cold compresses (whichever gives best relief). Antibiotics will only be necessary if all these methods have not dispersed the lump within 24 hours.

If a blocked duct is caught early, it will not go on to become infected and form a proper abscess (a walled-off, pus-filled structure within the breast). Once an abscess does form through it will probably (like abscesses elsewhere) need to be incised by a doctor to allow the pus to escape. If you have a breast abscess you should not feed the baby from that breast, but continue to feed from the other one. Once the abscess has cleared up you can feed again from both breasts. In the meantime, express milk from the affected breast frequently and discard it. It may be possible to avoid incision by catching the abscess early and treating it with antibiotics. Your doctor will prescribe a suitable drug should it be indicated.

Breast lump

Lumps in he breast are fairly common and have most often nothing to do with cancer. But with one woman in twenty dying of breast cancer in the UK today, breast lumps must be taken seriously. If you feel a lump, go to your doctor within 24 hours or to the first surgery on Monday if you find the lump over the weekend. He will feel it and tell you if he thinks it feels like a 'normal' lump that many women have in their breasts or if he thinks it needs a specialist opinion. Any breast lump associated with a recent (as opposed to a long-standing) inturning of the nipple or bleeding from the nipple must be seen by a doctor without delay.

One of the ways of saving yourself a lot of worry is to get into the habit of examining your breasts regularly every month. Do this after your period and get used to the feel of your breasts so that you will pick up a lump early on, should one occur. Early treatment makes a difference to the outcome. Do not delay going to your doctor because you are afraid. Delay can only make things worse.

Bronchitis

An inflammation of the large air tubes in the chest. There are two different conditions covered by this term and they need different treatment. Acute bronchitis comes on after flue and colds and produces a dry, painful cough and tightness in the chest. Later on, yellow, brown or green phlegm may be coughed up. The best treatment for this condition is to keep the room air moist by having a kettle steaming away in a corner. Coupled with steam inhalations (available from chemists) this can reduce chest tightness and help bring up the phlegm. Hot drinks also help bring up the phlegm. Most people get better but some will need antibiotics. If you bring up yellow, brown or green phlegm, tell your doctor. Antibiotics may not be necessary.

Chronic bronchitis is a long term illness seen in cigarette smokers and those who have lived in polluted air. These people will know they are 'bronchitics' and should have been told that there is no cure. The condition can be prevented from getting worse by (1) stopping smoking; (2) moving away from polluted air; (3) losing weight; (4) getting medical treatment for even trivial chest infections; and (5) doing regular breathing exercises.

Colds

There is no cure for the common cold, but the symptoms of headache, runny nose, fever aches, pains and weakness are worth treating. The best treatment for a cold is still bed rest. A day in bed does more good than anything else. Take aspirin in the recommended dose for a headache or fever; drink plenty of fluids; and take 1g of Vitamin C twice a day (it may do some good and will do no harm). If you are going to use nasal decongestants to help you breathe more easily, follow the instructions carefully — never overdo them.

If you get breathless or cough up green or yellow phlegm, seek medical help.

Colic

An intermittent pain caused by the contraction of a hollow organ or tube in the body. In adults, colic is typically caused by gall stones or kidney stones but most of us have suffered from abdominal pains that 'come and go' at some time, without having stones. The cause of these pains in hardly ever found, but the condition often improves once the person has had his bowels open. Any severe pain that comes and goes and is bad enough to make you feel sick or put you to bed must be assessed by a doctor. While waiting for the doctor, apply gentle warmth to your abdomen.

In children, 'three month' or evening colic is a term used to explain the screaming sessions that occur usually in the early evenings up to the age of about three months. The usual remedies of food, comfort, drink and nappy change seem to make little difference. A baby may cry at this time of day because of tension (mother is getting tired and is especially busy) or boredom (because he has been sleeping and eating all day and is ready to be amused).

If you are breast feeding, let your baby suck on and off all evening on your lap, if necessary. Cut out all cows' milk and milk products from your diet for a few days because some babies get colic from the traces of cows' milk in their mother's breast milk.

Colic in babies is in most cases no longer thought to be due to 'wind'. Anti-colic medicines are of little help and your baby will benefit most from being carried around (perhaps in a sling) and comforted.

Conjunctivitis

An inflammation of the membrane covering the eye. Usually caused by bacteria, it can be secondary to grit or even trauma. The eye becomes pink and the eyelashes stick together with yellow discharge especially on first waking. Bathe the eye with boric acid solution several times a day and tell your doctor as soon as practicable. He will give you drugs or an ointment which cure the conditions very quickly. Do not share face flannels or towels whilst you have this condition as it is easy to pass on. Wash your hands after touching your eyes and change your pillowslip daily.

Contraceptive failure

There are three crises that can occur with contraceptives. The first is forgetting the pill, the second is the failure of a barrier method and the third, the falling out of your coil (IUD).

Pill failure is relatively common because unless you are absolutely rigid about when you take it each day, it is easy to forget. If you discover that you have forgotten a pill within 24 hours of when you should have taken it, take another immediately and then take the next one at the normal time.

If you discover your mistake between 24-48 hours after you should have taken a pill, take two pills together immediately and then catch up with your old routine.

For any gap of more than 48 hours, take two pills per 24 hours until you have made up the deficit and are back on schedule again as judged by taking the right pill on the right day marked on the pack. In this case you should also use another method such as a diaphragm or a sheath together with contraceptive jelly to be sure you are safe. Your next cycle should see you back to normal again, so do not worry.

Should your IUD (coil or loop) fall out, there is nothing you can do yourself, so simply tell the doctor or clinic that fitted it and go and have it replaced as soon as you can. You are not protected at all, of course, while it is out, so use some other method in the meantime.

If a sheath bursts or comes off while the penis is in the vagina, if you find your diaphragm has a hole in it or if you think you may have got some sperms in your vagina during the withdrawal method, you can do one of two things. First, you can go to certain family planning clinics or hospital specialist clinics for a 'morning after' pill (your will need to phone around a bit to find one that offers it) or you can do something at once for yourself at home. (1) make up a solution of vinegar and water (half and half) and crouching over a bowl in the bath, splash the liquid up into your vagina vigorously; (2) using the vinegar and water mixture, thoroughly soak a tampon and push it high up into your vagina. A combination of 1 and 2 is a good idea. Neither of these methods is foolproof, of course, but they are worth trying and may be better than doing nothing.

Lastly, do not panic if you think you have a contraceptive failure. Bear in mind that except for the days around the middle of your cycle you are most unlikely to conceive anyway and that might put your mind at rest.

❒ NO HEART BEAT OR PULSE

How to tell

1. Person unconscious.
2. Person looks pale or blue-grey.
3. The pupils of the eyes (the back part in the centre) are very large.
4. No pulse over the carotid artery (left in the groove at the side of the Adam's apple).
5. No heartbeat heard on applying your ear to the left side of the breast bone.

What to do

1. Lie the person on his back on a hard surface. If on a bed, quickly but carefully lift him on to the floor.
2. Give one sharp, hard blow with the side of the hand over the lower left side of the breastbone. This may 'shock' the heart into re-starting spontaneously. Send someone else for an ambulance or doctor while you :

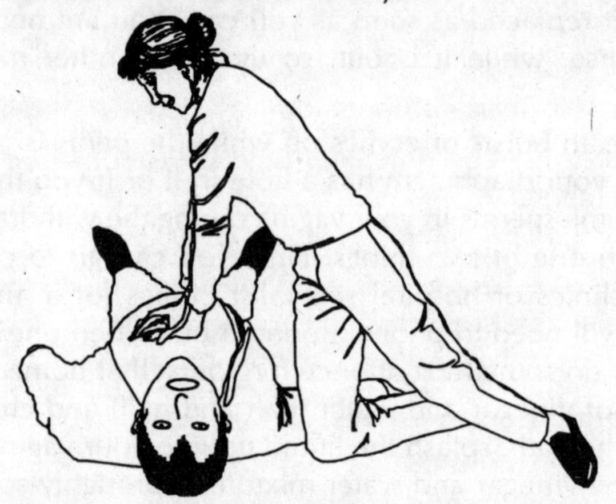

3. Start cardiac massage — but only if you are sure the heart is not beating.
4. Kneel on the person's right side facing him.
5. Put the heel of one hand over the lower half of the breastbone (not on its lower end). The rest of your hand should not exert pressure on the chest at all.
6. Place the heel of the other hand on the back of the first hand.
7. Keep your arms straight and rock backwards and forwards. Do not apply pressure by bending your arms or you will be exhausted within no time — let your body weight do the work. Keep your hands in position all the time.

   In **adults** : Depress the chest wall about 5 cm (2 in), 60 times per minute.

   In **children** : Use one hand only at 80 times per minute.

   In **babies** : Use two fingers only at 100 times per minute and press higher up the breastbone so as not to damage the liver which is large and easily ruptured.

How long to continue

1. Until the person looks a better colour.
2. Until his pupils reduce to normal size.
3. Until the neck pulse returns or he starts to recover.

If any of these signs is apparent, stop and check for the heartbeat or pulse.

If you are alone

1. Inflate the lungs quickly twice.
2. Do 15 heart compressions (as detailed above).

Repeat this circuit time after time while someone goes for help or an ambulance.

Do not go on compressing the chest of someone whose pulse has returned. Although breathing may stop on its own, the heart stopping also causes breathing to fail. So with someone whose heart has stopped you have a double problem.

When another person arrives

One person should do mouth to mouth resuscitation (the kiss of life) while the other does cardiac massage.

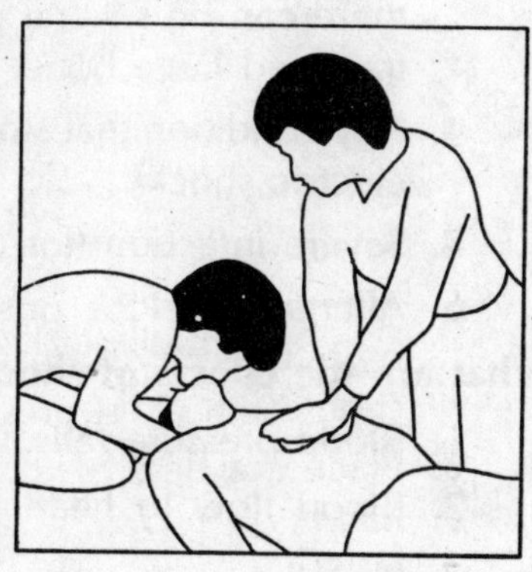

Keep the sequence as follows :

You breathe one breath — he does five heart compressions — you do one breath — he does five heart compressions and so on until successful or until professional help arrives. The person doing the breathing part should also check the neck pulse.

Why heart massage works

Contary to popular belief, the heart lies almost centrally in the chest and not under the left nipple. If the breastbone is depressed sufficiently (about 5 cm (2 in) in an adult) the heart will be physically compressed between the breastbone in front and the spine behind. This is not the way the heart normally performs but is a useful first aid procedure. This is why when you do cardiac massage you must only press in the centre of the chest, over the breastbone. If you press over the ribs you may break them but worst of all you would not be doing anything useful to the heart so the whole thing will be a waste of time.

❐ SHOCK

Emotional Shock — feeling faint or weak, even to the point of fainting. Brought about by unpleasant sights, emotional trauma, etc. This comes on quickly. True shock — a condition with many causes that affects body functions severely. It may end in death.

What causes it?

1. Severe loss of blood — usually more than 850 ml ($1\frac{1}{2}$ pints). Do not forget that a person can lose pints of blood internally.
2. Loss of body fluid through the surface of burns or from prolonged diarrhoea and vomiting.
3. Severe bruising — even with no outward sign of blood loss, there can be several pints of blood in the tissue around a fractured large bone.
4. Any condition that stops the heart beating (e.g. heart attack, electric shock).
5. Severe infection (for example, a burst appendix).
6. Allergic shock.

What are the effects of shock ?

1. Blood pressure falls.
2. Blood flow to heart is decreased so that the heart beats faster.
3. The blood vessels in the periphery constrict, so that most of the available blood is supplied to the vital organs of the body like the heart, brain, and kidneys. This ensures better supply of oxygen and nutrients to these structures.
4. As the shock progresses, the blood supply to the internal is shut off so that they undergo necrosis and lose their function.
5. If the shock is not treated in time, even the vital organs do not receive blood and the shock becomes irreversible.
6. The final stage is of death.

What are the factors affecting the degree of shock ?

1. Pain : Neurogenic shock increases in severity with the severity of pain.
2. Fatigue : It increases severity of shock.
3. Chronic diseases : Persons having chronic diseases develop shock easily.
4. Physical condition : People who are starved or exposed to extremes of heat or cold develop shock more easily.

Signs of a shocked person

Pale or even grey, Cold to touch, Eyelids are half open, pupils are dilated, Sweaty, Breathing in a rapid, shallow way, Pulse is fast and weak, Restless and anxious, Thirsty, Urine output is low or absent, blurring of vision, Nauseated and may vomit, Unconscious or may be in coma.

Action

If most of the above list are present, the victim is in a bad way and needs urgent medical help. Get some one to call an ambulance or doctor.

Try to help the shock victim before he gets this bad.

For any severe injury, start preventing shock even before signs appear.

1. Stop bleeding. Press over the area.
2. Remove him only from serious hazard — otherwise do not move him. If he is in the road — treat him there — and get others to keep traffic clear.
3. Place him in the recovery position.
4. Cover up and dress any wounds to reduce distress.
5. Loosen tight clothing.
6. Keep him from getting chilled with a blanket or other light covering.
7. Do not apply heat or lots of blankets.
8. Reassure him; keep crowds away (give them things to do).
9. Never give anything by mouth to anyone in a severe state of shock (even if he is thirsty) or to anyone who is

unconscious. Wet his lips with a damp cloth or your fingers dipped in water if he asks for a drink.

10. Never give alcohol or use hot water bottles — both draw blood (which is needed elsewhere for the vital functions of the body's organs) to the skin.
11. Watch breathing — resuscitate if it stops.
12. Feel pulse rate at neck. As shock develops, the pulse can double in rate (normal is around 70 beats per minute).

❐ HEART ATTACK

What is it ?

Sudden damage to the heart's muscle which renders it less able to carry out its function as a pump. Some heart attacks are so severe that they stop the heart altogether; others render the person severely ill for a time, but allow him to recover later; and others are so minor that they may cause only slight discomfort in the chest.

Signs

1. Severe sudden pain in the chest. Usually the pain is central and described as 'crushing', 'gripping', or 'a tightness'. It is rarely sharp or knife-like.
2. Pain down the arms or into the neck.
3. The person looks pale, sweaty, anxious and has a rapid and perhaps irregular pulse.
4. Breathlessness.
5. If the heart attack is very severe, there may be no pulse or heartbeat.

Any person complaining of any of these things, even in isolation, (except for breathlessness) needs urgent medical help.

Action : Is the person conscious and cooperative ?

If yes :

1. Sit him up at an angle of 45° in a bed or armchair or against a wall if out of doors.
2. Send for a doctor or ambulance, or get someone else to.
3. Get him to take his prescribed tablet if he carries them around with him for angina.

4. Loosen his clothing so that he breathe easily.
5. Dry his face of sweat.
6. Do not fuss around — keep people away.
7. Sit and talk reassuringly to him until professional help arrives.

If no :

1. Lie him down flat.
2. Loosen his collar and other restrictive clothing.
3. Feel for a pulse in the neck or place your ear on the left side of the breastbone and listen for the heartbeat. If none is heard, start resuscitation. If the heartbeat is present, keep a close watch while someone else goes off for help.

After a heart attack

1. Always take your medicines as prescribed — no more and no less.
2. Keep your weight to a level that is right for your height. If in any doubt, ask your doctor.
3. Never overeat — an overfull stomach can cause pressure on the heart.
4. Do not rush around after meals.
5. Cut down, or preferably stop smoking altogether.
6. Take regular, controlled exercise, but stop if you get chest or arm pain. Some people take up jogging after a heart attack with beneficial results.
7. Do not think of yourself as a cardiac cripple — millions of men are leading happy and fruitful lives after a heart attack.
8. Do not give up sex. Studies slow that the vast majority of heart attack patients can indulge in sexual activity without any fear of overstraining their hearts. But wait for 8 weeks after your heart attack before you start !
9. Get good restful sleep.

❒ HEART ATTACK : HOW TO PREVENT

Heart attacks kill an increasing number of people every year. One in three middle aged men today dies of a heart attack and the victims are getting younger and younger.

Certain factors seem to increase the risk :

(1) cigarette smoking; (2) high blood pressure; (3) high blood cholesterol (open to debate); (4) obesity; (5) lack of exercise; and (6) stress.

What to do

1. Stop smoking. If you smoke 20 or more cigarettes a day, you double your chance of having a heart attack.
2. Have your blood pressure checked by your doctor and keep to his treatment if it is high.
3. Cut down on fatty meat; use soft margarine instead of butter; use corn or sunflower oil for cooking; avoid cream; eat fewer than 3 eggs per week; cut down on pastries, cakes and biscuits; eat more fruit and vegetables; and eat wholemeal bread and wholemeal flour products. The advice here on cutting down on cholesterol-rich foods is currently under scrutiny, but it will do no harm to reduce cholesterol-containing foods. Do not cut them our altogether though.
4. Get your weight down to what your doctor suggests. Start by cutting your sugar intake by half and eventually cutting it out altogether. This alone will reduce your weight surprisingly quickly.
5. Sedentary people have 3 times the chance of having a heart attack than active ones, so take regular exercise. Active people have 3 times the chance of surviving their first heart attack compared with inactive ones. Walk or jog regularly (2-3 times per week) in such a way as to raise your pulse to 120 beats per minute or more. Anything less than this cannot be considered to be 'protective' exercise. Having said this, take care not to exercise too much too soon, but work it up gradually.
6. Stress, especially in the presence of other risk factors, can be an important trigger. Avoiding stress can be difficult, but it is worth trying to steer clear of the things that upset you or cause tension at work.

Remember A heart attack does not just happen to other people — it could happen to you.

❐ CHOKING

It is obstruction of the pharynx by a foreign body. Foreign bodies found in the throat are usually fish bones, some pieces of food, artificial teeth, coin, buttons, pins etc. Usually they are accidently swallowed. A child may swallow things during play. Unless treated promptly the victim can die of asphyxia.

Adults usually choke on food, children also on foreign bodies such as coins, buttons and boiled sweets.

How to tell : *Children* —

The child chokes, coughs violently and possibly his face becomes blue. He cannot breathe or speak.

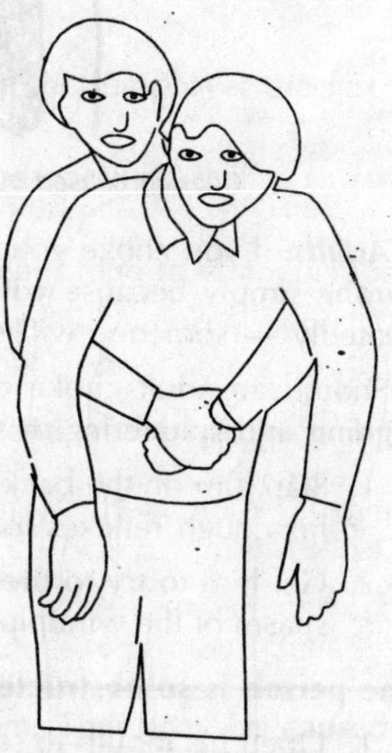

***Action* :**

1. A very small baby can be held upside down and smacked on the back.
2. For an older child, lie him over your knee or over a chair and slap him hard on the back with flat of the hand between the shoulder blades. This should dislodge the object and make him cough it up. If this does not work at once, try the Heimlich method :

   (*i*) Get behind the child and place your arms around his waist.

   (*ii*) Clench one of your hands into a first over the child's stomach between the navel and the rib cage.

   (*iii*) Grip the clenched first with the other hand.

   (*iv*) Press your hands strongly against the abdominal wall, pressing slightly upwards. This sharp pressure drives the air our of the lungs suddenly and carries the obstructing object up through the windpipe.

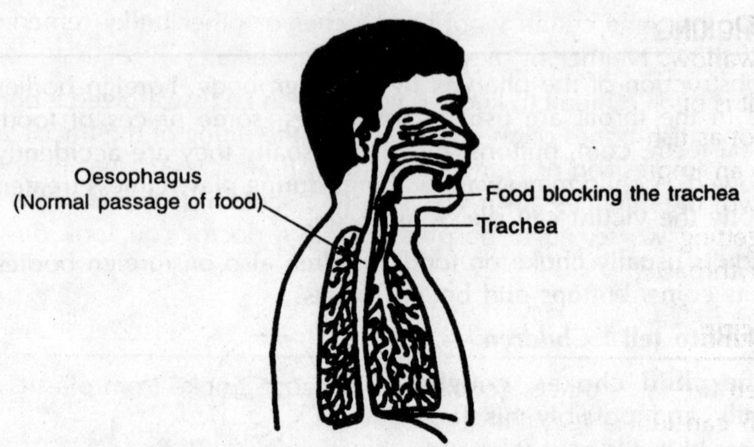

Choking caused by food entering the windpipe.

Adults. If you choke yourself it is very difficult to explain what is wrong simply because your cannot speak. Point to your throat repeatedly — someone will soon get the message.

Should an adult choke on something, decide if he is simply coughing and spluttering. If so

1. Slap him on the back if he wants help, but otherwise leave his cough reflexes to cope — they usually do.
2. Get him to try to breathe slowly and deeply. This reduces spasm of the windpipe and will release the choking object.

If the person is so obstructed that he is going blue

1. Open his mouth to see if you can hook out the obstruction with your finger. It is usually too far back for this, but it is worth looking quickly.
2. Get him on the floor and turn him on his side.
3. Slap him firmly on the back between the shoulder blades. This will almost always dislodge the foreign body.

If this does not work, use the Heimlich method.

Fishbone in throat

If the person is choking really seriously, treat as adult choking. If not :

Do not try to reach into the throat to pick the bone out.

Do not give cotton wool sandwiches or other bulky remedies to swallow. Neither of these procedures works.

It is often difficult to know if you have in fact swallowed a bone or not as fish-bones often simply scratch the lining of the throat yet give an impression of being stuck there. If all is well after an hour or two, the chances are it was simply a scratch. If things seem to be getting worse, go to hospital so that a doctor can look down your throat.

❒ FIRE

When fire takes place, get out fast, because smoke from plastic or foam can kill in less than two minutes.

The Fire Brigade should be called for any fire, however small.

If fire breaks out

At Home

(i) If the house catches fire

1. Get everyone in the house to a safe place on the ground floor so that they can get out quickly and safely. OR leave the house altogether, closing doors, windows, fan, lights, etc. so that draughts do not feed the fire.

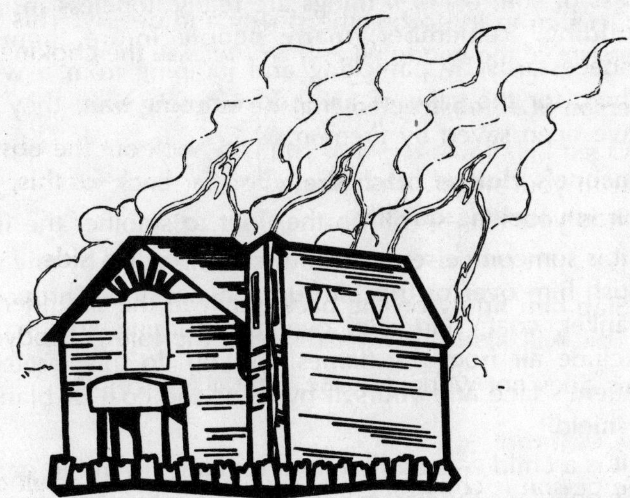

2. Do not assume that someone else has called the fire brigade — do it yourself.

3. Only when everyone is safe should you start to tackle the fire, but only if you can do so without taking personal risks.
4. Use your fire extinguisher if you have one.
5. Wait for the fire brigade.

(ii) If you are trapped by a fire

1. Close the door of the room.
2. Block up the gap under the door with bedding, towels, clothes, etc., wetted if possible.
3. Attract attention at the window by shouting or waving a highly coloured article outside.
4. Should the room fill with smoke, go to the window and lean out for fresh air. If you cannot do this, lie flat on the floor face down until help arrives or the situation gets desperate.
5. Should the room begin to burn or you cannot breathe because of the smoke, tie sheets or other strong material together, secure one end to a heavy piece of furniture and use this 'rope' to lower yourself from the window.
6. Never jump out of a window. Lower yourself until you are hanging by your hands from the window sill and then drop, but do this only if (*a*) you can land safely, preferably on grass or soil, or (*b*) if things are really hopeless inside the building. Remember, many people injure themselves unnecessarily by panicking and jumping from a window when, for the sake of another minute's wait, they could have been saved by firemen.

(iii) If someone's clothes catch fire

1. If it is yourself — roll on the floor to smother the flames.
2. If it is someone else — get him to the ground by any means (push him over or trip him up if necessary). Throw a rug, blanket, coat, skirt, etc. over the burning area so as to exclude air from the flames. As you do this, protect the patient's face and yourself by using the coat or blanket as a shield.
3. If it is a child — stop him from running around in panic (as this only fans the flames). Roll him in a blanket, etc. to put out the flames as above.

Smouldering clothes should not be smothered because the hot fabric will be forced on to the patient's skin and so cause more damage. Carefully pull smouldering clothes off by unburnt parts. Put them in a fireproof bowl or other container or throw them on the floor and stamp on them. Call an ambulance. If the person is not seriously burnt, take him at once to a hospital.

Never try to remove clothes that are charred or burnt firmly on to a person. Leave this to experts.

(iv) If an oil heater catches fire

Stand atleast 6 ft (2 m) away, and throw on buckets of water.

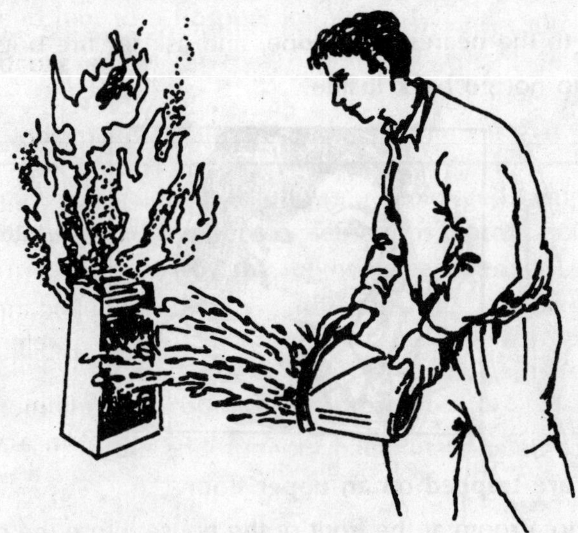

(v) If a foam sofa or armchair catches fire

Burning plastic foam gives off choking black smoke that can overcome you in one minute. Do not try to put out the fire.

(1) Get out of the room and close the door to prevent the smoke from spreading.

(vi) If you smell burning at night

1. Alert everyone in the house.
2. If the fire is too big to deal with safely get everyone outside. If you think the fire is well alight in a closed room, do not open door to find out.

3. Shut all doors behind you to restrict the spread of flames and smoke.

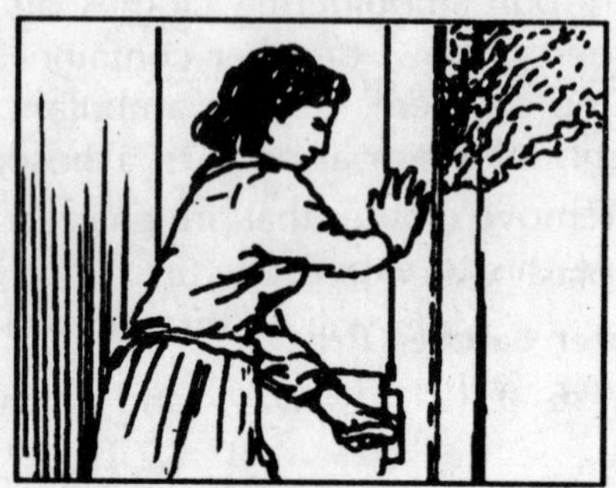

4. Go to the nearest telephone, and ask for fire brigade.
   – Do not go back inside.

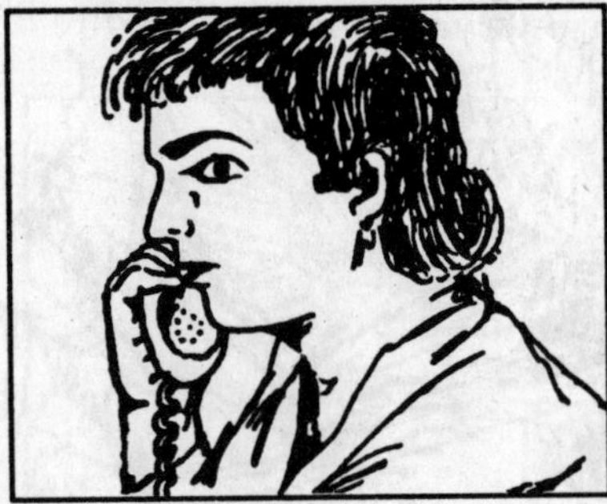

(vii) If you are trapped on an upper floor

1. Go to a room at the front of the house, close the door and block up cracks with bedding or clothes.

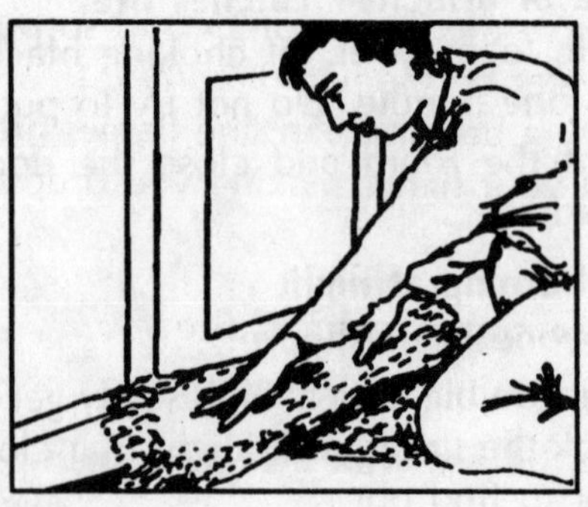

2. Open the window and call for help.

Do not jump out of the window, except as a last resort.

(vii) If a chimney catches fire

1. Remove the hearth rug and anything around the hearth that might burn.
2. Gently splash water on to the fire in the grate. Do not flood the fire or the water will be thrown back at you as a cloud of scalding steam.
3. If you have a fine meshed fire-guard, put it around the fire. If not, stand by with a bucket of water and a shovel to remove any burning soot that falls down the chimney and bounces back on to the carpet.

(ix) If a chip pan or frying pan catches fire

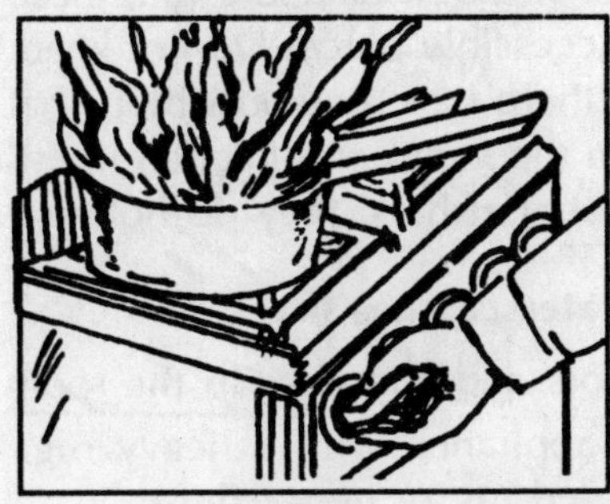

1. Turn off the heat (oil, gas or electric).
2. Cover the pan with its lid, a tray or a damp towel. All of these starve the flames of air and so put them out. Do not throw water on the pan or carry it to a sink or window. As you carry a burning pan, the flames are forced back on to you and your hand, making you drop the pan and spread the fire.

(x) If a TV or Computer catches fire

1. Pull out the plug or switch off at the main fuse box.
2. Smother the fire with a blanket or rug or a fire blanket.

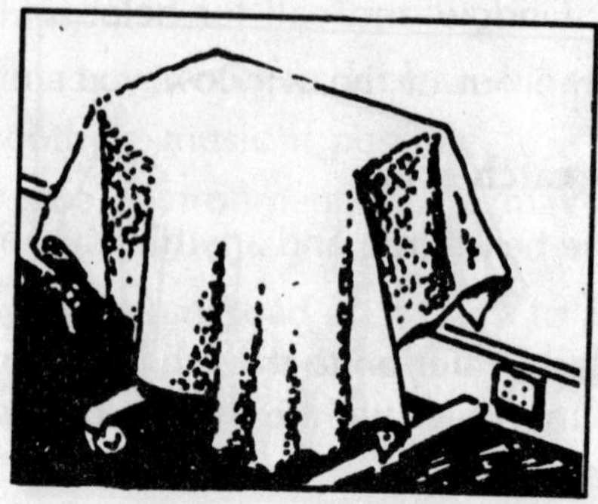

– Do not use water or a fire extinguisher, because residual electricity may remain in the set.

(xi) Fire extinguishers

Every home should have a domestic fire extinguisher and preferably a fire blanket too. Make sure that these are kept in the hall or other easily accessible place. Do not keep them under the kitchen sink because there's a strong possibility that you will not be able to get to them in the event of a kitchen fire. Keep a check on the expiry date on extinguishers, they do not last for ever.

(xii) If a stove or heater catches fire

1. Close the doors and windows in the room.
2. Smother the appliance with a heavy rug, towel, blanket, etc.
3. Unless the fire goes out at once, get everyone out of the building.

(xiii) Electrical fires

1. Switch off the source of the electricity supply and pull out the plug.
2. Smother the appliance with a heavy rug, towel, blanket, etc.
3. Unless the fire goes out at once, get everyone out of the building.
4. **Never throw water on to an electrical appliance.**

(xiv) In the shed or garage

1. Remove the car.
2. Remove any cans of petrol, cans of paint, creosote, etc.
3. Close all doors and windows.
4. Use a fire extinguisher if you have one.

IN A CARAVAN

1. Try simple measures to smother the fire or put it out with an extinguisher.
2. Turn off the gas cylinder outside and if possible disconnect it and roll it away.
3. Stand well clear.
4. Never leave children alone in a caravan.

If the fire is not immediately controllable, get out of the vehicle quickly as fires spread very rapidly in cars and caravans.

IN THE CAR

1. Stop the car.
2. Get everyone out.
3. Use a fire extinguisher if you have one and the fire is not too bad.
4. If engine compartment catches fire, open the bonnet a little only and push the nozzle of the fire extinguisher into the gap.
5. For a serious fire — stand well clear because the petrol tank may explode or poisonous fumes from burning plastics may harm your lungs.
6. If you see someone in a burning car, try to drag him free if you can do so without endangering yourself. Speedy action can prevent the inhalation of killer fumes. These are just as likely to kill as the flames.

Remember the fire brigade should always be called to any fire however small.

❐ BURNS AND SCALDS

Burn is defined as tissue damage caused by dry heat of open flame, hot object, molten metal or electricity.

Burn : Classified according to the area and depth of the injury.

Degree of burns : This classification indicates degree of damage to the tissues.

First degree : Reddened skin.

Second degree : Blisters on the skin.

Third degree : Destruction of deeper tissues and charring.

Scald : Wet heat such as steam, hot water, hot oil etc. produces scalds. The scald is superficial but often extensive. Blisters and red areas are in the surface.

Assessment of burn

The danger from burns depends on the area of the burns rather than the degree. Superficial burns over a large area are more dangerous than the complete charring of a part.

Any burn more than 30% should be hospitalised. Calculation for the percentage of the burn is to be done in the following manner as shown in the figure.

The skin area involved in a burn case is more important than the depth. Even a superficial burn involving more than 5% of the body surface is serious. If more than 15% the patient may suffer from shock. By following the "Rule-of-Nine", the percentage of skin area is to be calculated.

Rule of nine

Head and neck	:	9%
Chest	:	9%
Abdomen	:	9%
Genital area	:	1%
Front of each leg	:	9%
Back of each leg	:	9%
Each hand	:	9%
Back	:	18%

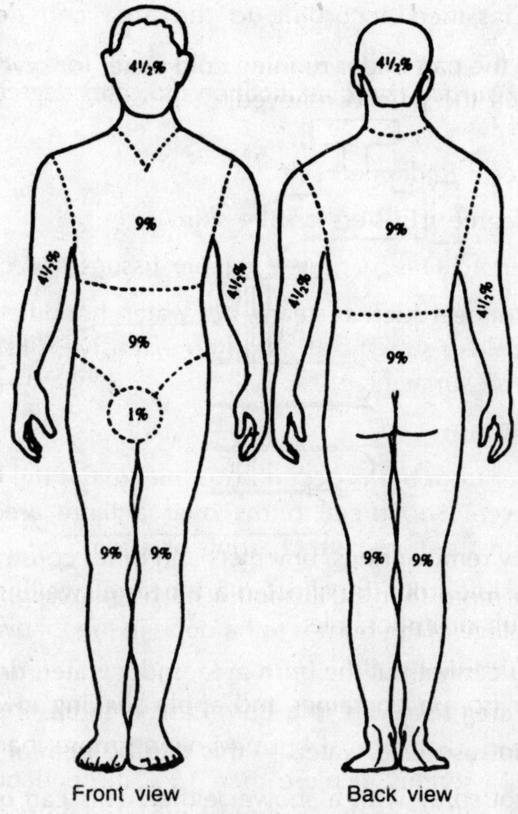

Rule-of-nine

General action

1. Remove the source of burning or scalding.
2. Cool the affected area at once.
3. Treat shock if present.
4. Get medical help if the person is severely ill.

Do not

1. Put cotton wool or any other fluffy dressings on to the burn (as they stick and are very difficult to remove).
2. Put grease, oily creams or butter on the wound. Leave blisters alone (if you burst them, you are encouraging infection).

What to do

1. Place the part under running cold water for several minutes, or until the pain is relieved.

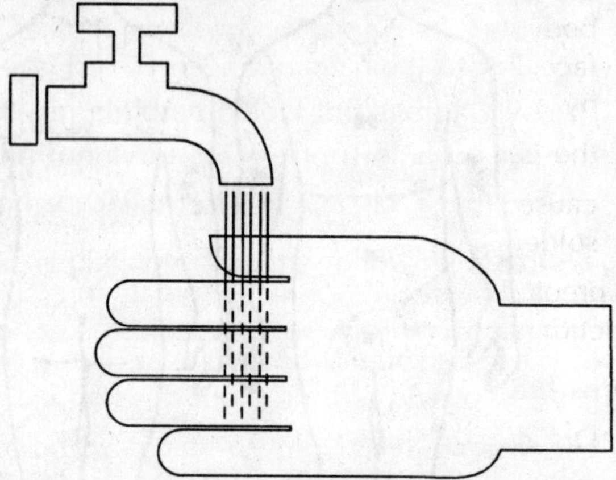

2. Gently remove rings, bracelets and other constricting things if possible from the affected are before swelling makes this difficult or impossible.
3. If you cannot put the burn area under water, drench it with water from a container and apply soaking towels.
4. Do not use iced water — this can be painful in itself.
5. Do not spray with a shower either. This can be extremely painful and may further damage the tissues.
6. Do not pull off any clothing around the burnt area unless the burn has affected only a small, confined area. Never pull away adherent charred clothes from flesh — this is an expert job.
7. Once the area has been cooled, you can gently remove clothing from the affected area around the scald. This goes for chemical burns too. Be careful not to burn yourself with chemical-soaked clothes.
8. Decide whether the person needs medical attention.

Is medical attention needed ?

No, if the scald or burn is small (less than 2.5 cm (1 in) across), shallow, easily covered by a dressing and the person is well.

Yes, if

1. the victim is a child;
2. the burn is large and especially if it involves areas of the body that move (around joints for example); affects the face; affects the palm or fingers or cannot easily be covered by a dressing.
3. the person is in shock or if you are at all worried;
4. caused by a chemical, electricity or molten metal (e.g. solder).

Be prepared to treat shock and to call an ambulance or doctor if the victim has 10 per cent or more of his body burned or scalded.

For burns that you can treat

1. Dry the area carefully.
2. Apply a dry dressing (not of cotton wool), preferably a non-adhesive burns dressing from your first-aid box.
3. Bandage the area lightly to hold the dressing in place.
4. Keep the burnt part elevated to reduce swelling.
5. Give the person a painkilling drug in the full recommended dose if the pain is bad.
6. If the burn gets infected (red, pussy, weeping or increasingly painful), get medical help. Infection will produce scarring later.

For burns you cannot treat

1. Lie the victim down and make him comfortable.
2. Give only tiny sips of water — any more may cause vomiting.
3. Keep calm and reassure him.

Some useful hints

1. Remove clothes drenched in boiling fat, water or steam as soon as possible.
2. Remove clothes drenched in chemicals. If necessary cut them to get them off quickly. Wash the area with plenty of running water.

3. Take any electrical burn to a doctor.
4. Treat severe friction burns as other burns.
5. Scalds in the month can be helped by sucking ice.
6. If chemicals enter the eye, wash it out with water at once. Get the person to hold his face under water and blink or put the eye under gently running water. Protect the uninjured eye. Go to hospital quickly.
7. Sunburn victims need cool, shade, fluids to drink (small sips) and soothing cream (or calamine lotion). Get medical help for severe cases.

❐ UNCONSCIOUSNESS

There are many causes of unconsciousness but you will not be able to sort them out. Leave the diagnosis to a doctor and in the meantime help the patient stay alive.

1. Make sure the person can breathe — before anything else.
2. Get someone to call an ambulance or doctor.
3. Suffocation is the greatest danger because the tongue can slip back and block the airway.
   Wipe out any vomit, blood, food, false teeth, etc. with your fingers (inside a handkerchief if available).
4. If he is not breathing, start resuscitation.
5. If he is breathing, lie him down in the recovery position, turn his head to one side and pull the jaw forward to clear the airway. If he makes gurgling or snoring noises you have not cleared the airway.
6. Give nothing by mouth until the person himself can hold a cup and then he should take only tiny sips or he may vomit.
7. While awaiting professional help — stop bleeding and prevent shock if present.
8. Keep him in the recovery position and keep people away.

The recovery position

Many people have died unnecessarily because they have choked on their own tongue or vomit. This can be prevented by placing the person in the recovery position.

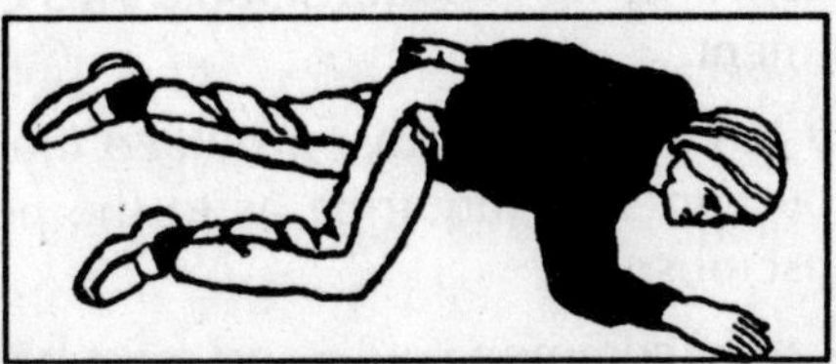

Always get an injured or unconscious person into this position as soon as possible except when you suspect a fracture, especially of the spine in which case do not move the person unless his life is threatened.

In such cases, stay by the head, turn it to one side and pull the chin forwards and upwards to clear the airway.

It is not easy to put someone into the recovery position if he is unconscious and much bigger than you. So follow the technique described below and you will not hurt yourself or him.

1. Kneel beside the casualty as he lies on his back.
2. Put both arms by his sides.
3. Bring his far leg across his near one and pull his far hip over so that his far leg can rest on the ground near your knees. His thigh should be at right angles to his hip.
4. Take care of his head during all this (with your right hand) so that it does not roll on to the ground and hurt him.
5. Bring his far arm (which is now near your knees) up towards his face and use it to prop the body up a bit so he does not lie flat on his face. His upper arm should end up at right angles to the shoulder. His other arm is behind him, out straight, close to his body.
6. Adjust the position of the head so that the chin is pulled forwards and the head tilted backwards to clear the airway.

   Do not use pillows. If the person is on a bed or stretcher, raise its foot.
7. Do not leave him alone. Watch breathing and feel for the neck pulse from time to time. At any sign of either failing, resuscitate, start heart massage or do both.
8. Look in his wallet to see if he carries a card or round his neck or wrist for a Medicalert or Talisman medallion which

night explain why he is unconscious. This could help in his later treatment.

9. Once you have done all this, provided the person is in no danger you can start inquiring as to the possible cause of the unconsciousness.

Head injuries are a common cause and must be taken seriously.

1. Any child who has been unconscious for however short a period must be seen by a doctor as soon as possible.
2. Anyone who has been 'knocked out' or suffered concussion should receive medical attention even if he feels all right. It is possible that there may be a fracture of the skull or other damage which is not immediately apparent yet which might cause danger later. A person who has bruising around the eye sockets or watery or blood-stained fluid from the nose or ears must have immediate medical help.
3. Anyone who has speech or coordination problems after a period of unconsciousness must be seen by a doctor at once. Severe headache, dizziness, vomiting or double vision are other important warnings of possible complications.

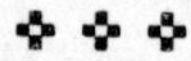

CHAPTER

10

Structure and Function of Human Body : You Must Know

The human body is an amazing combination of different systems that are well coordinated for smooth functioning as a unit. All the systems are equally important for health, and no particular system can be called as more important that other systems. a first aider

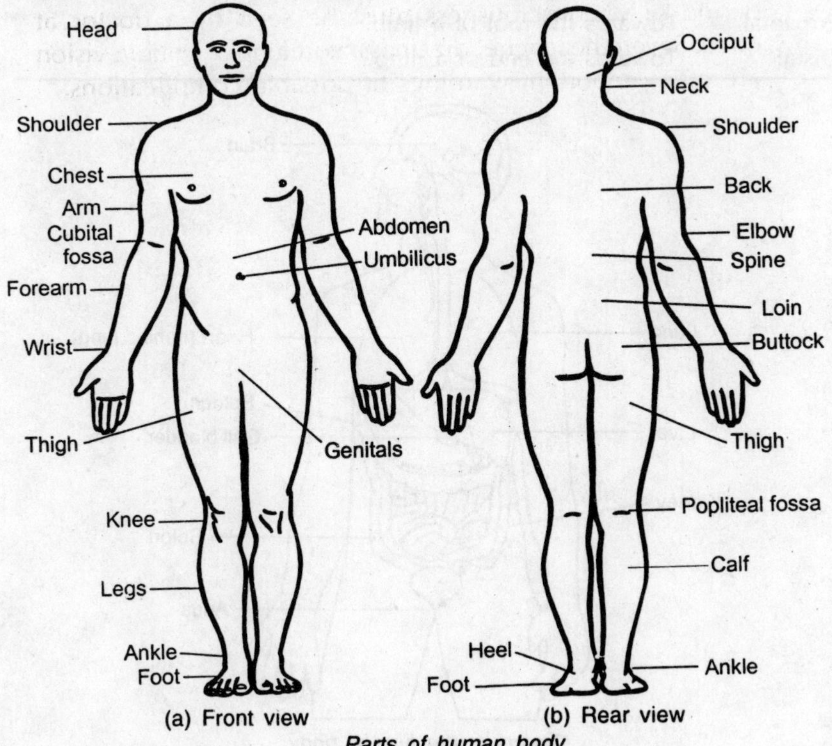

Parts of human body

needs to have knowledge of the structure and function of various systems so as to be able to clearly understand sickness and effects of injury on the body.

❒ THE BASIC STRUCTURE OF THE HUMAN BODY

We all know that the smallest functioning unit of every living being is a cell. A group of cells together form a tissue. Various tissues together form an organ. There may be a number of organs in a system that serve a specific purpose.

Term	Meaning
Midline	It divides the body into right and left halves with a vertical line.
Lateral	Anything away from the midline is said to be lateral.
Superior	Towards the head end.
Inferior	Towards the foot end.
Posterior	Back of the body.
Anterior	Front of the body.
Proximal	Towards the root of a limb.
Distal	Towards the end of a limb.

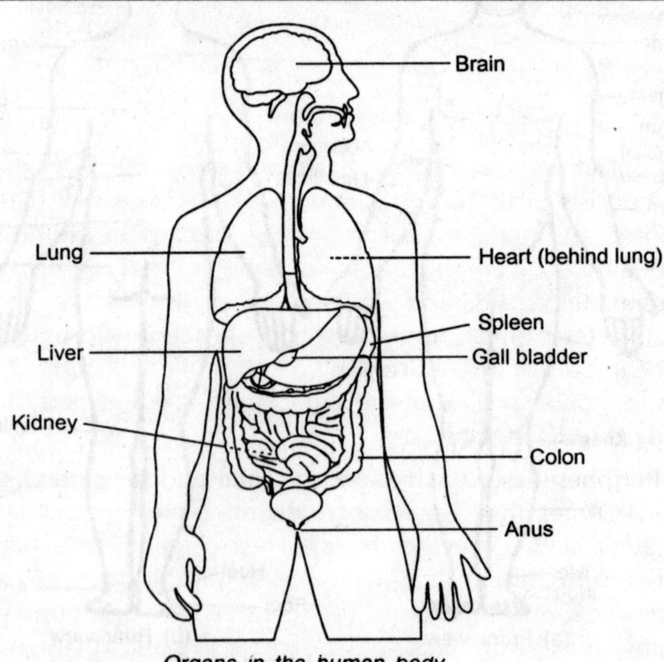

Organs in the human body.

❐ NERVOUS SYSTEM

The basic unit of the nervous system is a nerve cell (neuron). Each nerve cell has a body and processes which connect it to adjacent or distant nerve cells. Smaller branched processes called dendrites carry impulses to the nerve cell body, while longer unbranched processes called axons carry impulses away from the body. The sites of contact are called synapses. Neurotransmitters like acetylcholine and noradrenaline help transmit impulses across synapses.

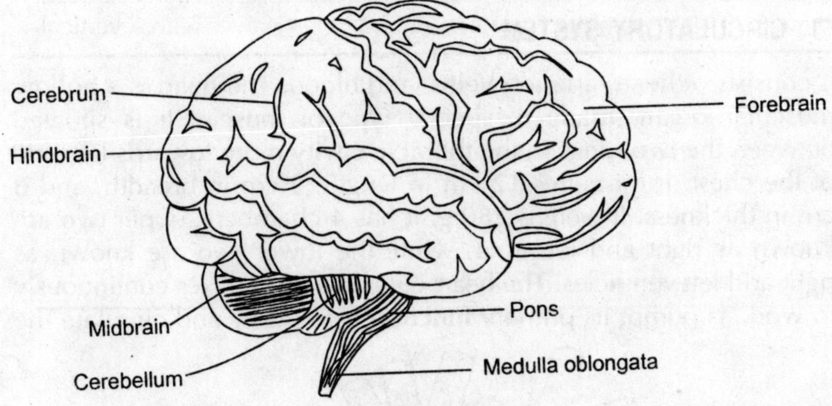

Parts of brain.

1. Central nervous system : brain and spinal cord. The nervous system consists of the brain, spinal cord, and nerves. It is divided into central and peripheral. The brain is situated in the hollow of the cranial bones. It comprises of two hemispheres. Each hemisphere has gray matter outside and white matter inside. The gray matter is responsible for storage, appreciation of sensations and generation of motor impulses. There are twelve cranial nerves coming out of various foramens in base of the skull. Brain is connected to rest of the body through spinal cord.

2. Peripheral nervous system : cranial and peripheral nerves. The nerve fibres may be sensory, motor, mixed, or autonomous (sympathetic and parasympathetic). They carry nervous impulses, motor fibers from the central nervous system to the muscles, sensory fibers from sense organs to the central nervous system, and autonomic fibers from autonomic centers to various systems.

Injuries to the head and spine can cause damage to the central nervous system. The brain takes care of thinking, receiving sensory input and giving motor output to bring about movements. It also controls vital functions like heart activity and respiration. The spinal cord is responsible for transmitting sensory impulses from skin and joints to the brain, and also for reflex actions of muscles. Injury to the skull could injure the brain, causing failure of vital body functions. Injury to the spine could cause paralysis of lower and/or upper limbs. If the damage is severe enough, the lost function may never recover.

❐ CIRCULATORY SYSTEM

It consists of heart, arteries, veins, and blood. The heart is a hollow muscular organ, made of special type of muscle. It is situated between the two lungs in the thoracic cavity more towards left side of the chest. It measures 12 cm in length, 9 cm in breadth, and 6 cm in thickness. It weighs 280 g. It has 4 chambers, upper two are known as right and left atria, while the lower two are known as right arid left ventricles. The heart contracts and relaxes continuously to work as pump. Its primary function is to purify and circulate the

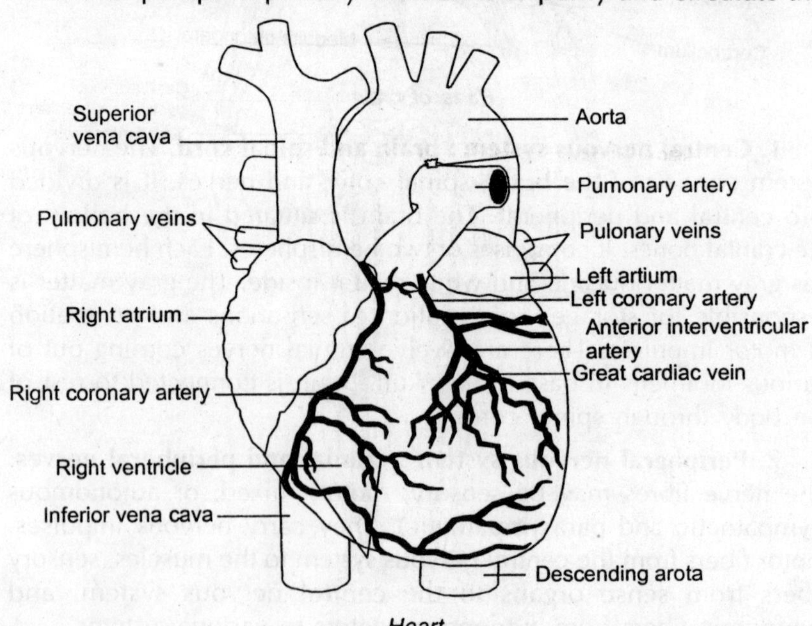

Heart

blood in the body and to help in distributing the nutrients and oxygen to the body, and waste material away from the sites of production to the organs of excretion.

Our Blood vessels are of three types. They are :

1. Arteries : They are the strongest of the blood vessels, owing to the presence of elastic tissue in their walls. They are red in colour and carry pure blood away from the heart. They branch to form arterioles and finally capillaries.

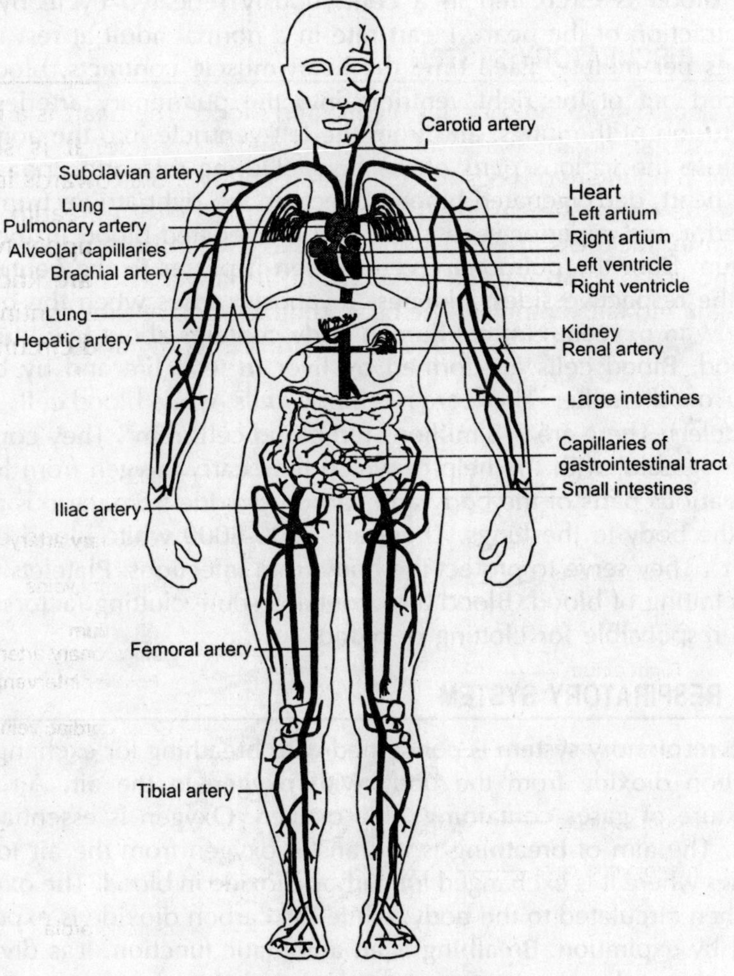

Arterial system of the body.

2. Capillaries : They are the result of the final branching of the arterioles. They are made of a thin layer of endothelial cells through which fluids and gases can pass to and from the tissue cells of the body.

3. Veins : They are not as strong as arteries due to less of elastic tissue in their walls. They are formed by joining of capillaries. They are bluish in colour. They carry impure blood back to heart. Blood coming from the digestive system also contains nutrients obtained by digestion of food.

Blood is circulated in a continuously repeated cycle by the contraction of the heart. Heart rate in a normal adult at rest is 72 times per minute. Each time the heart muscle contracts, blood is forced out of the right ventricle into the pulmonary arteries for perfusion of the lungs, and from the left ventricle into the aorta to perfuse the various parts of the body. During relaxation phase of the heart, deoxygenated blood collects in the right atrium from the inferior and superior vena cava, and oxygenated blood in the left atrium from the pulmonary veins. Then it passes to the ventricles of the respective sides. Blueness (cyanosis) arises when the blood is low in oxygen. Normal human body contains about five litres of blood. Blood cells are formed by liver in fetal life and by bone marrow thereafter. There are red blood cells, white blood cells, and platelets. There are 5-8 millions red blood cells/mm^3. They contain hemoglobin, with the help of which they carry oxygen from lungs to various parts of the body and carbon dioxide from various parts of the body to the lungs. There are 5000-8000 white blood cells/ mm^3. They serve to protect the body from infections. Platelets help in clotting of blood. Blood also contains some clotting factors that are responsible for clotting of blood.

❐ RESPIRATORY SYSTEM

The respiratory system is concerned with breathing for exchange of carbon dioxide from the body with oxygen in the air. Air is a mixture of gases containing 21% oxygen. Oxygen is essential for life. The aim of breathing is to transfer oxygen from the air to the lungs where it is exchanged for carbon dioxide in blood. The oxygen is then circulated to the body, while the carbon dioxide is expelled out by expiration. Breathing is an automatic function. It is divided into three phases.

1. Inspiration : breathing in.
2. Expiration : breathing out.
3. Pause.

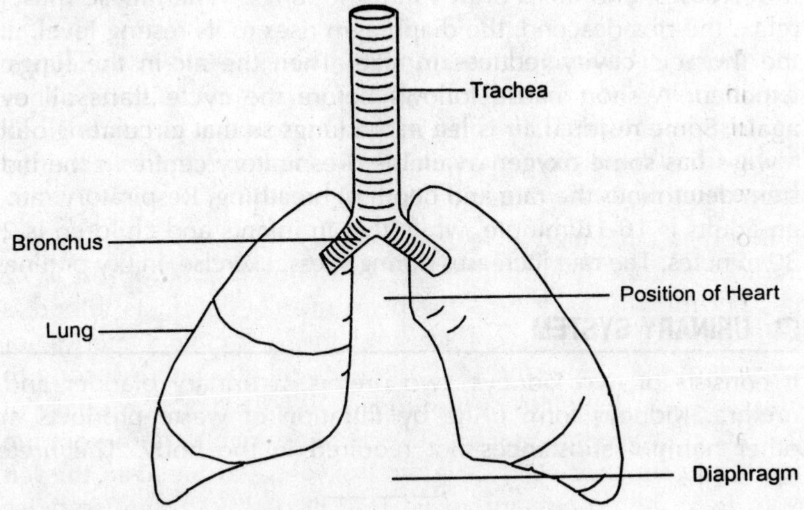

Important respiratory organs.

Structure	Features
Nose	Outermost primary way for air to enter and leave the system.
Mouth	Outermost secondary way for air to enter and leave the system.
Larynx	Connects the upper airway to the trachea.
Trachea	A cartilaginous tube made of many incomplete rings. It is a passage way for air flowing from larynx to the bronchi.
Bronchi	They form by branching of the trachea. Final small branches are bronchioles, to which alveoli are attached.
Lungs	Elastic organs, one on each side of the heart, containing microscopic air sacs called alveoli, where exchange of oxygen and carbon dioxide takes place between blood in alveolar capillaries and air in the alveoli.

There are muscles between the ribs that form the thoracic cage. There is a strong muscular partition between the chest cavity and the abdominal cavity called diaphragm. When one breathes in the chest muscles pull the ribs upwards while the diaphragm moves downwards. Thus the thoracic cavity expands, the pressure within it decreases, and air is drawn into the lungs. When these muscles relax, the ribs descend, the diaphragm rises to its resting level, and the thoracic cavity reduces in size. Then the air in the lungs is expelled. A short pause follows before the cycle starts all over again. Some residual air is left in the lungs so that circulating blood always has some oxygen available. Respiratory centre in the brain stem determines the rate and depth of breathing. Respiratory rate in an adults is 16-18/minute, while that in infants and children is 20-30/minutes. The rate increases during stress, exercise, injury or illness.

❒ URINARY SYSTEM

It consists of two kidneys, two ureters, a urinary bladder and a urethra. Kidneys form urine by filtration of waste products and other harmful substances not required in the body. The ureters

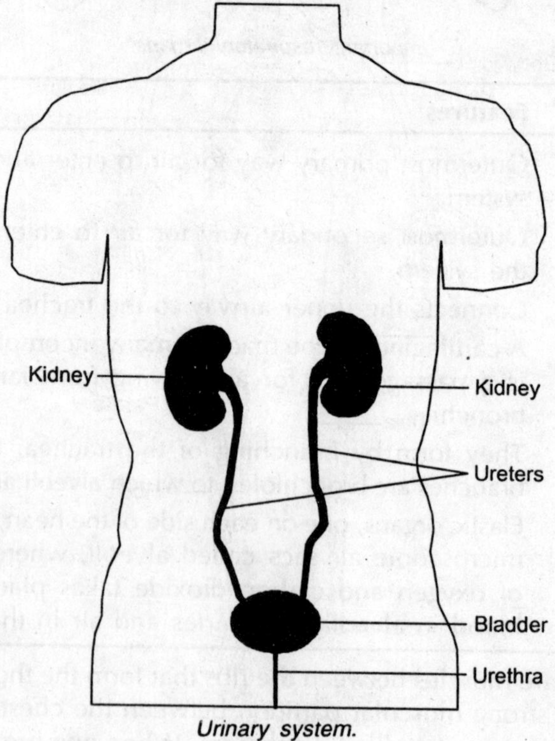

Urinary system.

conduct the urine to the urinary bladder, which is an expansible muscular bag for collecting urine. When it fills to about 200 to 250 ml, one gets a sensation of full bladder, and then expels the urine by voluntary contraction of the bladder muscle.

❐ SKELETAL SYSTEM

The skeletal system consists of 206 bones joined together by ligaments, cartilages and muscles. Its various parts are as follows.

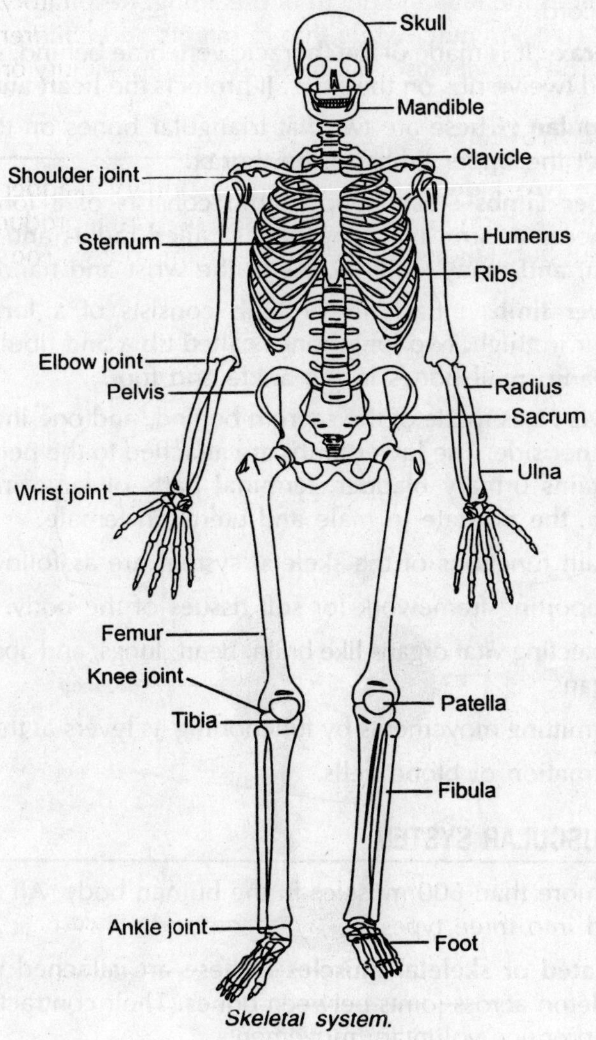

Skeletal system.

1. Skull : It is made up of many flat bones jointed together so that no movement is allowed in between the bones. It holds the brain. Eyes are located in bony cavities on the front of skull. The nose is made up of small bones attached to skull.

2. Spine : It consists of 33 bones. There are seven in neck (cervical), twelve in chest back (thoracic), five in lumbar region, five in sacrum, and four in the coccyx. These are small bones with central cavities which joined end to end form a canal that contains the spinal cord.

3. Thorax : It is made of the thoracic vertebrae behind, sternum in front, and twelve ribs on the sides. It protects the heart and lungs.

4. Scapulae : These are two flat triangular bones on the back that connect the upper limbs to the thorax.

5. Upper Limbs : Each upper limb consists of a long bone called humerus in arm, two long bones called radius and ulna in the forearm, and many small bones in the wrist and hands.

6. Lower limbs : Each lower limb consists of a long bone called femur in thigh, two long bones called tibia and fibula in the leg, and many small bones in the ankle and foot.

7. Pelvis : It is made of the sacrum behind, and one inominate bone on either side. The lower limbs are attached to the pelvis. The pelvis contains urinary bladder, terminal parts of large intestines and rectum, the prostate in male and uterus in female.

The main functions of the skeletal system are as follows.

1. Supporting framework for soft tissues of the body.
2. Protecting vital organs like brain, heart, lungs, and abdominal organs.
3. Permitting movements by functioning as levers at the joints.
4. Formation of blood cells.

❒ THE MUSCULAR SYSTEM

There are more than 600 muscles in the human body. All muscles are divided into three types.

1. Striated or skeletal muscles : These are attached to some part of skeleton across joints between bones. Their contraction and relaxation produce voluntary movements.

2. Smooth muscles : These are small and delicate. They are found in the walls of bowel, respiratory tract and blood vessels. They are known as involuntary because one does not have direct control over their activity.

3. Cardiac muscle : Its fibers show some striations under a microscope, but it is involuntary in nature.

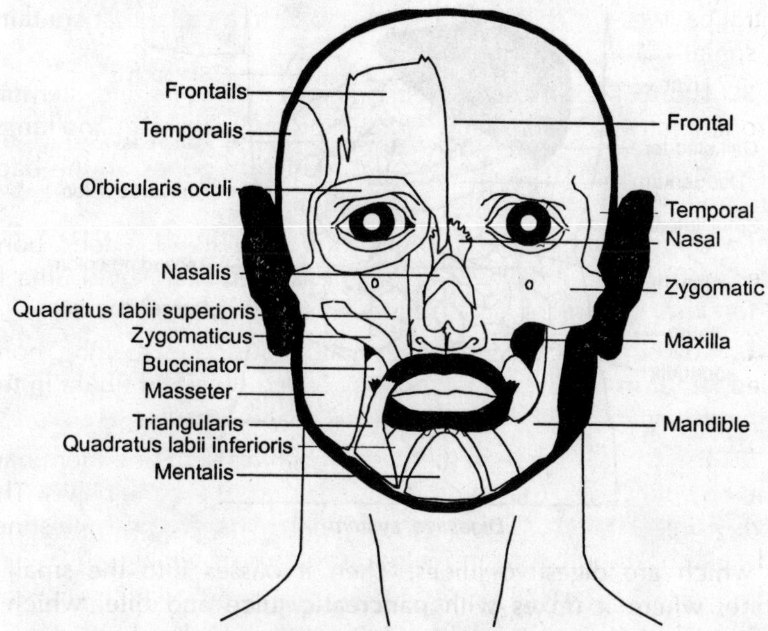

Bones and muscles of the head.

❐ THE DIGESTIVE SYSTEM

Our digestive system consists of the digestive tract and various glands that secrete digestive juices into the tract. The tract includes mouth, pharynx, esophagus, stomach, small intestine, large intestine, rectum and anus. The accessory glands include the salivary glands, liver, gall bladder, and pancreas. Teeth are used to tear the food to pieces and chew (masticate) it. Saliva is produced by salivary glands. Dry food is mixed with saliva to moisten it. Ptylin in the saliva digests some carbohydrates. Food reaches the stomach through the esophagus. There it mixes with rennin, pepsin, and hydrochloric

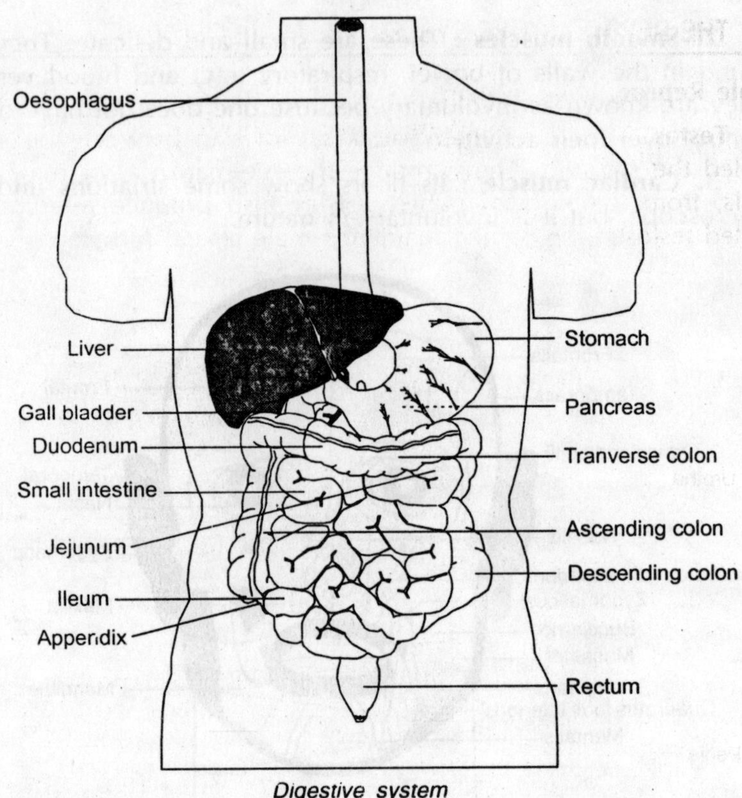

Digestive system

acid, which are digestive juices. Then it passes into the small intestine, where it mixes with pancreatic juice and bile, which digest the food further. Products of digestion are absorbed in the small intestine. Undigested food passes into the large intestine. Water is absorbed from it there, and the residue is thrown out of the rectum and anus as feces.

❐ THE EXCRETORY SYSTEM

The function of the excretory system is excretion of waste products present in the body. The following organs perform this function.

1. Skin : perspiration.
2. Lungs : through respiration.
3. The urinary system : as discussed before.

❒ THE REPRODUCTIVE SYSTEM

Male Reproductive System

Testes. They are situated in a sac of skin between the legs, called the scrotum. They produce the spermatozoa, or male sex cells, from the time of puberty. They also produce a hormone called testosterone, which maintains male sexual function.

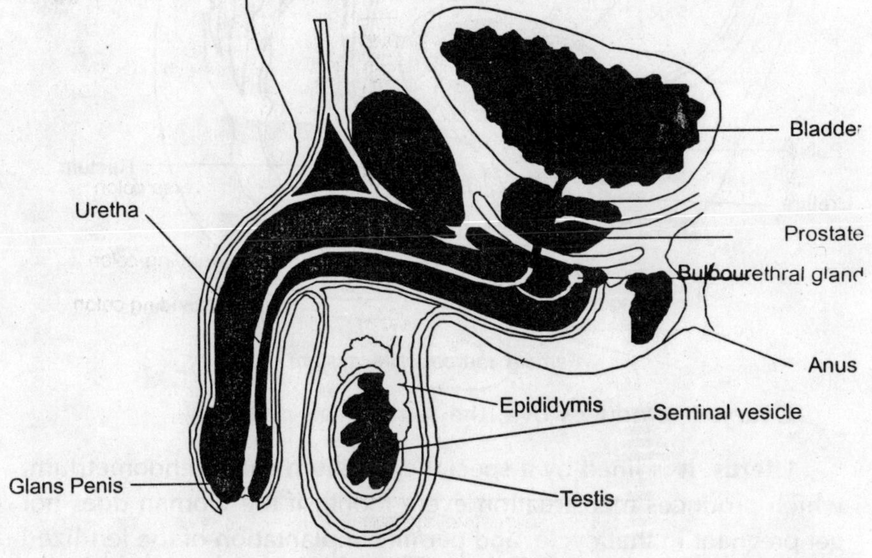

Male reproductive system

Vasa deferentia. They carry sperm from testes to the seminal vesicles.

Seminal vesicles. They function as reservoir for sperm, and also produce a secretion required for survival of sperm.

Prostate. It produces a secretion required for survival of sperm.

Ejaculatory ducts. They carry semen into the urethra. Semen is a mixture of sperm, and secretions of seminal vesicles and prostate.

Penis. It is the external genital organ for copulation. The urethra passes through it to open at its tip.

Female Reproductive Sustem

Fallopian tubes. They collect ova and transmit them to the uterus. They also permit transfer of sperm to the ova for fertilization.

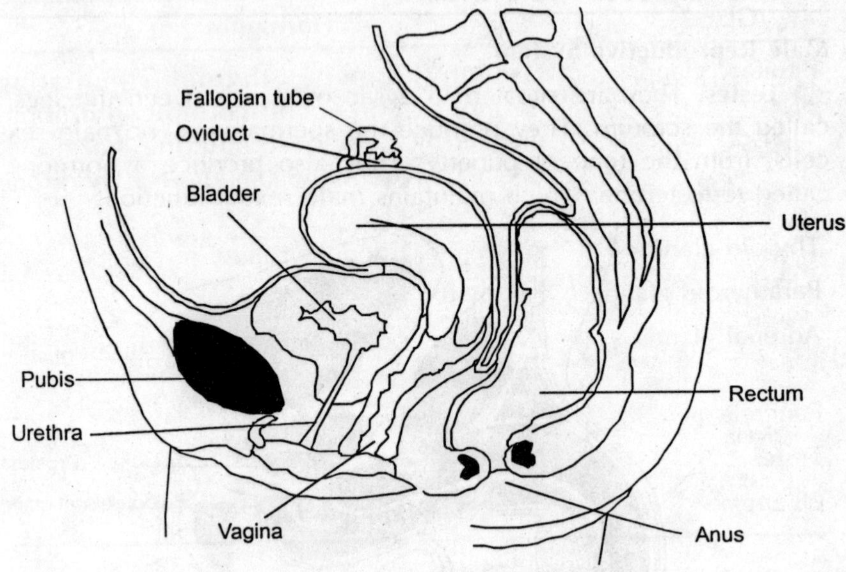

Female reproductive system.

Ovary. It produces ova, the female sex cells.

Uterus. It is lined by a special epithelium called endometrium, which produces menstruation every month if the woman does not get pregnant in that cycle, and permits implantation of the fertilized ovum and its growth if she gets pregnant.

Vagina. It is the lower end of the female genital tract. It is the organ of copulation.

Vulva. It is the external genitals of a woman. It includes the clitoris, labia minora, and labia majora.

❒ ENDOCRINE SYSTEM

Endocrine glands are ductless glands. Their secretions called hormones are poured directly into the blood stream. The blood carries them to distant sites for action. The hormones regulate a number of physiologic and metabolic functions of the body. Various endocrine glands and their secretions are as follows.

Gland	Hormones
Pituitary gland	Growth hormone, thyroid stimulating hormone, adrenocorticotropic hormone, prolactin, follicle stimulating hormone, luteinizing hormone, antidiuretic hormone and oxytocin.
Thyroid gland	Thyroxine, triiodothyronine.
Parathyroid glands	Parathormone.
Adrenal glands	Glucocorticoids, mineralocorticoids, sex steroids, adrenaline, noradrenaline.
Pancreas	Insulin, glucagons.
Testes	Testosterone.
Ovaries	Estrogen, progesterone.

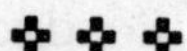

CHAPTER

11

General Management Needs Attention

The first aider has to act decisively, quickly, calmly and correctly in order to give efficient first aid. This is achieved by following the measures given below :

1. A calm and controlled approach.
2. Giving one's identification before taking charge of the situation if there are no doctors, nurses or other trained persons.
3. Avoiding placing oneself in danger when approaching the casualty.
4. A quick assessment of the situation and the casualty.
5. A correct diagnosis of the condition based on the history of the incident, symptoms and signs.
6. Immediate and appropriate treatment of any conditions.
7. Proper disposal of the victim depending on his condition.

❐ HOW TO ASSESS THE SITUATION ?

Any further damage to the victim and any risk to self and to bystanders are minimized as follows.

Situation and Measures

Road accidents. (1) Instruct a bystander to control the traffic, keeping it away from oneself and the victim. (2) Switch off the ignition of the vehicles concerned. (3) Watch out for risk of fire from petrol spillage.

Electrical contact. (1) Break the contact. (2) Take the necessary measures to prevent further contact.

Gas and Poisonous fumes. Cut off the source.

Fire. Move the victim to a safe place immediately.

Collapsing building. Move the victim to a safe place immediately.

❒ HOW TO OBTAIN HELP FROM OTHERS ?

Bystanders should be asked to perform the following tasks.

1. Control traffic.
2. Stand with their backs to the victim to give her privacy and keep others away.
3. Telephone for assistance.
4. Telephone for ambulance to shift the victim.
5. Perform tasks outlined under assessment of situation.
6. Help control bleeding or apply splints.

❒ HOW TO DETERMINE THE PRIORITIES OF TREATMENT ?

The following checks should be done immediately.

Airway. The airway is checked to confirm that it is not blocked.

Breathing. The victim's breathing is checked to see that it is normal.

Circulation. Presence and adequacy of the pulse and heart beat are confirmed.

Consciousness. If the victim is unconscious, he is placed in the recovery position, unless there is risk of spinal injury.

Hemorrhage. Any severe bleeding is looked for and controlled.

Based on the findings of the history, these factors, and clinical examination, the priority list is as follows :

1. Vital parameters : temperature, pulse rate, respiratory rate per minute. Temperature is judged by touching the victim's forehead with the back of the hand. Respiratory rate is counted by observing the chest wall movements. Pulse rate is counted by feeling the pulsations at the wrist.
2. Level of consciousness.
3. Paleness (pallor) : indicates anemia or acute blood loss.

4. Ability to move the limbs.
5. Features of injury : bleeding, external wounds, features of fractures and dislocations.
6. Pupils : size, equality on both sides, reaction to light. The pupils should be equal, small, and should constrict when light is shone over them.

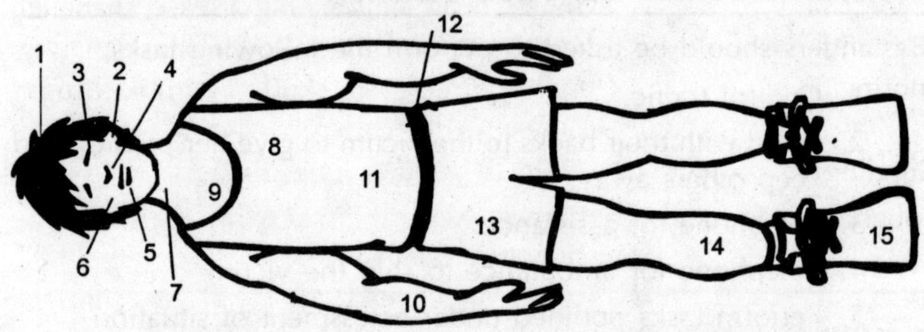

1. Scalp : bleeding, swelling, depression; 2. Response to speech in each ear, bleeding, watery discharge; 3. Eyes : appearance, movements, pupils; 4. Nose : bleeding, watery discharge; 5. Breathing : rate, depth, regularity; 6. Skin : colour, temperature, state; 7. Neck : pulsations, tracheostomy hole, warning medallion, spine tenderness; 8. Chest : expansion with breathing, rib fractures; 9. Collar bone and shoulders : tenderness, deformity; 10. Upper limbs : movements, tenderness, deformities; 11. Lower back : swelling, tenderness; 12. Abdomen : swelling, tenderness, guarding, rigidity; 13. Pelvis and hips : tenderness, bleeding from orifices, hip movements; 14. Lower limbs : movements, tenderness, deformities; 15. Toes : movements, feeling, colour.

TOP-TO-TOE SURVEY

❐ ABNORMAL PULSE RATE

Abnormality	Causes
Rapid, good volume	Anxiety, fear, heat stroke, overexertion, early stage of hemorrhage.
Slow, good volume	Stroke, fracture of skull.
Rapid, weak	Severe hemorrhage, shock, diabetic coma.
Absent	Cardiac arrest.

❒ ABNORMAL RESPIRATION

Observation	Causes
Rapid, shallow	Shock, heart disease, heat exhaustion, insulin shock.
Deep, gasping	Airway obstruction, chest injury, lung injury, heart failure, lung disease, diabetic coma.
Snoring	Stroke, fractured skull, alcohol, drugs abuse.
Gurgling	Fluid in airway, lung diseases.
Coughing blood	Chest wound, fractured rib, lung puncture, heart disease.

❒ ABNORMALITIES OF PUPILS

Abnormality	Causes
Unequal	Head injury, hemorrhage within skull, stroke.
Dilated	Alcohol intoxication.
Dilated, not responding to light	Coma, cardiac arrest, drug toxicity.
Constricted, not responding to light	Damage to brain, drug toxicity.

Various levels of consciousness are as follows :

1. Conscious : normal.
2. Restless.
3. Stuporous : apparently sleeping, but can be woken up by giving painful stimuli.
4. Coma (unconsciousness) : apparently sleeping, but cannot be awakened even by giving painful stimuli.

❒ ABNORMALITIES OF SKIN

Abnormalities of skin colour may be due to any of the causes shown in the following table.

Abnormalities of Skin Temperature

Abnormality	Causes
Hot, dry	High fever, heat stroke.
Hot, moist	Infection.
Cool, dry	Exposure to cold.
Cool, clammy	Shock.

Abnormalities of Skin Colour

Abnormality	Causes
Red	High blood pressure, heart attack, heat stroke.
Cherry red	Carbon monoxide poisoning.
Blue	Heart failure, airway obstruction, lung diseases.
Pale	Shock, bleeding, heart attack, fright.

❐ INABILITY TO MOVE

Type	Causes
All four limbs	Injury to cervical spinal cord.
Lower limbs	Injury to thoracic or lumbar spinal cord.
Single limb	Fracture of the limb bones.
One side limbs	Stroke.

❐ HOW TO REMOVE CLOTHING

Footwear

1. Support the ankle and remove the shoe carefully.
2. Slit long shoes down the back seam with a sharp knife.

Socks

1. Pull them off gently.
2. If that cannot be done, lift each one away from the leg with a finger passed into it and cut it with scissors.

Trousers

1. Pull up the trouser leg gently and expose the calf and knee.
2. Pull the trouser down from the waist to expose the thigh.

Sweater

1. Remove the victim's uninjured arm from its sleeve.
2. Ease the sweater from his head without disturbing the injured arm.
3. Support the injured arm and slip off the sweater.

Shirt or coat

1. Unbutton it.
2. Remove the uninjured arm from its sleeve first.
3. Pull the shirt/coat round the injured side.
4. Support the injured arm and slip the shirt/coat off the arm.

❐ HOW TO REMOVE PROTECTIVE HELMET

If the victim can do so, get him to remove it himself. If he cannot do so, it is best left on, and is removed only if absolutely necessary, e.g. for performance of artificial ventilation. Two persons are required to remove it. One should support the victim's head and neck. The other should remove the helmet.

Open-face helmet

1. Align the victim's head with his spine in neutral position.
2. Unfasten the buckle or cut through the chinstrap.
3. If the helmet has sides, grip it from above and force the sides apart to take the pressure off his head.
4. Lift the helmet upward and backwards gently and remove it.

Full-face helmet

1. Align the victim's head with his spine in neutral position.
2. Unfasten the buckle or cut through the chinstrap.
3. Working from the base of the helmet, ease the fingers of both of your hands under the rim.
4. Support the neck with one hand and hold the lower jaw firmly.
5. Ask your helper to work from above. Get him to tilt the helmet backwards without moving the head and lift the front clear of the chin gently.

6. Continuing to support the neck and jaw, get the helper to gilt the helmet forwards slightly so that it can be passed over the back of the head. Then get him to lift it straight off the victim's head.

After observation of these important abnormalities, a detailed examination should be done from the head to toe. Any abnormalities should be noted and recorded carefully. Based on the diagnosis, appropriate treatment should be given. An observation chart should be made as shown below.

❒ FIRST-AID RECORD

Name :	Date :	Time :
Parameter	Time and Observation	
Temperature (every 10 min)		
Pulse (every 10 min)		
Respiration (every 10 min)		
Consciousness (every 10 min)		
Pupils Size Reactivity		
Limb movements		
Body movements		
Speech		
Temperature (every 10 min)		
Skin colour (every 10 min)		
Fractures		
Dislocations		
External injuries		
Hemorrhage		
Urinary incontinence		
Fecal incontinence		
Burns		
Treatment given		

CHAPTER

12

"Life Saving" Resuscitation

Resuscitation is a vital emergency technique for the restoration of life or consciousness of the person whose respiration and cardiac activity have ceased. Cessation of these functions results in cessation of oxygenation of blood and pumping of the oxygenated blood to tissues. Since oxygen is essential for survival, resuscitation is done to reestablish tissue oxygenation until respiratory and cardiac functions are restored.

❐ CAUSES OF A CARDIAC ARREST

1. Electric shock.
2. Heart attack.
3. Asphyxia.
4. Drowning.
5. Allergic reaction.
6. Severe injuries.

❐ SIGNS OF A CARDIAC ARREST

The carotid pulse is felt in the hollow between the windpipe and large neck muscles. It is absent in cardiac arrest.

1. Unconsciousness.
2. Absence of a pulse.
3. Absence of breathing. Put your cheek against the person's mouth and feel for breaths.
4. Absence of heart beat (Look for chest movement)
5. Dilated and fixed pupils.
6. A bluish colour of skin, lips or nail beds.

❐ ABC OF RESUSCITATION

Sign	Function
A	CLEAR AIRWAY.
B	RESTORE BREATHING
C	RESTORE CIRCULATION

❐ HOW TO CLEAR THE AIRWAY ?

Clear airway by keeping the head tilted back and sweeping a finger around the mouth.

The airway may be blocked in an unconscious patient due to loss of cough and gag reflexes. That allows the tongue to sag back and block the airway. Mucous or foreign bodies like regurgitated solid food particles may also block the airway. That makes breathing difficult and noisy. Airway is cleared as follows.

1. Use the index finger to hook out any material in the mouth and pharynx, such as broken teeth, vomit, broken dentures, foreign body or mucous.
2. Remove constrictions around the neck, if any.
3. Hyperextend the neck by placing one hand under the neck and the other hand on forehead to tilt the head back. Lift the chin forwards. That pulls the tongue forwards and opens the airway at the back of the throat and he may restart breathing soon. Put him in recovery position and stay with him.

❐ HOW TO RESTORE BREATHING ?

Mouth to mouth ventilation (Kiss of Life)

After the airway is cleared, listen for five seconds with your ear close to the victim's nose and mouth. If breathing has not been reestablished, perform mouth to mouth breathing by the following technique.

1. Put the person on his back.
2. Tilt the head back as far as possible (nostrils then point directly upwards at you).

3. Cup one hand under his chin.
4. Put the heel of the other hand on his forehead so that the fingers of that hand can pinch his nose.
5. Use both hands together to leen the head back.
6. Pinch and compress nose to close nostrils.
7. Make sure the person's mouth is open.
8. Take a deep breath.
9. Place your mouth over the victim's mouth, making an airtight seal.

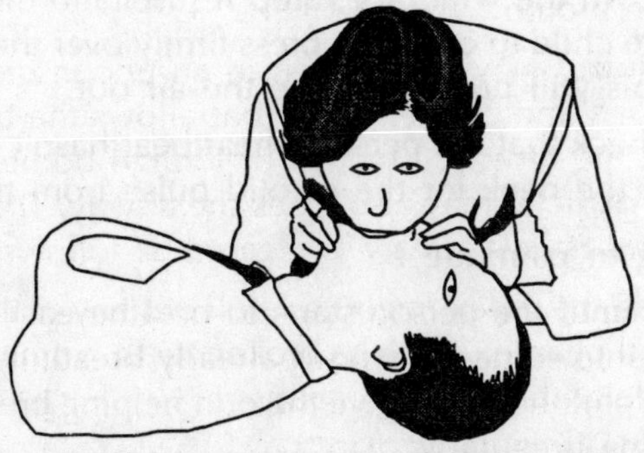

10. Breathe into victim's mouth firmly and quickly, taking quick breaths in between to refill your own lungs with fresh air.
11. Allow patient to exhale passively by elastic recoil of his chest between two breaths.
12. Try to 'blow' a breath into the patient about every six seconds. Be guided by common sense on this. For example, the first few breaths can be given much more quickly to try to get some oxygen into the patient.
13. Stop when the patient shows clear signs of starting to breathe but even then keep a close eye on his chest movements until professional help arrives.

Some useful hints

1. Don't blow too hard as this may send air into the stomach and make the person vomit, which is dangerous for him and unpleasant for you.

2. Should he vomit, turn his head to one side and let the vomit dribble out of his mouth. Clean out the mouth and carry on with resuscitation.
3. If a child is the victim, seal your lips over both nose and mouth after positioning the head as before. **Only blow gently**. Be guided by what procedures a rise and fall of the chest wall. In babies, use only the amount of air you can hold in your cheeks — **don't blow** from your lungs.
4. If the abdomen starts swelling up, you'll know you're blowing air down the gullet into the stomach instead of down the windpipe. Stop resuscitation for a moment, turn the child to one side, press firmly over the swollen stomach. This will probably force the air out.
5. Check that the person's heartbeat hasn't stopped by feeling in the neck for the carotid pulse from time to time.

How long to continue ?

Either until the person starts to breathe easily again. Never try breathing into someone who is already breathing spontaneously. It can be helpful though to give the odd helping breath if he is gasping or breathing irregularly.

Or until professional help arrive. This may take time, so get others to help you. Keep going until a doctor says the person is dead. Don't give up too readily, especially in cases of drowning or electric shock.

Calling an ambulance

1. Dial '102' or any other number available for your local area ambulance.
2. When the operator answers give him your telephone number so that he may ring you back, should your be cut off.
3. When you get through to the ambulance officer, tell him briefly what the emergency is.
4. Give directions to guide the ambulance to your home, especially if it is difficult to find, or has a name of the place and no number etc. It would be helpful to go out to the nearest road intersection, or to a major landmark to meet the ambulance, if you live in an out-of-the-way place, which they might not find easily.

5. When he ambulance arrives, describe what has happened.
6. Get someone to look after the children or other relatives while you go off. If your child is the patient, always try to go with him.
7. Take your money with you and your front door key. Ambulance are under no obligation to deliver you back home. You will need money for a taxi or bus to come back.

Mouth to nose ventilation

Mouth to nose ventilation has to be used in situations such as mouth injuries making a good seal impossible or rescue from water.

1. With the victim's mouth closed, form a tight seal with your lips around the victim's nose.
2. Breathe into his nose four times quickly.
3. Open the mouth to let the breath out after every breath in.
4. Watch victim's chest movement for rise and fall of chest with each breath to confirm adequacy of your ventilation. If the chest does not rise, check that your have a firm seal around the victim's nose and you have close the mouth completely.

❒ MANUAL METHODS OF ARTIFICIAL VENTILATION

In certain situations, mouth to mouth respiration cannot be given e.g. when the face is damaged, the lower jaw is fractured, or the lips and mouth have been burned by a poison. In such cases, manual methods are used.

Arm-lift/back-pressure method (Holger Nielsen)

1. Place the victim on the ground, face down, the forehead resting on the back of the overlapping hands.
2. Keep the head straight, so as to keep air passages completely open and free.
3. Kneel near the victim's head, placing one knee near his head and the opposite foot by the side of the corresponding side elbow. The knee and foot may be alternated from time to time.

4. Place both hands over the lower parts of the victim's shoulder blades, the fingers spread and the thumbs near midline. Keep the arms and forearms straight, lean forward so as to apply pressure by the weight of the upper part of the body.
5. Count one-two and then lean back, sliding hand to just above elbows of the patient, as you count three.
6. Grasp the arms of the victim near the elbows and lift them up, keeping upper limbs straight. Count four-five and then lower patient's arms back to original position as you count six.
7. Then start all over again.

This method is not suitable if the patient has injuries of the chest wall or fractures of the arms.

Hip lift back pressure method

1. Place the victim face down, forehead resting on the back of the uninjured hand.
2. Keep the head straight.
3. Straddle the patient at the level of his hip, placing one knee and the other foot on the ground.
4. Then bend forwards and catch the bony pelvis with both hands.
5. Bend backwards keeping the upper limbs straight, such that the hips are lifted 10-15 cm above the ground, while you count one-two-three.
6. Lower the hips to the ground and slide the hands to the middle of the back just up to the tips of the shoulder blades, fingers spread and thumbs near midline, as you count four.
7. Rock forwards keeping your upper limbs straight so as to apply pressure till resistance is felt. Count five-six-seven.
8. Release the pressure gradually and slide the hands back beneath the hips again as you count eight.
9. Repeat the whole process 10 times a minute.

Arm-lift / chest pressure method (Silvester)

1. Place the patient face upwards.
2. Place a folded blanket under his shoulders to raise them so that the head falls backwards.
3. Kneel near the head.
4. Grasp his forearms near his wrists, cross them over to the lower part of the chest and then lean forward to press the crossed arms for 2 seconds.
5. Then pull the arms upwards and outwards with a sweeping movement and place them on the ground by your own knees for 3 seconds.
6. Repeat the cycle 12 times a minute.

This method is useful when the victim cannot be placed face down. It is more effective than the prone pressure method.

Prone pressure method (Schafer)

1. Place the victim in prone position, head turned to one side, resting on the back of over lapped hands.
2. Kneel by his side at the level of the hips.
3. Place the hands on the lower part of the back, the wrists almost touching, thumbs forward and fingers opposed.
4. Keep your upper limbs straight as you lean forwards so as to apply pressure by the weight of the body.
5. Then rock backwards to release the pressure.
6. Repeat the cycle 12 times a minute.

Tilting or rocking method

1. Place the victim on a stretcher or a plank and strap him to it. Rock him alternately in 45° head low and 45° head high positions.
2. Perform this 12 times a minute.

Rocking can be done on a high bench, a fence or piled up rocks. This method is particularly suitable for infants and children who can be manually rocked.

Bag and mask ventilation

The patient can be artificially ventilated using a face mask and an Ambu bag. After clearing the airway, hold an anaesthesist's mask firmly over the victim's nose and mouth with the left hand, the angle of the lower jaw held forwards to prevent the tongue from falling back. The bag is alternately compressed and released by the right hand. The valve in between the bag and the mask permits air to pass into the victim's airway when the bag is compressed and allows it to flow to the atmosphere when the bag is released.

Resustitube

Johnson and Johnson's resustitube can be used instead of mouth to mouth ventilation. It is a 17.5 cm long plastic tube with a diameter of 1.8 cm. There is a plastic cover 8.75 cm in diameter. It fits snugly over the mouth and prevents escape of air during artificial ventilation. Lower part of the tube is curved to fit over the tongue and thereby prevents the tongue from falling back. The tube is placed in the victim's mouth and mouth to tube ventilation is done.

❒ HOW TO RESTORE CIRCULATION ?

Precordial thump is the first measure to be taken except for patients known to have myocardial disease. Make a sharp thump over the midsternal region with a closed fist. It may restore normal cardiac activity especially in electric shock cases.

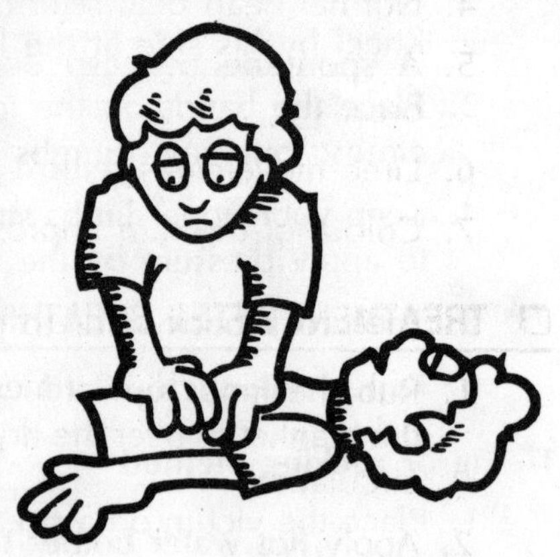

External cardiac massage is given if precordial thump fails to restore normal cardiac activity. Its technique is as follows.

1. Place victim on a hard surface.
2. Kneel by his side.
3. Place heel of one hand over the sternum 1-2" above xiphoid process.
4. Place the other hand on top of it.

5. Interlock fingers so as to keep them off the victim's ribs.
6. Compress downward making full use of your body weight to depress victim's sternum by 1.5 to 2".
7. Relax pressure completely without lifting your hands from the victim's so as not to lose correct hand position.
8. Repeat all steps.
9. After every 15 chest compressions give 2 quick lung inflations by mouth-to-mouth breathing.
10. If there are two first aiders, one person can give the external cardiac massage, while the other gives the artificial ventilation. It is necessary to stop the cardiac massage when the ventilation is done.

❐ SIGNS OF SUCCESSFUL RESUSCITATION

1. Chest expansion occurs with each breath.
2. A pulse is felt every time the sternum is compressed.
3. The pupil appears normal and reacts to light.
4. Normal heart beat returns.
5. A spontaneous gasp occurs, followed by spontaneous breathing.
6. Limb movements return.
7. Colour of the skin improves.

❐ TREATMENT AFTER BREATHING HAS BEEN RESTORED

1. Rub the limbs upward with firm grasping pressure under the blanket or over the dry clothing to promote warmth and circulation.
2. Apply hot water bottles to promote warmth of the body.
3. Let there be free and fresh air in the room.
4. A teaspoonful of warm water may be given if the ability to swallow has returned. If the patient tolerates that well small quantities of coffee or tea may be given.
5. Keep the victim in bed and encourage him to sleep.

❒ HOW TO RESUSCITATE A CHILD ?

Cardiopulmonary resuscitation can be performed in older children just as in an adult, except that the rate must be slightly faster, and the pressure must be lighter. The technique for small children and babies is as follows.

1. Open the airway by gently lifting the chin and tilting the head.
2. Support the head slightly.
3. Watch for breathing.
4. Clear any obstruction with a finger without touching the back of the child's throat.
5. Check for the circulation by placing your index and middle fingers on the inside of the arm, and pressing lightly towards the bone. This allows feeling for the brachial pulse.
6. Give artificial ventilation at twice the rate used for adults, using similar technique.
7. If you cannot detect a pulse or, in infants, if it is very slow (less than 60) give external cardiac massage over the lower half of the sternum breastbone. Press at a rate of 100 compressions per minute, to a depth of 1.5-2.5 cm.
8. Combine with artificial ventilation, giving five compressions to one breath.

Cardiopulmonary resuscitation in children

Age (years)	Chest compression	Artificial ventilation
<1	5 (with 2 fingers)	1 (on mouth and nose)
1-7	5 (with 1 hand)	1 (on mouth only)
≥ 8	15 (with 2 hands)	2 (on mouth only)

❒ WHAT IS RECOVERY POSITION ?

Any unconscious victim should positively be placed in the recovery position. The head is slightly lower than the rest of the body to allow liquids to drain from the mouth, reducing the risk of the victim inhaling regurgitated stomach contents. The head, neck, and back are kept in a straight line, while the limbs are kept bent to keep the body in a secure and comfortable position. An unconscious victim may be left unattended in this position, if necessary. This method can also be used to transport a casualty on a stretcher. The advantages of a recovery position are as follows.

1. It maintains open airway.
2. Tongue cannot fall to the back of the throat.
3. The head and neck remain extended so that the air passage is widened and any vomiting or other fluid in the victim's mouth drains freely.
4. Necessary stability is provided to keep the body propped in a safe and comfortable position.

The technique for placing a victim in the recovery position is as follows.

1. Remove spectacles if worn, and bulky objects from the victim's pockets, if any.
2. Kneeling beside the casualty, open the airway by tilting the head and lifting the chin.
3. Straighten his legs.
4. Place the arm nearest you uppermost.
5. Bring the arm furthest from you across the chest, hold the hand, palm outwards, against the victim's cheek.
6. With your other hand, grasp the thigh furthest from you and pull the knee up, keeping the foot flat on the ground.
7. Keeping his hand pressed against his cheek, pull at the high to roll the casualty towards you and on to his side.
8. Tilt the head back to keep the airway remains open.
9. Adjust the hand under the cheek, so that the head stays in this position.
10. Keep the hip and knee bent at right angles.

The recovery position may have to be modified to avoid making injuries worse.

1. An unconscious victim with spinal injury needs extra support for the head and neck during turning, and in the final position, to keep the head and trunk aligned at all times.

2. If limbs are injured and cannot be bent, or if the victim is lying in a confined space extra helpers are required or a rolled blanket has to be placed against the victim's body to prevent it from toppling forward.
3. A heavy victim has to be turned using both hands. The clothing may be grasped at the shoulders and hips to pull the victim against you thighs. Another person should support the head while the victim is being turned.

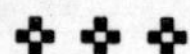

CHAPTER

13

Wounds Are A Pain

A wound is an injury or an abnormal break in the continuity of the skin or other tissues. In an external wound, there is danger that germs will enter the wound and cause an infection. If the wound is deep, severe bleeding may occur or there may be serious damage to structures within the body, such as the bowel, heart, lungs, or brain.

❒ TYPES OF WOUNDS

A wound may be open or closed. In the open wound skin is broken and blood escapes out. In a closed wound skin is not broken.

❒ TYPE OF WOUND

Abrasion/Graze

Cause. Friction or pressure of a rough object.

Features. A superficial injury involving only the outer layers of the skin. It is painful, but bleeds slightly or oozing.

Bruise

Cause. Blunt force, e.g. stone, stick, or fist.

Features. It is red due to infiltration of blood into tissues. Skin over it is intact. It becomes blue, black, green, yellow and finally disappears with time.

If the area of bruising is very large, get medical help. Generally rest and local warmth are helpful in small bruises.

Laceration

Cause. Blunt force, e.g. fall of roof, fall of a house, fall on a rough surface, rough spikes.

They aare much more difficult to treat and need medical attention. Stop bleeding by applying pressure. Only remove large and loose pieces of glass or other debris—otherwise leave this to the experts. This sort of injury particularly calls for tetanus protection.

Features. The skin and underlying tissues are torn. It has irregular edges and abrasion / jagged.

Incised wound

Cause. A weapon with a sharp cutting edge e.g., knife, razor, glass, etc.

Features. The edges of the wound are clean cut. It bleeds more than a laceration.

If less than 1 cm long, will probably heal well if you stop bleeding, pull edges together and apply adhesive dressing. Do not fiddle about with disinfectant. Wash your hands, clean the area around the wound, ensuring that no water gets into open wound, dry it carefully, then apply the dressing. Other incisions need stitches. Stop bleeding by applying pressure. Apply a dressing and bandage if you have them. Go to a doctor, if the bleeding is severe.

Punctured wound (stab wound)

Cause. A pointed weapon driven in through the skin, e.g. knife, nail, sharp tool, arrow, spear, dagger, bullet, needle etc.

Features. The opening is small, but the wound may be very deep. The vital organs of body may be injured through it. It is called a penetrating wound when there is only a wound of entry. It is called a perforating wound when there is a wound of exit too, as in the case of a gun-shot wound.

This wound may sometimes, seem trivial with very little bleeding.

Avulsion

Cause. Excessive force.

Features. A part of the body is completely torn away, e.g. finger, toe, hand, arm, foot, ear, nose, and penis.

❐ FIRST-AID

1. Place the victim in a supine position.
2. Cover the wound with sterile gauze pad.
3. Apply pressure to control bleeding.
4. Apply a tourniquet if necessary.
5. Immobilize the part.
6. Treat shock.
7. Do not remove an object impacted in the wound.
8. Preserve avulsed part, as it may be possible to reattach it to the body by surgery.
9. Cover protruding organs like eyeball or bowel with a sterile sheet. Do not try to replace them.

❐ HOW TO MANAGE AN INFECTED WOUND ?

Any wound that has not begun to heal after 48 hours is infected. It contains bacteria, dirt, and may contain a foreign body. The infection may spread elsewhere in the body and cause further damage. Features of an infected wound are as follows.

1. Pain and soreness in the wound.
2. Swelling and redness around the wound.
3. Pus in the wound.
4. Fever, chills.
5. Pain, swelling and tenderness over lymph nodes draining the area.

First-aid

1. Hold the soiled dressing at a dry and clean corner and remove it.
2. Wash hands with soap and water.
3. Clean the wound with sterile swabs soaked in an antiseptic solution.
4. Apply a new dressing over the wound.

❒ WOUNDS OF PALM OF THE HAND

These wounds tend to bleed profusely. There is also the risk of injury to the nerves and tendons in the palm. In such cases, there is a loss of sensation in the affected fingers, and inability to move the fingers.

First aid

1. Control the bleeding by placing a pad of sterile gauze over the wound and applying pressure.
2. Ask the victim to clench the first to maintain the pressure.
3. Elevate the injured hand.
4. Apply a firm bandage over the fist.
5. Support the arm in an elevated sling before transport to a hospital.

❒ ABDOMINAL WOUND

An abdominal wound may be quite serious because there can be internal bleeding as well as serious injury to intra-abdominal organs. The bowel may protrude out of the wound. Escape of intestinal contents can cause peritoneal infection (peritonitis).

Before discussing the treatment of abdominal wounds, it is necessary to know the organs present inside the abdomen or belly.

Abdominal organs

Organs in the abdomen are : (i) Stomach (ii) Liver (iii) Gall bladder (iv) Pancreas (v) Spleen (vi) Small Intestine (vii) Large intestine (viii) Appendix (ix) Kidney (x) Urinary baldder (xi) Ureter.

Abdominal wounds are of two types. Those are either closed abdominal wounds or open abdominal wounds. The treatment differs with the types.

(A) Closed Abdominal Wounds

On the approach of the patient :

- Get a correct history and time of accident.
- Find the level of consciousness. (e.g., Fully conscious, partly conscious or totally unconscious)

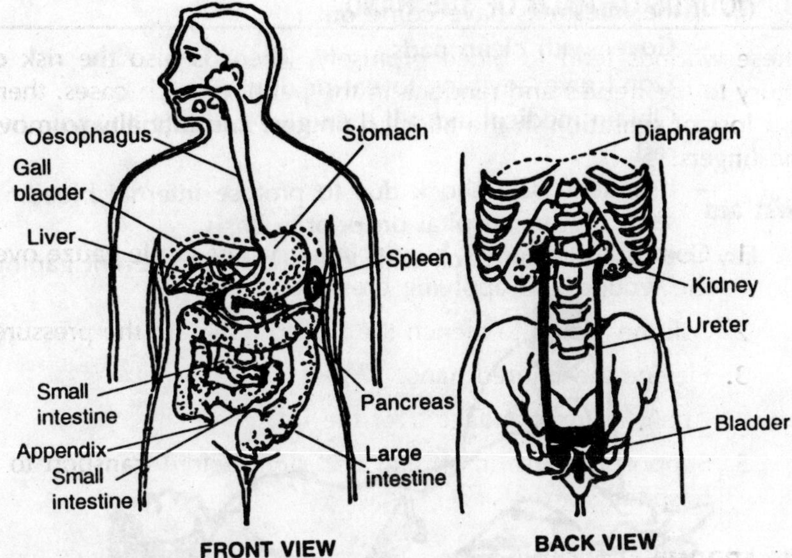

Signs and Symptoms

- Pain over the site of injury which is increased by movement of breathing.
- Swelling of the area.
- Shock and its symptoms (e.g. Pallor, cold or calmy skin, rapid pulse, shallow breathing, nausea and vomiting).

First-Aid

- Control external bleeding, if any.
- Do not give any food or drink.
- Note pulse and respiration every half an hour or earlier.
- Loosen tight clothes.
- Cover the body with light blanket.
- Quickly transport to a docor or hospital.

(B) Open Abdominal Wounds

First-Aid

(1) Adjust the patient's position so that the wound does not gap e.g., if the wound is horizontal place him on his back with head and shoulders raised and a pillow under his knees.

(2) If the intestines have come out :

- Cover with clean pads.
- Don't give anything to eat or drink.
- Obtain medical aid, till then give casualty absolute bed rest.
- If patient is in shock due to profuse internal bleeding, send him to hospital on priority basis.

Lay the casuality on back with knees bent to prevent gaping.

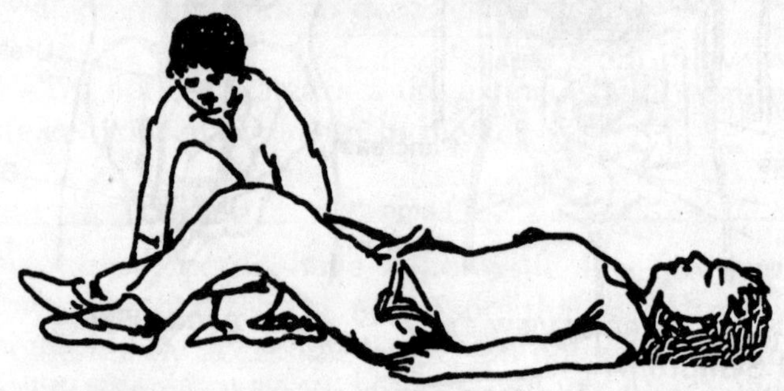

Apply sterile dressing or gauze and a clean pad over the wound and secure with a bandage or adhesive strapping.

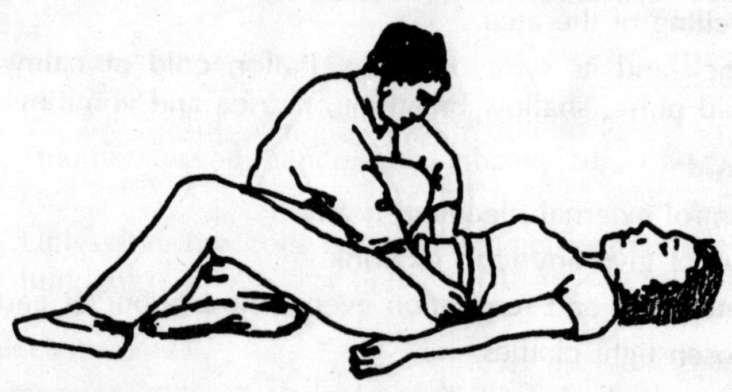

❒ SKIN INJURY

First-Aid

Dust off solid and water flush

- Dust off the solid immediately and then flush the skin with water.
- If the solid has penetrated through the clothings, promptly remove the clothing and flush the skin with water.
- Arrange for medical attention.

Soap Wash

- Soap or mild detergent washing for the skin area.
- Continue for some time so that irritation vanishes.
- If irritation persists, take medical advice.

Petro-Product Rinse

- Rinse the contaminated area immediately with kerosene or similar petroleum product.
- Then wash the area with soap or mild detergent.
- Now wash the area with water.
- Get medical attention.

❒ WOUNDS TO CHEST AND BACK

This commonly occurs in traffic accidents and assaults with knife or gun. These are serious wounds as there is the grave danger of injury to the heart, lungs, and major blood vessels. Heart injuries may be fatal. Injuries to the lungs allow air to escape out, by the pressure of which the lungs collapse and the victim gets hypoxic. Injury to major vessels causes shock, and death if not treated in time. Multiple fractures of chest wall result in the area losing its rigidity and prevent its breathing movements. Broken bones may damage other internal organs or penetrate the skin causing a sucking wound. There may be coughing of bright red frothy blood if lung is injured.

First aid

1. Seal the would immediately with the palm of your hand, and then place a tight, leak-proof dressing over it.
2. Resuscitate the victim.
3. Treat shock.
4. Place him in recovery position with his body inclined towards the injured side so that uninjured lung is uppermost.
5. Shift him to a hospital immediately.

❒ CRUSH INJURIES

These are due to severe pressure of a heavy object over a part of the body. There may not be much of an external injury. But there can be extensive damage to the tissues underneath, e.g. muscles and bones. Internal hemorrhage is possible. Toxic materials released from the damaged tissue can enter the blood stream and cause failure of the kidneys.

First aid

1. Release the trapped part from under the heavy object.
2. Place the victim in a head-low position.
3. Treat hemorrhage and shock.
4. Splint fractures. Elevate the injured limb if possible.
5. Shift him to a hospital immediately.

❐ BLAST INJURIES

Explosions can result from a bomb blast or from accidental ignition of explosive gases. Explosions generate waves of high pressure that can damage lungs and other organs of the body. That can rupture ear drums, cause fractures, and cause embedding of glass pieces in tissues.

First aid

1. Do not move the victim unless it is necessary to get him away from further danger at the site of the explosion.
2. Reassure the casualty.
3. Place him in a half-sitting position, supporting the head and shoulders.
4. Loosen any constricting clothing that may impair breathing movements.
5. Treat bleeding and shock.
6. Treat wounds and burns.
7. Treat fractures.
8. Shift him to a hospital immediately.

❐ INJURIES TO MUSCLES

Muscles are of two types, voluntary and involuntary. Injuries occur to the voluntary or skeletal muscles. These may be due to overstretching, or tearing due to violent or sudden movements. Muscle injuries are of the following types.

Muscle Injuries

Type	Features
Strain	There is a partial tearing of the muscle, often at the junction of the muscle and its tendon.
Rupture	There is a complete tearing of the muscle in its fleshy part or tendon.
Deep bruising	It occurs when there is severe injury to a large bulk of the muscle.

The condition is diagnosed by the following features.

1. There is severe and sharp pain over the site of injury to the muscle.
2. The victim is unable to move the part. On making an attempt at moving it, there is sharp pain locally.
3. The muscle may be swollen and stiff.

First aid

1. Give rest to the injured part.
2. Apply an ice pack locally to reduce swelling and pain.
3. Apply an elastic crepe bandage over the affected part.
4. Elevate the injured part.
5. Give paracetamol for pain.
6. Send him to hospital whenever it is possible to do so.

❐ HEAD INJURIES

Head injuries are always grave injuries because they can be associated with serious injury to the brain within the skull. These may be accompanied by skull fractures. They may be caused by road accidents, mining accidents, sports accidents, fall from a height etc. Various manifestations of head injuries are as follows.

1. Scalp wounds.
2. Skull fractures.
3. Concussion : there is a temporary disturbance of the function of the brain. The victim becomes unconscious. However he

recovers fully after some time. He may not remember nothing of the previous happenings.

4. Intracranial hemorrhage : it may be due to tear of the meninges producing extradural hematoma, subdural hematoma, subarachnoid hemorrhage, or intra-cerebroventricular hemorrhage. External pressure on the brain damages it. The increase in the intracranial tension may make the victim unconscious. If the brainstem gets pushed down the vertebral canal, the vital centers may get damaged and produce cardiorespiratory arrest and death.

The condition is diagnosed by the following features.

1. The victim may be unconscious.
2. The pupils may be dilated, not responding to light, or of unequal size.
3. Respiration may be labored or noisy.
4. Pulse may be slow and bounding.
5. Neurological signs may be present, e.g. paralysis of one side of the body.

First aid

1. Place the victim in recovery position.
2. Monitor his vital parameters every 10 minutes.
3. Do not give him anything orally.
4. Shift him to a hospital immediately.

❒ EAR INJURY

It is caused by a direct blow to the ear. A hematoma forms due to accumulation of blood between the external ear cartilage and perichondrium.

First aid

1. Apply an ice pack locally.
2. Apply compression over the injured ear.
3. Send him to a hospital immediately.

❒ UNDER WATER DIVING INJURY

With under water diving, there is increase in pressure on the ear drums from outside, while the eustachian tube is unable to equalize pressure. The ear drums may rupture below the depth of 3 meters. It causes severe pain in the ear.

First Aid

Send him to a hospital immediately.

❒ MAXILLOFACIAL INJURIES

A blow to the upper jaw causes injuries to the maxilla and zygomatic bone, as in boxing. The condition is diagnosed by the following features.

1. One half of a cheek may feel numb.
2. There is pain and tenderness over the affected bones. Swelling may be present over the side of the injury.
3. Teeth may be out of alignment.
4. Chewing or biting on a folded cloth causes pain.
5. Bony deformity may be seen by looking at both cheekbones from the top of the patients head.

First aid

1. Apply ice locally to relieve pain.
2. Give paracetamol for pain.
3. Send him to a hospital immediately.

❒ NASAL INJURIES

A blow to the nose causes nasal injuries, as in boxing bout. The condition is diagnosed by the following features.

1. There is pain and tenderness over the nasal bones. Swelling may be present over the site of the injury.
2. There is bleeding from the nose.
3. A deformity is felt on running a finger down the front of the nose.
4. The nasal bones may be deviated to one side or depressed.

First aid

1. Control local hemorrhage by pinching the nose between fingers, the head held forward.
2. In case if bleeding is severe a cotton ball or compress may be placed inside the nostril.
3. Send him to a hospital immediately.

❒ DENTAL INJURY

A direct hit generally knocks out anterior teeth. If the teeth are hit but not knocked out, soft tissue damage is only minor. The teeth and mouth are sore. The tooth is not displaced. It may be loose and tender and there may be some gum damage.

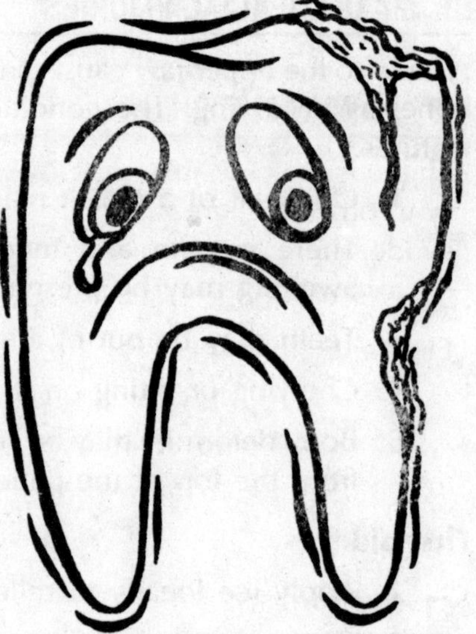

First aid

1. Ask the victim to hold the tooth in its socket firmly using a towel.
2. Send him to a dentist immediately for reimplantation of the tooth.
3. If the tooth has totally fallen off and cannot be replaced, treat hemorrhage by pressing the bleeding socket with a wad of gauze.

❒ BLISTERS

They occur as due to shearing or compression of the skin. Loose sports shoes may cause blisters over the heels. A narrow toe shoe may cause blisters on the fifth toe.

First aid

1. Use petroleum jelly between toes.
2. Use powder or astringent to dry the foot.
3. Send him to a hospital for drainage of acute blisters.

❒ BURSITIS

There are 14 bursae around the knee joint. Any of them can get inflamed. Prepatellar bursa is usually injured by falling onto the anterior aspect of knee or by prolonged kneeling. It is painful when compressed. Septic bursitis may result if it gets infected. In semimembranosus bursitis, there is pain on the lower posteromedial aspect of the knee.

First aid

1. Give paracetamol for pain.
2. Send him to a hospital for orthopedic treatment.

❒ PAIN IN THE SHIN

There is pain in he anterior lower leg in anterior compartment syndrome. It increases on dorsiflexion of the foot. It is due to a sudden increase in training intensity, especially jumping or running on a hard surface.

First aid

1. Give rest.
2. Give paracetamol for pain.
3. Send him to a hospital for orthopedic treatment if these measures fail.

❒ TENNIS LEG

Tennis leg is a strain of the gastrocnemius muscle. Women over the age of 30 are generally affected. The condition is diagnosed by the following features.

1. The athlete often feels something giving way in the back of the leg or as if she has been hit from behind, just after forceful jump.
2. Pain and spasm occur rapidly so that she cannot put her foot on the ground.
3. Swelling and bruising develop distal to the injury site, reaching maximum after 48 hours.
4. There is local tenderness at the junction of upper and middle third of the calf.

5. There is pain at that point on passively stretching the muscle, worse when the knee is straight than when it is flexed.

First aid

1. Immobilize the leg to prevent further damage.
2. Apply a compression damage to the calf to limit the size of the swelling.
3. Give paracetamol for pain.
4. Send him to a hospital afterwards.

❒ ACHILLES TENDINITIS

Achilles tendon is the tendon of the calf muscles attached to the heel of the foot. Its inflammation is diagnosed by the following features.

1. Pain around the tendon.
2. Swelling around the tendon.

First aid

1. Initial treatment is aimed at reducing local oedema. Give rest and apply ice packs locally to reduce pain and resolve inflammation.
2. Give paracetamol for pain.
3. Use a heel raise to reduce the stretch of the tendon. It should initially be non-weight bearing.
4. Send him to a hospital afterwards.

❒ RETROCALCANEAL PAIN

It is seen in adolescents during the rapid growth spurt between the age of 11 and 15 years. There is tenderness on compression of the medial and lateral aspects of the heel.

First aid

1. Give total rest initially to allow the pain to subside.
2. Give paracetamol for pain.
3. Advise use of shock absorbing heel pads in all shoes.
4. Send him to a hospital afterwards.

❒ TENNIS ELBOW

It occurs mainly in tennis players. It is characterized by soft tissue pain between shoulder and wrist. Repeated activity causes multiple small injuries of the common extensor origin. The condition is diagnosed by the following features.

1. There is pain over the region of the lateral epicondyle.
2. It extends distally.
3. It increases with extension of the wrist against resistance.

First aid

1. Give total rest initially to allow the pain to subside.
2. Give paracetamol for pain.
3. Advise stretching exercises after the pain subsides.

❒ WRIST PAIN IN GYMNASTS

It is common in gymnasts. It is due to repetitive forced extension of the knee. It causes compression and impaction forces on the wrist. The condition is diagnosed by the following features.

1. There is pain over the dorsum of the wrist.
2. The range of flexion and extension at the wrist are limited.

First aid

1. Give total initially to allow the pain to subside.
2. Give paracetamol for pain.
3. Advise exercises after the pain subsides.

❒ BLEEDING

Some helpful thoughts

1. For every stone of body weight we have approximately one pint of blood.
2. The average healthy adult can lose up to 850 ml without serious effect. In children, half a pint can be critical.
3. When you cut yourself the amount of blood lost always looks a lot more then it actually is, so do not panic.

4. Severe bruising can remove more blood from the circulation than may a fair sized cut. For example, a fractured thigh can cause a loss of up to three pints of blood yet there is no visible bleeding.

5. Forget whatever you have been told about pressure points — they are hard to find in dressed people and even harder to keep pressure on for long periods.

6. Mild bleeding stops of its own accord because the body has a 'plugging up' mechanism that comes into play when the blood vessels are damaged. Simply apply firm pressure over the area until bleeding stops.

7. Stopping severe bleeding is essential, life-saving, and should be done as follows :

   (*i*) Do not delay, do something at once. Get someone else to call a doctor or an ambulance.

   (*ii*) Raise the bleeding part where possible. This reduces the blood flow to some extent simply by reducing the effect of gravity. If you think the part might be fractured, do not raise it.

   (*iii*) Apply pressure to the wound. Use your fingers and thumb to close the edges of the wound together. Grab it hard — do not be afraid of hurting the person. **Do not waste time washing your hands.**

   (*iv*) If this does not seem to be producing results, ask someone to get you a freshly laundered cloth of any kind make it into a pad large enough to cover the wound and press it firmly on to the would for 10 minutes. If you are on your own, use your handkerchief and tie it on as a dressing.

Could there be internal bleeding?

Any serious accident can be complicated by internal bleeding even though the injured person seems and feels well (at first anyway).

Invisible bleeding can be just as serious as visible bleeding.

Symptoms : 1. Bruising — especially over a large area or over the trunk 2. Dizziness 3. Cold, clammy, sweaty skin 4. Rapid, weak pulse 5. Difficult breathing 6. Frothy blood being coughed up 7. Severe abdominal pain 8. Evidence of a fracture.

Action : Treat for shock, get professional help quickly.

Some special bleeding problems

Nose bleed

1. Sit down, preferably at a table. Put a bowl under your nose on the table.
2. Grasp the soft part of your nose firmly between your thumb and index finger.
3. Lean your head forwards and hold your nose for 10 minutes — this cures the vast majority of nose bleeds.
4. Never ignore a nose bleed in someone who has hit his head or had a fall, especially if the nose is discharging clear fluid as well as blood. This is a sign of a fractured skull and needs immediate medical attention.
5. Once a nose bleed has stopped, do not blow or sniff. You will dislodge the clot and have to start all over again.
6. If you have lots of nose bleeds, tell your doctor.

Bleeding from the back passage

This is almost always caused by piles. See your doctor for advice. Never ignore bleeding from your back passage. If the bleeding is accompanied by a sharp pain, you may have torn the skin because you are constipated. Eat plenty of high fibre foods (vegetables, whole meal bread, bran-containing breakfast cereals) and you will not be troubled again. This is also good treatment for early piles.

Bleeding tongue

Sit as with a nose bleed. Grasp the tongue with a freshly laundered handkerchief. Press for 10 minutes.

Bleeding tooth socket

Usually happens after a tooth extraction.

Do not wash out the mouth or you'll disturb clot formation. Sit up as for nose bleeding. Put a thick wad of gauze or similar material over the socket area and bite hard on it. Do this for 10 minutes and then gently remove the dressing. If bleeding persists, telephone the dentist who did the extraction.

Bleeding into the urine

If your urine is bloody there is nothing you can or should do except tell your doctor. It can be caused by trivial or serious conditions but needs thorough investigation. (Beetroot, some sweets and some constipation medicines can make your urine red).

Bleeding from the stomach

Most likely caused by a bleeding ulcer. Blood in vomit can be red, brown or black like coffee grounds. The colour indicates how long it has been in the stomach. (It darkens with time.)

Keen the person lying down. Watch for shock and get medical help.

Beware of red foods when worrying about blood in vomit. It is usually easy to tell beetroot, red peppers and tomatoes from vomited fresh red blood if your look carefully.

Bleeding scalp

The scalp is especially rich in blood vessels and bleeds profusely even from small cuts. Apply pressure to the cut area for 10 minutes using a freshly laundered handkerchief. If the bleeding does not stop (and it might well not, unlike other areas of the body) go to hospital for stitches. **Remember** that any wound of the scalp may be accompanied by a fracture of the skull. If you feel peculiar in any way, have difficulty with speaking or coordination, feel drowsy or have any watery or blood stained fluid from your nose or ears, get medical help at once.

Bleeding from the lungs

The strain of repeated coughing can cause tiny streaks of blood to be coughed up. Heavier bleeding from disease or injury to the chest needs medical attention and is usually pink and frothy. If bleeding is heavy, go to hospital at once or call an ambulance.

Bleeding from the ear

Any bleeding from inside the ear must be treated with respect. In any person who has fallen or possibly hit his head, think of a fractured skull if blood comes from the ear, especially if it is accompanied by clear, watery fluid. Get medical help.

Bleeding varicose veins

Press over the bleeding point with or without a dressing. Raise the leg on a stool or chair as you lie on the floor, remove stockings and garters and bandage a dressing or freshly laundered handkerchief over the area. Talk to your doctor about long term treatment of the various veins.

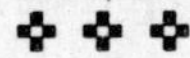

CHAPTER 14

Dressings and Bandages are Crucial

The first rule in any treatment modality for wounds is cleanliness. Prevention of infection is the only assurance that a wound will heal well.

- In wounds caused by accidents where dirt and dust is spread around, e.g. road accidents, earthquakes, train collisions etc., there are greater chances of infection.
- Wounds caused by metal, burns or neat incised cuts acquired through glass injuries are generally clean wounds.
- Open wounds always carry the risk of infection.

❒ DRESSINGS

A dressing is a material or fabric piece applied to a wound or to an injured part and is primarily used for three purposes :

- To control bleeding.
- To protect a wound from further infection.
- To prevent or lessen infection.

❒ TYPE OF DRESSINGS

1. Prepared sterile dressing

This is the ideal dressing for all wounds and consists of a sterilised (germ-free) piece of gauze or lint to which sometimes a pad or roller bandage is stitched. This dressing is enclosed and sealed in a protective covering. Before using a sterile dressing, hands must be thoroughly washed with a disinfectant preferably chlorhexidine 7.5% or with soap and water. Loosen the protective covering and remove

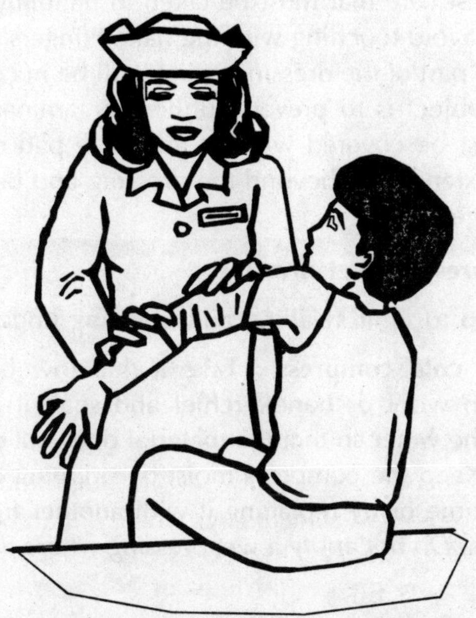

the dressing. Expose the dressing as little as possible to the air. Do not breath or cough over it. Avoid fingering the surface of the dressing which is to be applied to the wound.

2. Gauze or lint

If a sterile dressing is not available, cover the wound with a piece of clean gauze or lint.

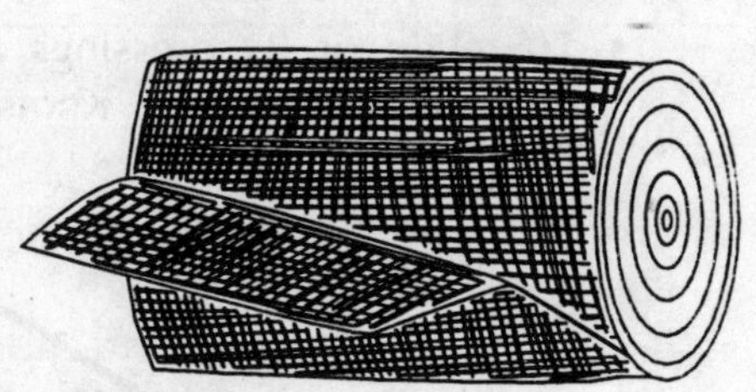

Do not use cotton wool or a fluffy fabric directly on an open wound as it will stick to the surface.

3. Emergency dressing

If a prepared sterile dressing or gauze or lint is not immediately available, soft old sari material, cotton bed sheets, table cover, sanitary pads, the inside fold of a clean handkerchief or freshly laundered towel, a piece of linen or even clean paper tissue can be used, but their use is only temporary until a prepared sterile dressing or gauze or lint is procured.

The greatest care that must be taken in handling and applying dressing is to avoid touching with the naked fingers any part of the wound or any part of the dressing which will be in contact with the wound. The object is to prevent further contamination by germs. Dressings must be covered with an adequate pad of cotton wool which must extend well beyond the dressing and be kept in place with a bandage.

4. Cold compress or wet dressing

It can help to limit swelling and bleeding under the skin.

Making a cold compress : Take a thin towel, piece of lint, flannel, cotton wool or handkerchief and soak it in cold water. Squeeze out the water so that the material does not drip but do not wring it dry. Keep the compress moist by dripping on more water from time to time or by replacing it with another freshly prepared cold compress. *Do not apply a wet dressing where there is an open wound.*

Note : A bleeding wound needs a pressure pad dressing.

❒ BANDAGES

Objective of bandaging

- To retain or fix dressings and splints in position and to immobilise tractures. Knots should never be tied over a fracture.

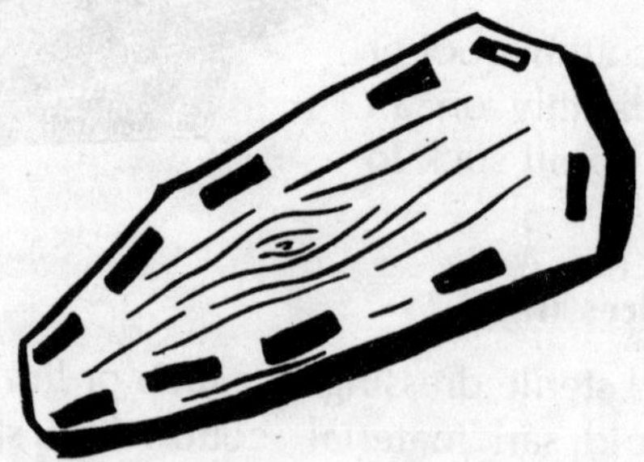

- To afford support to an injured part (e.g. sprained ankle) or to form a sling.

- To prevent infection
- To control bleeding.

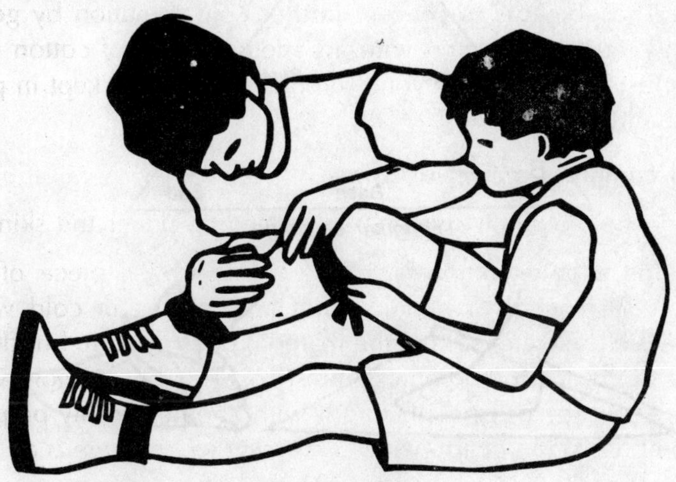

- To reduce or prevent swelling.
- To assist in lifting and carrying casualties.
- To increase the temperature of the injured part.

Signs and Symptoms of tight bandage

- Skin distal to bandaging, may became bluish.
- Numbness and tingling.
- Nail beds become blue.

Treatment

- Immediate loosening of the bandage.

Types of bandages

There are generally three types of bandages :

1. Triangular bandage : most useful multipurpose bandage for a first-aider.
2. Roller bandage.
3. Adhesive bandage and dressing.

Triangular bandage : It is made by cutting a piece of linen or fabric, not less than 38 inches square, diagonally into two pieces.

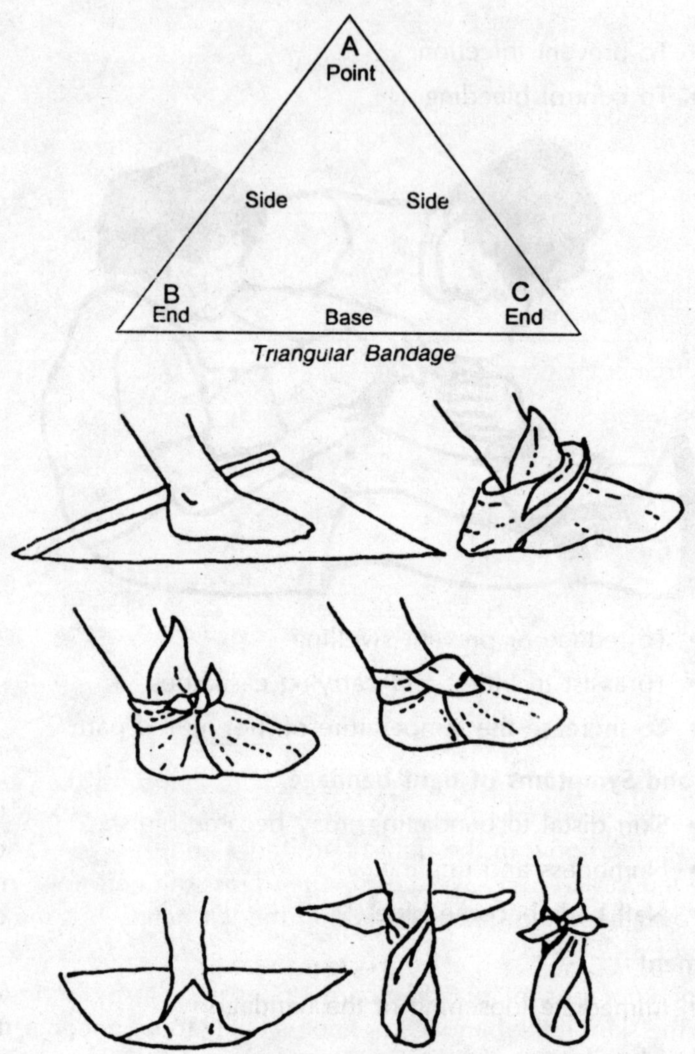

Triangular Bandage

Triangular Bandage on foot

The bandage may be applied :

As a whole cloth : This can be spread out to its full extent, e.g., chest bandage.

As a broad bandage : This can be done by bringing the point down to the centre of the base and then folding the bandage again in the same direction.

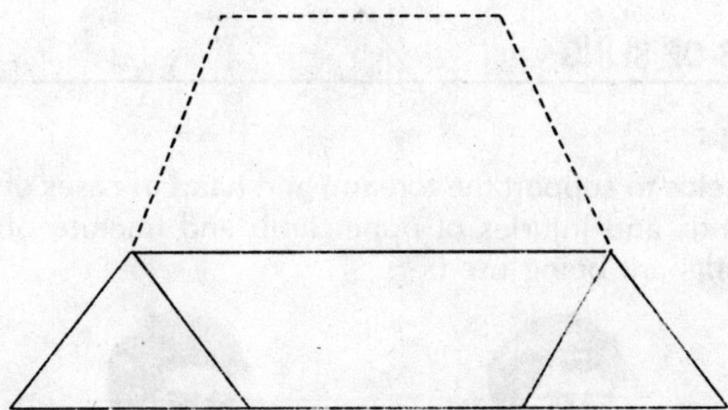

A triangular bandage secures dressings or pads in place.

As a narrow bandage : This is made by folding the broad bandage, once again in the same direction.

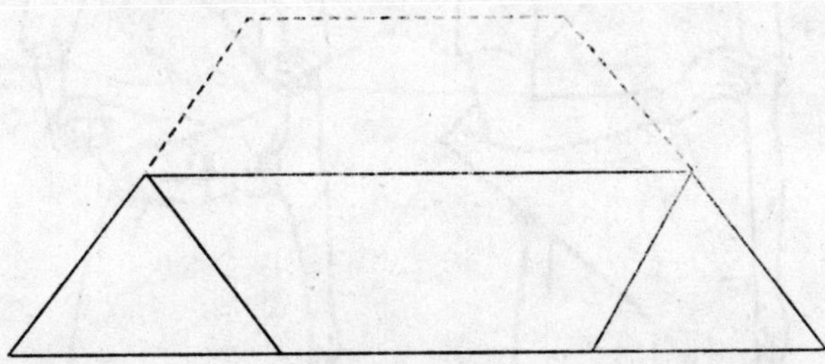

To secure the ends of a bandage a reef knot must be used. To make a reef knot, take the ends of the bandage, one in each hand. Cross the end now in the right hand under and then over the end in the left hand thus make a turn. Then cross the end now in right hand over and then under the end in the left hand, thus making a second turn.

The knot must be placed where it does not cause discomfort or chafe the skin. if the bandage or knot is likely to be uncomfortable, a pad is placed between the bandage or knot and the body. Granny knots are apt to slip and must not be used.

❐ SLINGS

Slings are used :

1. To afford support or rest to an upper limb.
2. To prevent the weight of an upper limb pulling on or moving the chest, shoulder or neck.

❐ TYPES OF SLING

Arm Sling :

This helps to support the forearm and hand in cases of fractured ribs, wounds and injuries of upper limb and fracture of forearms when splints are being used.

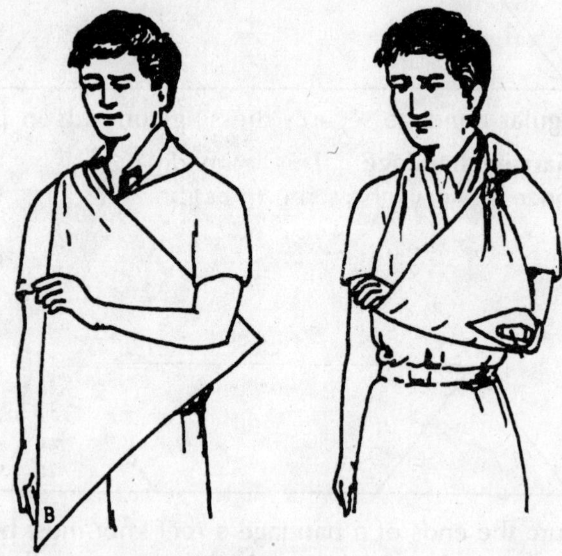

Application of an Arm Sling : Face the casualty and put one end of a spread out triangular sheet or bandage over his shoulder on the sound side with the point towards the injured side. Pass it around his neck so that it appears over the shoulder of the injured side and let the other end hang down in front of the chest. Carry the point behind the elbow of the injured limb and place the forearm over the middle of the bandage so that it is at right angles of the upper arm; then carry the second end up to the first and tie them in the hollow just above the collar bone. Tuck the bandage into the back of the elbow, bring the point forward and secure it with a safety pin to the front of the bandage.

The base of the bandage should be at the root of the little finger so that all the finger nails are exposed. A bluish tinge of the finger nail indicates that their is a dangerous constriction interfering with the circulation in the upper limb.

Collar and Cuff Sling :

It helps to support the wrist by clove hitch bandage. To apply a collar and cuff sling bend the casualty's elbow and lay his forearm across the chest with his fingers touching his opposite shoulder. Pass a "clove hitch" around his wrist and tie the ends of the bandage in the hollow just above the collar bone on the injured side.

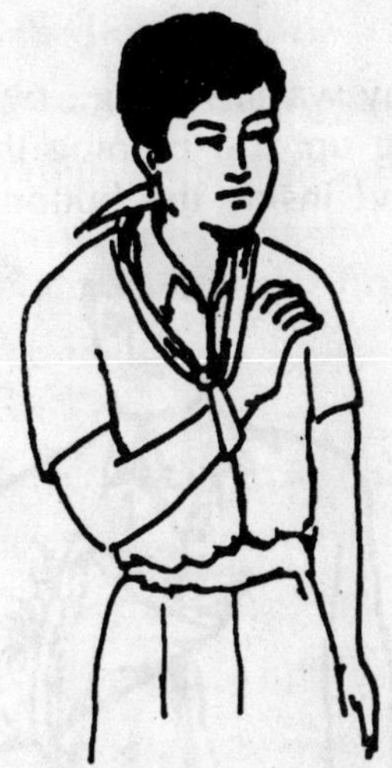

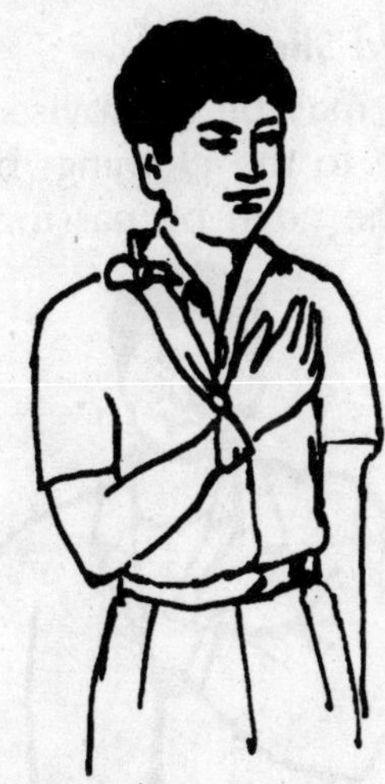

A "clove hitch" is made by taking a narrow bandage and making a loop. Make a second loop and lay it on top of first, then lay the top loop behind the first without turning.

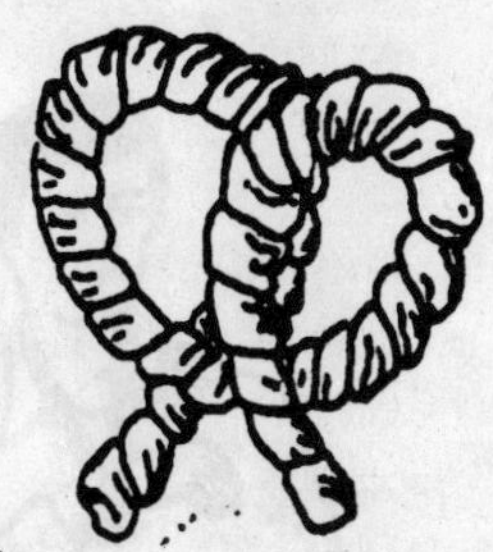

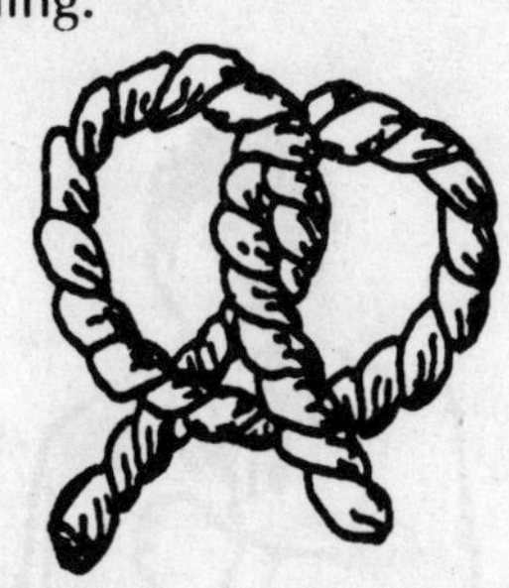

Triangular Sling

It helps to keep the hand well raised and is applied in cases of fractured collar bone. Place the casualty's forearm across his chest so that his fingers point towards the shoulder and the centre of the palm rests on the breast-bone. Lay an open bandage over the forearm with one end over the hand and the point well below the elbow. Steady the limb and tuck the base of the bandage well under the hand and forearm so that the lower end may be brought under the bent elbow and then upwards across the back to the uninjured shoulder, where it is tied in the hollow above the collar bone. The loose point of the bandage is then tucked well in between the forearm and bandaged in front and the fold thus formed is turned backwards over the lower part of the upper arm and pinned.

Improvised Slings

Slings may be improvised in many ways; for e.g., by pinning the sleeve to the clothing; by turning up and pinning the lower edge of the coat; by passing the hand inside the buttoned coat,

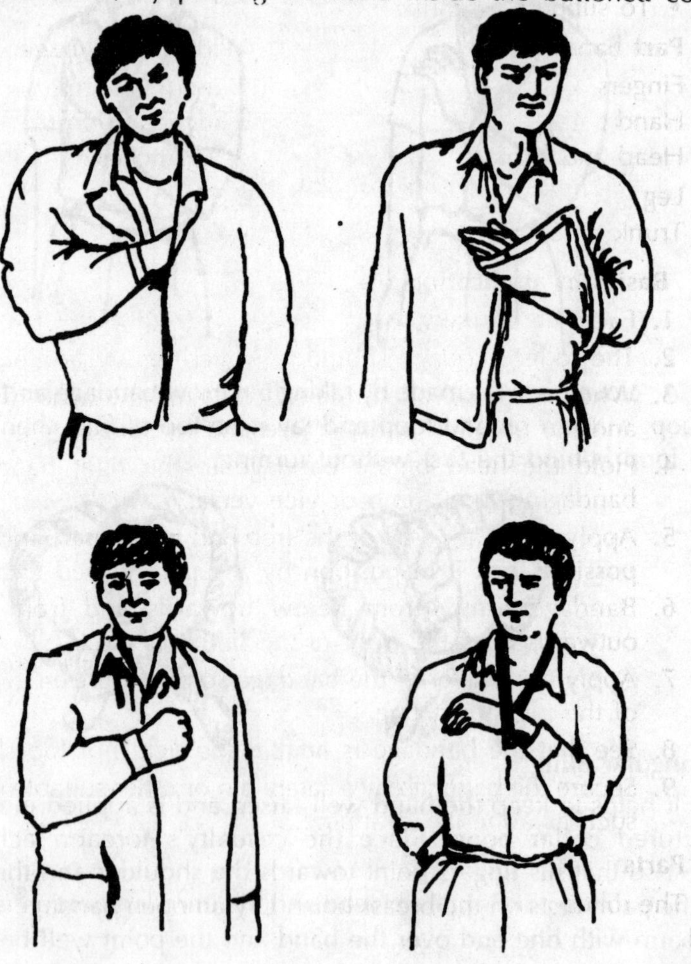

jacket or waistcoat. Scarves, ties, belts or tights etc. can also be used as slings.

Roller Bandage

Roller bandages are made of various materials like cotton or linen with loose mesh and are of various lengths and widths according to the use to which they are put. They are used in hospitals and first-aid posts.

Use of Roller Bandage

- To keep dressing in position.
- To apply pressure to control bleeding.
- To support a sprain.

Part bandaged	Width of bandage
Fingers	1 inch (2.5 cm)
Hand	2 inches (5 cm)
Head and Arm	2-2$\frac{1}{2}$ inches
Leg	3-3$\frac{1}{2}$ inches
Trunk	4-6 inches

Basics of application :

1. Face the casualty.
2. The roller bandage should be rolled tightly and evenly.
3. When partly unrolled, the roll is called the head (or drum) and the unrolled part the free end (or tail).
4. Hold the head of the bandage in the right hand when bandaging a left limb or vice versa.
5. Apply the outer side of the free end to the part and where possible lock it in position by a superimposed turn.
6. Bandage firmly from below upwards and from within outwards over the front of the limb.
7. Apply each layer of the bandage so that it covers two-third of the preceding one.
8. See that the bandage is neither too tight nor too slack.
9. Secure the bandage by a safety pin or other suitable method such as adhesive strapping.

Parts

The rolled part is called Head and the unrolled portion is called Tail.

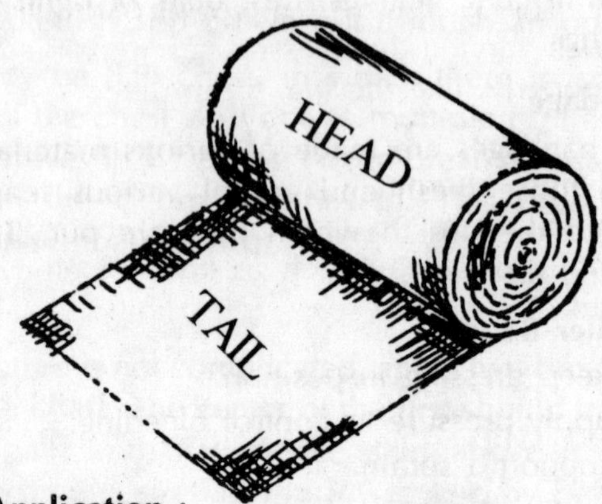

Methods of Application :

There are four major methods of application of roller bandage :

Simple Spiral : This can be used when the part to be bandaged is of uniform thickness as, for instance, the finger or wrist and a short portion of the forearm above it. The bandage is rolled in a spiral direction.

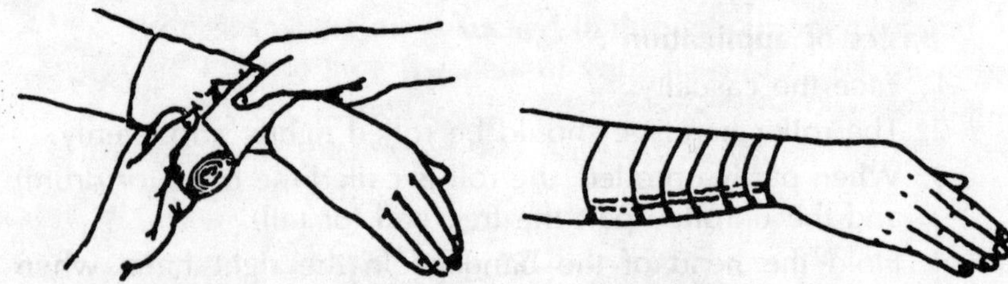

Reverse Spiral : This is done by a number of spiral turns in which the bandage is reversed downwards upon itself at each circuit

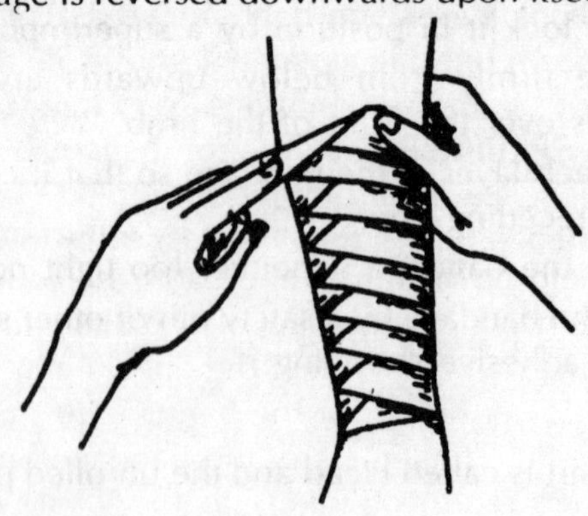

of the limb. This is used in bandaging parts of the limbs, where, owing to their varying thickness, it is impossible to make a simple spiral lie properly, like the leg, forarm etc.

Figure of Eight : It is applied by passing the bandage obliquely round the limb, alternately upwards and downwards, the loops resembling the figure 8. It is used for bandaging at or in the neighbourhood of a joint such as knee or elbow. It can also be used instead of a reverse spiral for a limb.

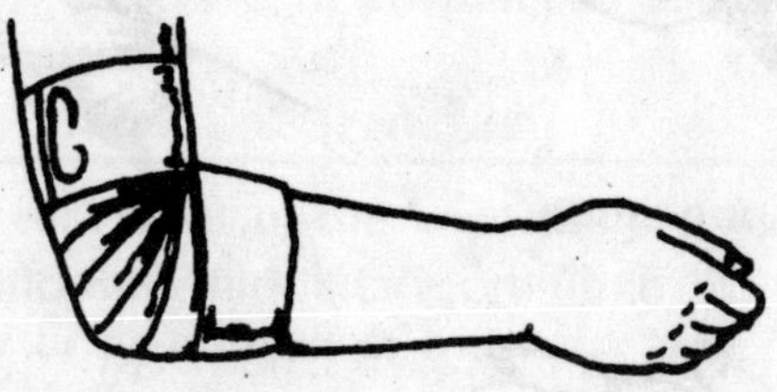

Spica : This is a modified figure of 8 used for bandaging the hip, shoulder, groin or thumb.

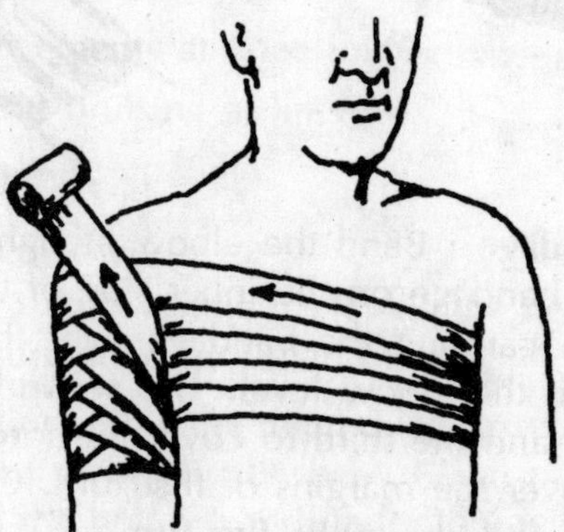

❒ BANDAGING SPECIAL BODY PARTS

1. Hand Bandage : Fix the bandage by a turn around the wrist, with the palm held downwards, and carry the roll obliquely over the back of the hand to the side of the little finger. Carry the bandage round the palm encircling the fingers with one horizontal turn, so that the lower border of the bandage just reaches the root of the nail of the little finger. Carry the bandage once more round the palm and then return obliquely to the wrist. The figure of 8 turns around the wrist and hand are repeated until the hand is covered and the bandage is then finished with a spiral turn round the wrist.

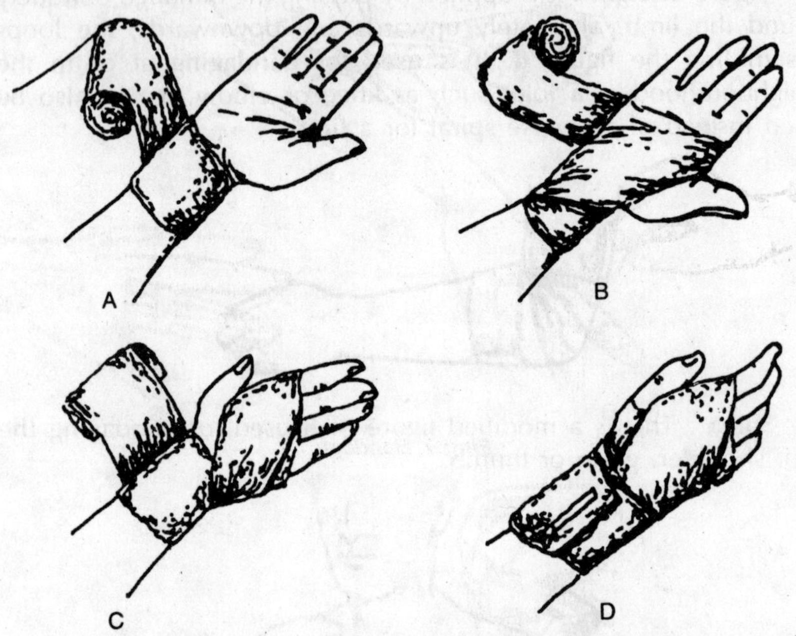

2. Elbow bandage : Bend the elbow at right angles. Lay the outer side of the bandage on the inner side of the joint and take one straight turn, carrying the bandage over the elbow tip and round the limb at the elbow level. The second turn is made to encircle the arm, and the third to cover the forearm, each of the turns made to cover the margins of first turn. Continue the turns alternately below and above the first turn.

3. Finger bandage : With the palm downward fix a one-inch bandage by two circular turns round the wrist, leaving the end free for tying off afterwards. Carry the bandage obliquely over the back of the hand to the base of finger to be bandaged, taking the fingers in order starting from the little finger side. Take one spiral turn to the base of finger nail and then cover the finger by simple spiral turns. Now carry the bandage across the back of the hand to the wrist and complete it with one straight turn round the wrist. Secure the bandage by a safety pin or by tying the two ends of the bandage together. If more than one finger is to be bandaged, take a turn

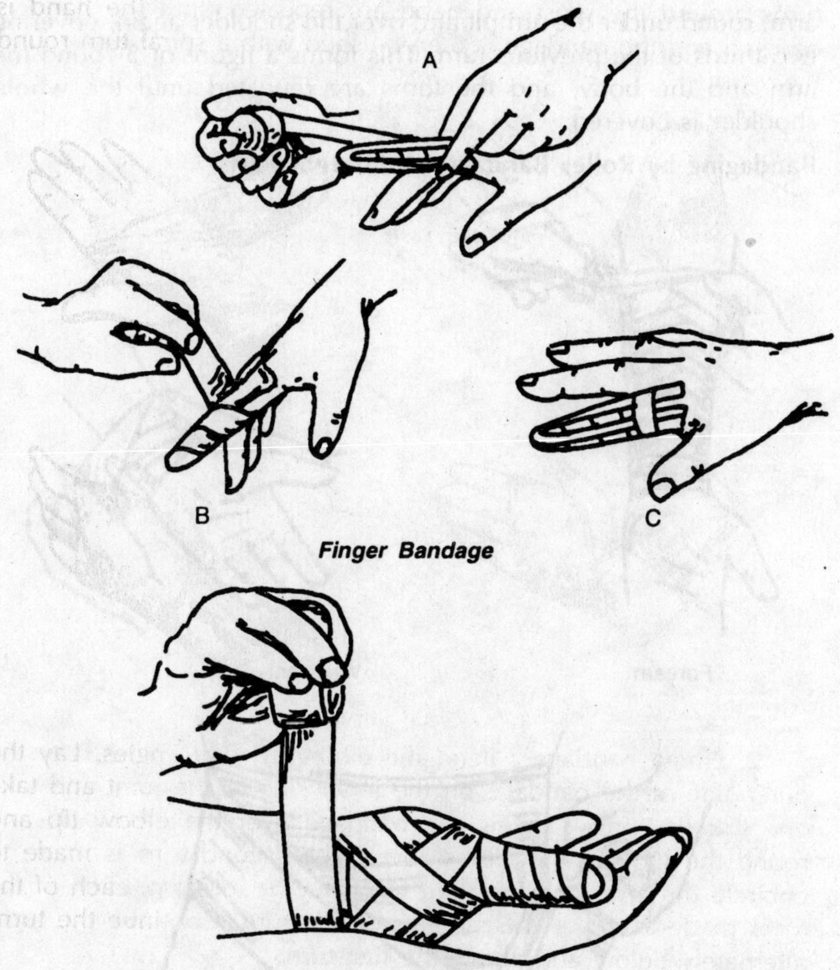

Finger Bandage

Thumb & Wrist Bandage

round the wrist between each two fingers, and continue as above until the bandage is complete.

4. Shoulder bandage : Place a small pad of cotton wool under each armpit. Take a 3-4 inch bandage and fix it with two spiral turns round the upper part of the arm. Make 2 or 3 reverse spiral turns round the upper arm until the bandage reaches spiral turns round the upper arm until the bandage reaches the point of the shoulder, then carry the bandage over the shoulder, across the back and under the opposite armpit. Bring it back across the chest and arm, round under the armpit and over the shoulder again, covering two-thirds of the previous turn. This forms a figure of 8 round the arm and the body, and the turns are repeated until the whole shoulder is covered.

Bandaging by Roller Bandage of different Parts

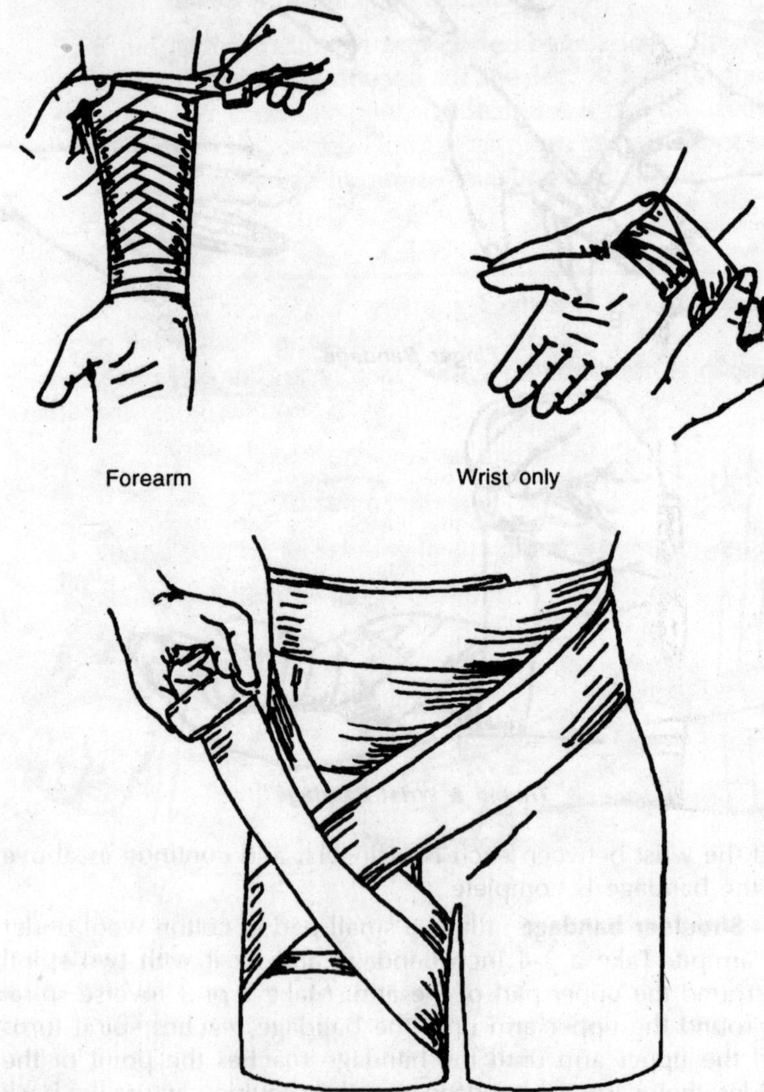

Forearm

Wrist only

Special bandage for hip and thigh

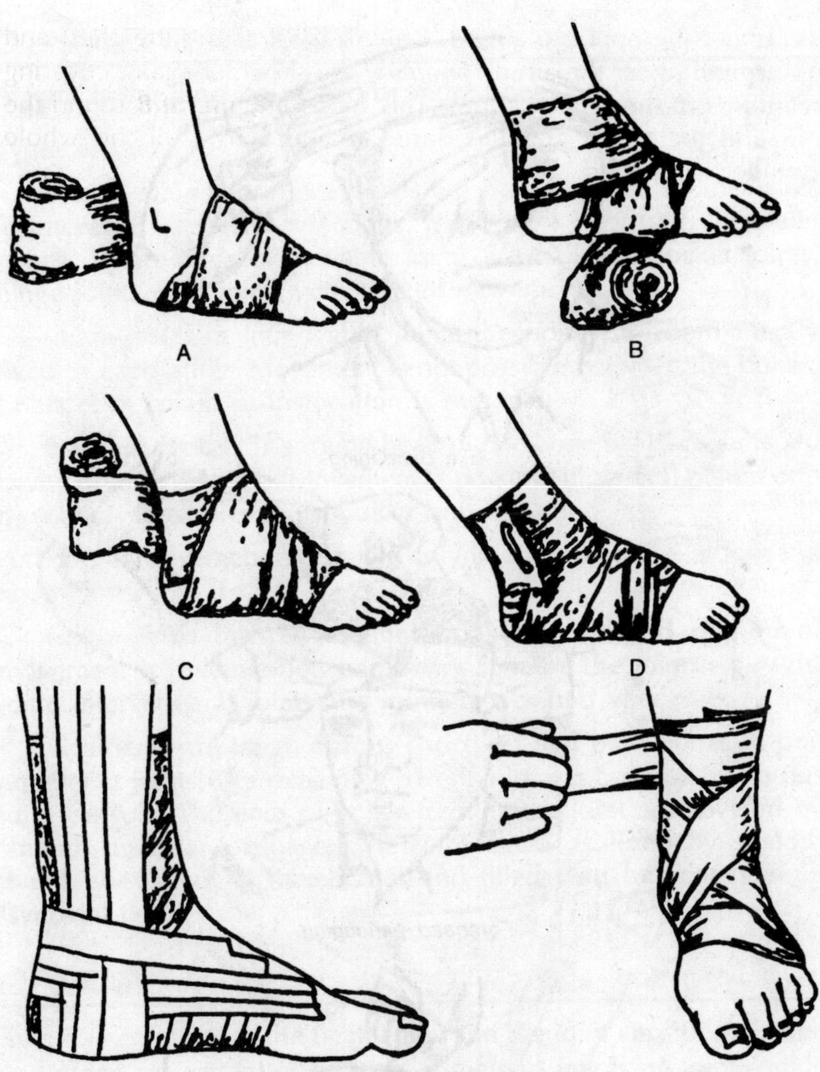

Bandages for ankle and foot

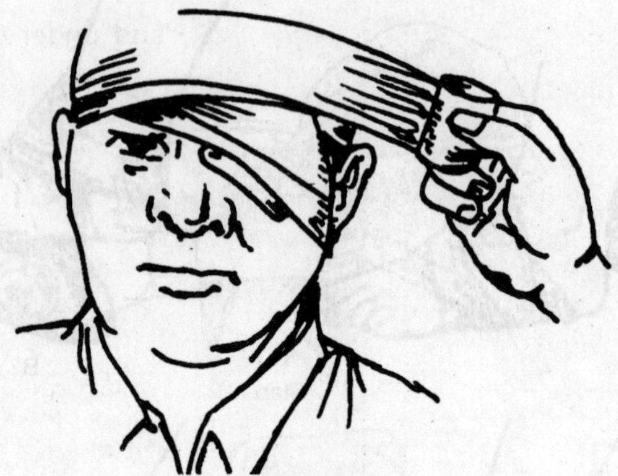

Eye bandaging

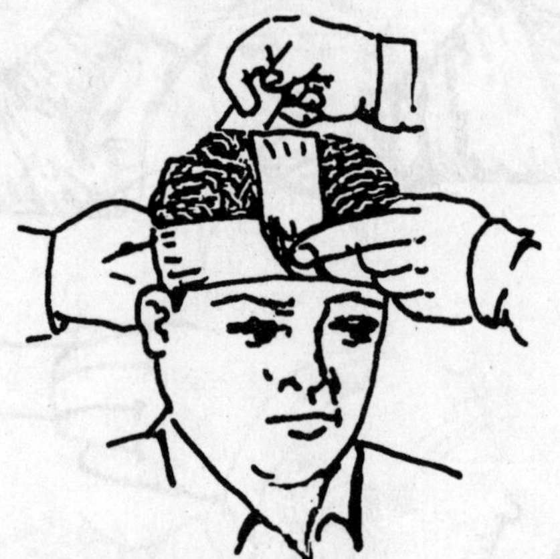

Forehead bandaging

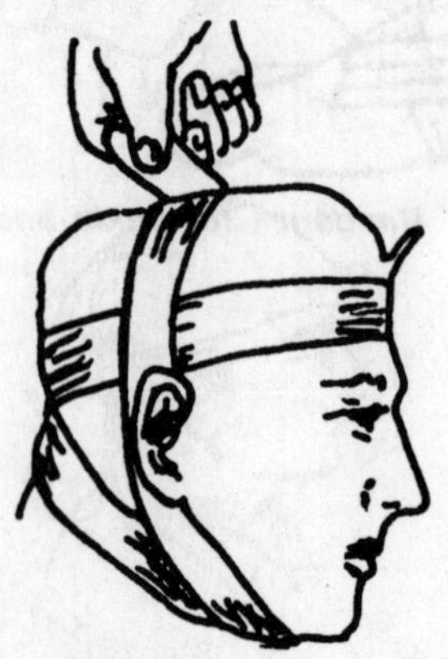

Jaw bandaging

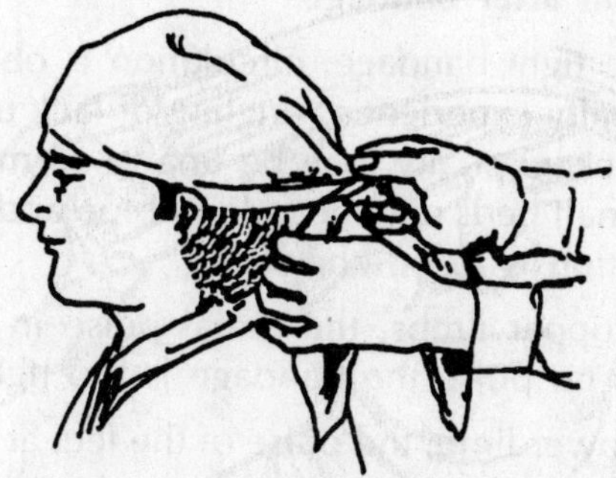

Step I

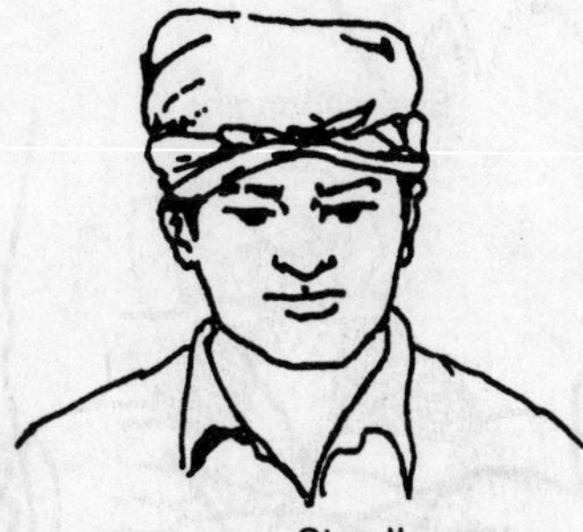

Step II

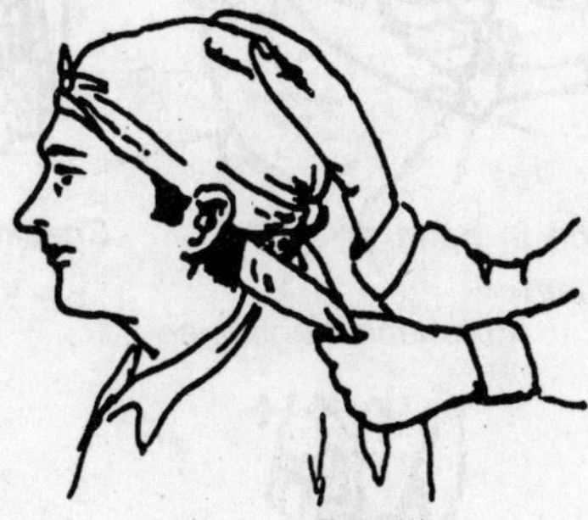

Step III

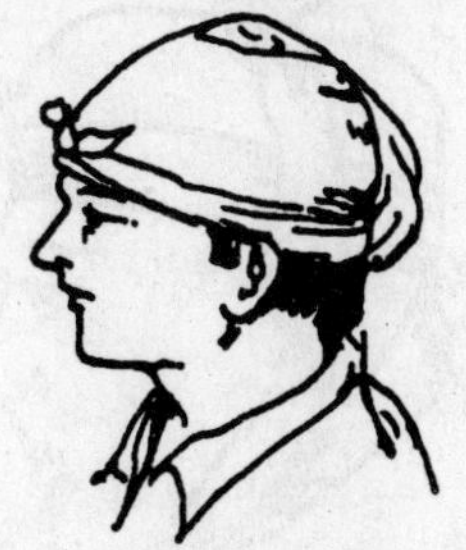

Step IV

Scalp bandage

To check circulation after bandage

Sometimes with tight bandage, circulation is obstructed down below and the casualty experiences tingling or lack of feeling in his or her fingers or toes. Casualty may be unable to move his or her fingers or toes, toe nail beds may be pale or blue and become cold. Hence, the circulation is to be checked.

(1) In case of upper limbs, the radial pulse in hand is to be checked. If no pulse the bandage is too tight.

(2) In case of lower limb, the pulse of the feet at the ankle joint on the inside of the leg to be felt. If no pulse the bandage is too tight.

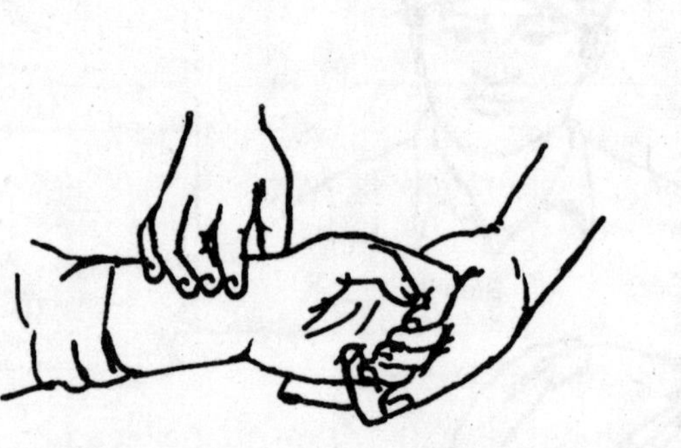

Checking circulation in hand (Radial pulse)

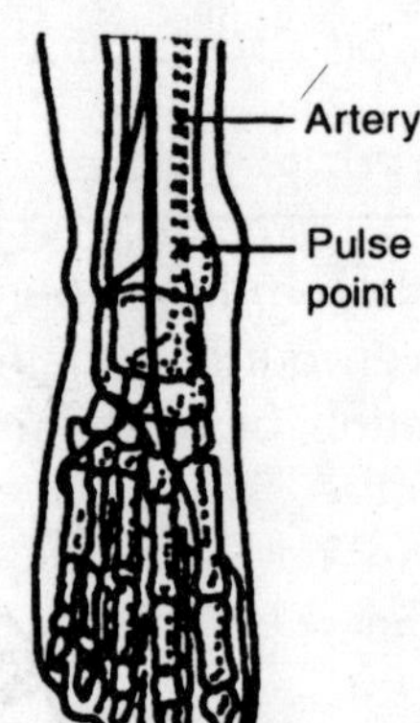

Checking circulation in the leg

CHAPTER

15

Nursing : A Noble Job

The first aider needs to know a few basic principles of nursing so as to be able to render first aid effectively.

❐ TEMPERATURE

Metabolism in the human body generates heat. It is given out by breathing, evaporation of sweat, excretion of urine and stools and by radiation from the skin surface. The temperature of the human body is maintained between 36°C and 37°C. When it goes above 37°C, the patient is said to have fever. When it is below 36°C the patient is said to have subnormal temperature. The fever may be constant, remittent (ups and downs without reaching the normal temperature), intermittent or irregular. The body temperature can be judged by the back of the hand. Accurate measurement of temperature is done using a thermometer, placing it under the tongue or in the dried axilla for 3 minutes. It is placed in the rectum of children. The patient must not have taken anything hot or cold orally for at least 30 minutes before recording oral temperature. The thermometer is shaken well so that the mercury column goes below the 35°C mark. After use it is cleaned with antiseptic solution and put dipping in a bottle with an antiseptic solution and a cotton swab at the bottom.

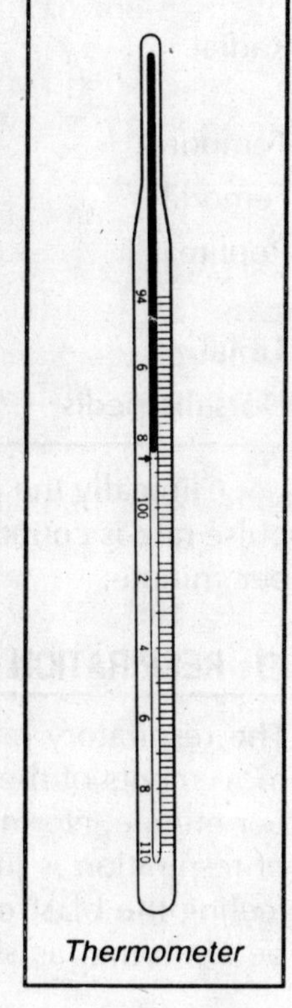

Thermometer

❐ PULSE

The pulse is felt over arteries where they lie over a bone and under the skin. It is felt due to the pulsatile flow of blood through the arteries as a result of contraction and relaxation of the heart rhythmically. The pulse rate, rhythm, and volume tell about the condition of the heart and circulation. The pulse can be felt at the following sites.

Sites of Peripheral Pulses

Vessel	Site
Carotid	Against the transverse process of 6th cervical vertebra in the side of the neck.
Axillary	Against the head of the humerus on the lateral wall of the axilla.
Brachial	Against the humerus on the medial aspect of the arm.
Radial	Against the lower end of the radius on the front of the wrist.
Temporal	Against the temporal bone in front of the ear.
Femoral	At the root of the lower limb.
Popliteal	Against the upper end of tibia on the back of the knee.
Tibial	On the medial aspect of the ankle.
Dorsalis pedis	On the front of the ankle.

Clinically the pulse is examined in the neck or at the wrist. The pulse rate is counted for 1 minute and is expressed in terms of beats per minute.

❐ RESPIRATION

The respiratory rate is counted by noting the outward and inward movements of the anterior chest wall and anterior abdominal wall per minute. Normal respiratory rate is 16-20/minute. The adequacy of respiration is judged by holding a hand in front of the nose and feeling the blast of air as the patient breathes out. Respiration can be abnormal as shown in the following table.

Respiratory Abnormalities

Type	Causes
Rapid	Lack of oxygen at the tissue level which might be due to low oxygen content in the inspired air, diseases of the lungs or heart, low hemoglobin level, or shock.
Slow	Depression of respiratory center.
Stridor	Partial airway obstruction during inspiration, expiration, or both.
Shallow	Painful conditions of chest wall such as fracture of ribs.
Granting	Pneumonia.
Gasping	Usually in a dying patient.
Cheyne-Stokes	The interval between successive breaths goes on increasing until the breathing appears to have ceased. Then it starts all over again.

❒ TEPID SPONGING

Sponging is the process in which the patient's body is cleaned with soap and wet cloth while the patient remains in bed. Ordinary sponging is never required by the first aider, but tepid sponging may be required. It is done so as to reduce the body temperature in cases of high fever. The method is as follows.

1. Check the body temperature.
2. Soak sponges with water, squeeze them and place two of them in the patient axillae, two in the groins, and one on the abdomen. Place an ice-bag on the head. Change the sponges periodically.
3. Wipe the patient's body with sponges soaked in the water. Do not dry the body entirely.
4. Complete the procedure in 18-20 minutes.
5. Check the body temperature $\frac{1}{2}$ hour later.

❒ COLD PACK

This procedure is done to lower body temperature in cases of high fever. The method is as follows.

1. Place a mackintosh and a bath-blanket under the patient.
2. Remove the patient's clothes.
3. Soak two bed sheets in water at 18°C and squeeze them moderately.
4. Turn the patient on one side and place one bed sheet under the patient. Then place the patient on this bedsheet and place the other bed sheet over him from neck to toes.
5. Place cold compresses or ice bag on his head.
6. Soak the bed sheet in water after it becomes less cool, squeeze and place it over the patient again. Do this for 10 to 15 minutes.
7. Check the patient's temperature after 30 minutes.

❒ ICE BAG

It is a rubber bag in which pieces of ice are kept. It is used to reduce body temperature in cases of high fever, to reduce hemorrhage into a hematoma, and toe relieve pain after blunt trauma. The procedure for its use is as follows.

1. Break ice into pieces of desired size. Place them in a bowl of water so as to remove sharp edges which could tear the rubber bag.
2. Put them in the bag with a spoon. Add some salt to it so as to lower the freezing point further. Do not fill the bag more than 2/3.
3. Place the bag on a flat surface, remove air from it and dry it.
4. Place a mackintosh below the part to be cooled with the ice-bag.
5. Place the ice bag over the part to be cooled.
6. Check periodically to see that the part does not become numb.
7. Do not leave very old or very young patients alone while the ice bag is being applied.

8. Check the patient's temperature periodically. Avoid overcooling.
9. After use empty the bag. Dry it well from inside as well as outside. Let some air into it and place in a cool, dry place.

❒ HOT WATER BAG

A hot water bag is used for varied problems such as :

1. To relieve pain.
2. To help resorption of a hematoma.
3. To help a patient with urinary retention to pass urine.
4. To keep a patient of hypothermia warm.
5. To keep a newborn baby warm in conditions like prematurity, birth asphyxia, hypothermia etc.

The procedure for the use of a hot water bag is as follows :

1. Fill the bag about 2/3 with water at 55-60°C.
2. Place the bag on a flat surface and remove all air from the bag.
3. Close the mouth of the bag.
4. Invert the bag to confirm that it does not leak. Dry the outer side of the bag.
5. Cover the bag with cloth or a cover.
6. Place it over the area to be warmed covered by a towel.
7. Change the water inside when it cools.
8. Empty the bag after use, dry it well from inside and outside, let some air in, and keep it in a cool, dry place.
9. Do not use water at a temperature more than 49°C when to be used for small children and patients with heart disease.
10. Do not place the bag under the body at any time.
11. Do not use a hot water bag if the patient is unconscious or paralytic with loss of sensation, as accidental burns can occur.
12. Change the position of the bag after 5 minutes.
13. Remove the bag if the site of application of the bag becomes red. Apply talcum powder locally.

❒ EYE WASH

Eye wash or eye irrigation is the procedure of washing the eye under aseptic precautions. It is done to remove a foreign body from the eye, to remove inflammatory discharge from the eye, and before an eye operation. The procedure of giving an eye wash is as follows.

1. Make the patient lie down or sit up as convenient. Tilt the head backward in sitting position. Put a mackintosh under the head in a lying down position and wrap a towel around his neck.
2. Ask the patient or an assistant to hold a kidney tray below the eye to be washed. Wash your hands thoroughly well with soap and water. Open the patient's eyelids.
3. Soak a swab of cotton in sterile normal saline and squeeze it into the patient's eye, first under the upper eyelid and then under the lower eyelid.
4. Repeat the procedure till the eye becomes clean.
5. Dry the eyelids from outside using dry cotton swabs.

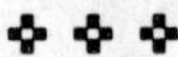

CHAPTER

16

Disinfection and Sterilization are A Must

❐ DISINFECTION

A disinfectant or a germicide is an agent used for killing micro-organisms and their spores which cause diseases. Various disinfectants are shown in the following table.

Disinfectants

Type	**Examples**
Natural	Sunlight, air.
Physical agents	
Dry heat	Burning hot air, hot air oven.
Moist heat	Boiling, autoclaving.
Radiation	Ultraviolet rays, gamma rays.
Chemical agents	
Solids	Zinc, bleaching powder, potassium permanganate.
Liquids	Formalin, gluteraldehyde, phenol, cresol, lysol, dettol, savlon.
Gases	Formaldehyde, ethylene oxide.

❐ COMMON DISINFECTANTS

1. **Dettol :** when used to clean the skin surface, it is applied in pure form and left uncovered until the skin becomes dry. When used as an antiseptic hand lotion, two to four teaspoonful of dettol is added to 500 ml of water.

2. **Savlon :** in a dilution of 1:200, it is used for general antiseptic purposes like washing hospital equipment, disinfection of soiled linen, and spraying the patient's room.

3. **Potassium permanganate :** it is an oxidizing agent. It is used as a general germicide, for gargles as a 1:60 solution, and for purification of water.

❐ WHAT ARE ANTISEPTICS ?

They are used for preventing the growth of micro-organisms. But they cannot kill microorganisms. Various antiseptics are shown in the following table.

Antiseptic	Features
Spirit	It is a 70% solution of alcohol in water. It kills bacteria effectively. It is used for disinfection of the skin, instruments and ampoules of injections. It is not used for disinfection of raw surfaces and wounds because it exposes tissue, aggravates injuries, and removes the coagulum formed that prevents bacterial entry into the wound.
Acriflavine	It is aniline derivative, soluble in water. It is orange in powder form and yellow in 1:1000 aqueous solution. It stains tissues yellow. It has a bacteriostatic and bactericidal action upon a variety of bacteria, especially gram positive bacteria in an alkaline medium. It is used in dressing of the wounds.
Boric Acid	It is available in the form of colourless and odourless crystals or white powder. Its solubility in water is 5% and in glycerin 25%. It is used as solution, dusting powder, or ointment.

	It is effective for mucosal inflammation such as eczema, burns, impetigo, fungal infections of skin and bed sores.
	Its solution is also used for mouth wash and irrigation of bladder.
Carbolic acid	It is a hygroscopic and highly corrosive substance.
	It is used as disinfectant for sharp instruments like scissors and knife blades.
	It is used topically to cauterize dog bites, snake bites and other small wounds.
Gentian violet	It is moderately soluble in water, alcohol and glycerin.
	Its 1% solution in 10% alcohol is used for superficial pyogenic infection of skin and mucous membranes, chronic and irritant lesions of the skin.
Glycerin	It is a colourless, odourless, hygroscopic, thick liquid.
	It is used with other substances mainly magnesium sulphate to reduce swelling in inflammation.
Hydrogen peroxide	It is used in cleaning of wounds. It breaks down into nascent (active) oxygen and water. The oxygen bubbles removes tissue debris from inaccessible parts of wounds. It also kills bacteria by oxidation.
Iodine	It is in the form of grayish-black, brittle plate-shaped crystals with a metallic luster. Its tincture contains 2% iodine and 2% potassium iodide in alcoholic solution.
	It is used for disinfection of skin and treatment of wounds.
	Its 0.5 to 1% aqueous solution is used for application to wounds, 0.1% solution for irrigation, and 2% solution in glycerin for application to mucous membranes.

Iodoform	It is a mixture of iodine, alcohol and potash. It has a penetrating, rather pleasant smell. It is a mild antiseptic. It relieves pain when applied to a raw mucous surface and prevents putrefaction in wounds discharging pus.
Merbromin (Mercurochrome)	It is an organic salt of mercury with weak antiseptic action. It is more bacteriostatic and less irritating and less toxic than inorganic salts of mercury. It is used as antiseptic over dressing.
Nitrofurazone	It is used as topical antibacterial agent in the treatment of mixed infections of skin wounds.
Povidone iodine	It is a complex of iodine with polyvinylpyrolidine and is available as 5 and 10% solutions for antiseptic use. It is less painful than tincture of iodine when applied to wounds.
Silver nitrate	It is in the form of colourless crystals freely soluble in water. It is caustic, antiseptic, and astringent. Its sticks are used for chemical cauterization of granulation tissue. Its 1:1000 solution is used for irrigation of bladder. Its 10% solution is used for application to infected oral ulcers.
Sulfur ointment	It contains 10% precipitated sulfur. It is fungicide and parasiticide. It is used for various skin disorders.

❒ STERILIZATION

It is the process of destroying all microorganisms. In first aid gauze, cotton wool, syringes, needles, and instruments have to be sterilized before use, so as to prevent wound infection. Various methods of sterilization for different articles are as shown in the following table.

Article	Method
Syringes	Boil for 15 minutes. Autoclaving.
Gauze and cotton	Autoclaving.
Metallic instruments	Boil for 15 minutes. Autoclaving.

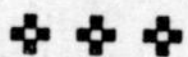

CHAPTER

17

"Deadly" Asphyxia (Suffocation)

It is deficiency of oxygen and increase in carbon dioxide in the blood and tissues. It occurs due to a failure of exchange of oxygen and carbon dioxide between the air and pulmonary capillaries.

❒ CAUSES OF ASPHYXIA

Airway obstruction due to

- Foreign body in the airway causing choking.
- Spasm of respiratory muscles as in tetanus.
- Drowning.
- Suffocation under bed.
- Suffocation due to a plastic bag over the head.
- Strangulation, hanging or throttling.
- Bronchospasm, e.g. bronchial asthma.
- Electric shock.

Lack of oxygen in the air inspired due to

- High altitudes with low atmospheric pressure.
- *Fire* : inhalation of smoke.
- *Gas leaks* : inhalation of gas (Coal gas, automobile exhaust fumes etc.)

❒ EFFECTS OF ASPHYXIA

1. First stage

- Respiratory rate increases.
- Breaths become shorter and noisy.

- Chest movements of breathing are reversed. The chest wall gets sucked in instead of moving out when the victim breathes in.
- The nostrils flare during breathing.
- Neck veins get distended.
- Cyanosis develops. The face, lips, nails, fingers, and toes turn blue.
- Pulse becomes faster and feeble.

2. Second stage

- Consciousness is lost.
- Frothing occurs at the mouth and nose.
- Convulsions may occur.
- Urine and feces are passed involuntarily.
- Death may occur if not treated in time.

First-aid

1. Remove the cause, if possible.
2. Place the victim on his back.
3. Clear the airway and provide warmth.
4. Loosen his collar.
5. Put a finger in the mouth and throat and remove a foreign body if present.
6. Remove denture, if present.
7. Hold the angle of the jaw forward and tilt the head backwards. This opens the airway.
8. Give artificial ventilation and external cardiac massage, if required.
9. Send him to a hospital after he settles down.

❐ DROWNING

A person who does not know how to swim can drown accidentally if he falls into water. It may also be homicidal. Persons who know how to swim may drown too, if under the influence of alcohol, or if there is head injury at the time of the fall and the person becomes unconscious. Water enters the airway so that asphyxia develops. A little amount of water enters the lungs too, and damages them.

Rescuing a drowning person

1. Do not swim out to rescue him unless you have been trained as a lifeguard.
2. If the water is not too deep, wade through it to get him out of it. Do not wade out if the nature of the bottom of the water is not known, because you may fall into a hole or a bed of quicksand.
3. If the victim is near the shoreline, extend a long stick or pole towards him. Pull him in when he grabs it.
4. If he cannot be reached by a stick, throw him a lifebuoy or a plank that he can float on. Tell him to keep his face above water.
5. Use a boat to reach the victim, if one is available easily. Tell him to climb in when you reach him. If he cannot do that ask him to hold onto the boat while you row him back to land.

First-aid

1. Put the victim on the ground, face down.
2. Clear the airway of any foreign body.
3. Elevate the middle part of his body with your hands under him to make any water in the lungs to drain out.
4. Do not try to force the water out from the stomach.
5. Give artificial ventilation until normal breathing is restored.
6. Remove wet clothes and put on dry clothes. Keep him warm with blankets and hot water bags.
7. Do not allow him to sit up.
8. Give him hot tea or coffee to drink.
9. Send him to a hospital as soon as possible.

❐ STRANGULTION

It includes hanging, strangling, and throttling. External pressure is exerted on the neck, which causes obstruction of the airway and cuts off flow of air to the lungs. Hanging and strangling may be accidental or homicidal. Throttling is homicidal.

❐ STRANGULATION

Type	Features
Hanging	Suspension of the body by a noose around the neck.
Strangling	Constriction around the neck.
Throttling	Squeezing the throat.

The condition is diagnosed by the following features.

1. The constricting article may be present around the victim's neck.
2. If it has been removed, its marks are found on the neck.
3. There are features of asphyxia.

Tiny red spots may be seen on the face or the whites of the eyes.

First aid

1. Remove any constriction present around the victim's neck. Support the body if you are cutting a noose around his neck while he is still hanging.
2. Place him flat on the ground, face up.
3. If he is not breathing, give artificial respiration.
4. Shift him to hospital soon and inform police.

CHAPTER

18

Medical Disorders are Troublesome

❒ INFLUENZA

It is a common virus infection characterized by running nose, cough, sore throat and sometimes fever or pain in the joints. There are constitutional symptoms like malaise and body ache. It reduces body resistance to other infections, so that serious disorders like ear infections, sinusitis, and pneumonia may develop.

First aid

1. Give enough rest.
2. Advise steam inhalation.
3. Avoid sour and cold foods and beverages.
4. Give plenty of water orally.
5. It usually gets cured without medicine. Paracetamol may be used if the fever is high.

Prevention

1. Avoid contact with a patient of influenza because it spreads by droplet infection.
2. Adequate sleep and nutritious diet containing tomatoes, oranges, other fruits, and vitamin C build up body resistance and prevent colds.
3. Avoid breeze over wet body and hair. Do not wear wet clothes.
4. After washing the hair, dry it well thoroughly.

❐ FEVER

Fever is elevation of the body temperature above 37°C. The temperature measured in the mouth and rectum is generally at least half a degree higher than that of the axilla.

Types of Fever

Continuous Fever. The temperature does not fluctuate by more than 1°C in 24 hours, and always above 37°C.

Remittent Fever. The temperature fluctuates by more than 2°C in 24 hours.

Intermittent Fever. Fever does not last for all of the 24 hours of the day.

Fever is not a disease itself, but just a symptom of a large number of illnesses. The commonest cause is infection. Acute pyogenic infections cause high fever with chills. Chronic infections like tuberculosis cause low grade fever, often without chills. The condition is diagnosed by the following features.

1. There may be prodromal symptoms like malaise and bodyache.
2. The patient feels chills and rigors.
3. The body becomes warm.
4. The face is flushed.
5. The pulse becomes rapid.
6. The patient may get delirious when the fever is very high.
7. Children below the age of 3 years may get convulsions when the fever is very high.
8. Appetite is lost.
9. The tongue becomes coated and furry.
10. Sweating is absent. Urine output increases.

First aid

1. Give complete bed rest.
2. Give plenty of oral fluids. Add a little sugar or jaggery to it to supply calories.

3. Do tepid sponging in high fever. Cold compresses or ice bag may be applied to the forehead and abdomen.
4. Give aspirin or paracetamol to lower the fever.
5. Shift him to a hospital immediately if he does not respond to these measures or if complications develop like convulsions in a child or delirium.

❐ HEADACHE

Headache is pain anywhere in the head. It may be constant, throbbing, or intermittent. It is a symptom of a disease and not a disease by itself. Various causes of headache are as follows.

1. Refractive errors.
2. Exhaustion.
3. Lack of sleep.
4. Anxiety.
5. Dental caries.
6. Sinusitis.
7. Constipation.
8. Common cold.
9. Hypertension.
10. Migraine.
11. Brain tumors.

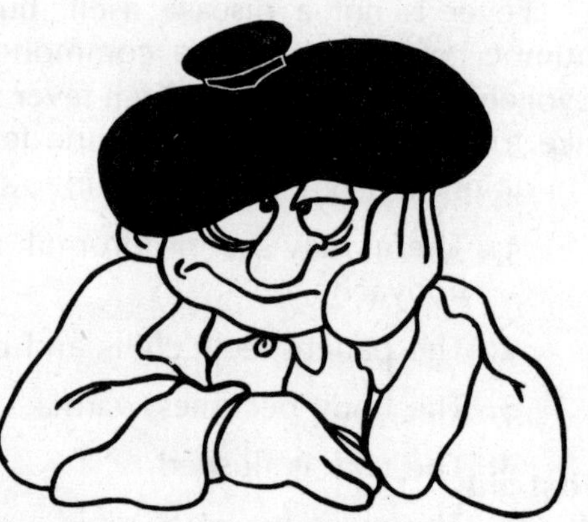

First-aid

1. Place the patient in a dark, quiet pace. Make him relax and not think about his problems.
2. Give aspirin or paracetamol orally.
3. Shift him to a doctor if these simple measures fail to relieve the headache or if it recurs.

❐ MIGRAINE

It is a disease in which there is unilateral headache. It may be precipitated by emotional disturbances or bright light. In many cases no cause can be found. The condition is diagnosed by the following features.

1. There is intense unilateral headache.
2. Flickering vision may precede the headache.
3. Nausea and vomiting are present.
4. There is intolerance to light or noise.

First-aid

1. Give aspirin or paracetamol orally to relieve the pain.
2. Send him to a doctor for evaluation and treatment.

❐ EARACHE

Earache is occurrence of pain in the ear. If may be due to any of the following conditions.

1. Dental caries.
2. Tooth abscess.
3. Middle ear infection.
4. Boil in the ear.
5. Wax in the ear.
6. Foreign body in the ear.
7. Under water swimming.
8. Air travel.

First-aid

1. Give aspirin or paracetamol orally to relieve the pain.
2. Send him to a doctor for check-up and treatment.

❐ BACKACHE

Backache is pain anywhere in the back. It may be in the upper back or lower back and may be constant or intermittent. It is a symptom of a disease and not a disease by itself. Various causes of backache are as follows.

1. Bad posture : standing or sitting in a bad posture, with the shoulders drooped.
2. Sprain of the joints of the back.
3. Prolapsed intervertebral disc.

4. Menstruation in women : low backache.
5. Pelvic tumors : low backache.
6. Kidney disease : pain in the middle of the back.

First-aid

1. Give aspirin or paracetamol orally. Local hot fomentation may be done.
2. Advise good posture when standing and sitting.
3. Advise him to sleep on a firm flat surface.
4. Send him to a doctor.

❐ TOOTHACHE

It is usually due to dental neglect resulting in dental caries. When the tooth decay reaches the canal in the root of the tooth, nerve endings get irritated and cause pain. An abscess may form around the apex of the root and cause further pain. The tooth may also hurt when its outer coating is worn off and hypersensitive inner part is exposed. In such cases contact with cold or very sweet substances produces pain.

First-aid

1. Give aspirin or paracetamol orally.
2. Insert a little cotton ball soaked with clove oil into the cavity of the tooth.
3. Send him to a dentist.

Prevention

1. Eat less food stuffs that are very sweet and sticky.
2. Brush teeth properly after every feed.
3. Have periodic dental check up.

❐ PAIN IN ABDOMEN

Abdominal pain is a symptom and not a disease by itself. It can be caused by a large number of causes like peptic ulcer, gastritis, gastroenteritis, appendicitis, indigestion, flatulence, intestinal obstruction, intestinal perforation and peritonitis.

First-aid

1. Place the patient in half sitting position with the head and shoulders well-supported and the lower limbs drawn up a little.
2. Apply hot water bottle or bag to the abdomen in the painful area.
3. Withhold all food.
4. Do not give a laxative.
5. Shift him to a hospital immediately.

❒ VOMITING

Vomiting is a symptom and not a disease by itself. It can be caused by a large number of causes like gastritis, indigestion, gastric ulcer, gastroenteritis, cancer of the stomach upset, peritonitis, and intestinal obstruction. It may be mild stomach upset and get cured by itself. However the serious disorders listed above require medical treatment.

First-aid

1. If it is a mild stomach upset, give the patient an antacid and an antiemetic tablet.
2. Shift him to a hospital immediately if he has severe disease, if the vomiting is persistent and progressively increasing in severity, if he vomits out blood, or if the vomit smells like feces.

❒ DIARRHOEA

It is passage of watery loose motions and can be mild or severe. It can be acute on onset and short duration, or chronic, lasting for many days. It is more common and more dangerous in young children, especially those who are malnourished. Infection due to consumption of contaminated food is the commonest cause. Indigestion, malabsorption, liver disorders, and misuse of drugs like ampicillin are other causes.

First-aid

1. Give oral rehydration therapy, which consists of water mixed with salts (1 liter of boiled water plus 2 tablespoons of

sugar or honey and 1/4 teaspoon salt and 1/4 teaspoon of sodium bicarbonate). It reestablishes the hydration and electrolyte content of the body.

2. Shift him to a hospital immediately if the diarrhoea is severe or there are signs of acute dehydration.
3. Breast feeding should be continued in children.

Prevention

1. Wash hands well before eating.
2. Use sanitary latrines especially in slums and rural areas.
3. Wash hands well with soap and water after defecation.
4. Do not eat exposed food or food purchased from unhygienic food handlers.
5. Control fly infestation.

❒ DYSENTERY

It is characterized by passage of motions with blood and mucus and can be mild or severe. It can be acute onset and short duration, or chronic, lasting for many days. It is caused by infection with ameba or bacilli. It may be due to conditions like chronic ulcerative colitis and also due to consumption of contaminated food.

First-aid

1. Give oral rehydration therapy, which consists of water mixed with salts (1 liter of boiled water plus 2 tablespoons of sugar or honey and 1/4 teaspoon salt and 1/4 teaspoon of sodium bicarbonate). It reestablishes the hydration and electrolyte content of the body.
2. Send him to a doctor for specific therapy.
3. Breast feeding should be continued in children.

Prevention

1. Wash hands well before eating.
2. Use sanitary latrines.
3. Do not eat exposed food or food purchased from unhygienic food handlers.
4. Control fly infestation.

❒ ASTHMA

It is an allergic condition characterized by attacks of difficult breathing and often begins in childhood and may last throughout life. It tends to occur in families. It tends to be worse at night and during winter. An acute attack may be caused by eating or breathing things to which the person is allergic. There is a spasm of the windpipe and its branches, so that breathing becomes difficult. The condition is diagnosed by the following features.

1. The patient is breathless.
2. A wheezing sound is heard during his breathing.
3. He cannot get enough air. So his nails and lips may turn blue.
4. The neck veins may be distended.

First-aid

1. Reassure the patient. Never panic and keep calm.
2. Ask him to take his usual medication, which may be in the form of an inhalation spray or tablets.
3. Make him sit at a place that is warm and airy. Loosen any tight clothing.
4. Steam inhalation may also help.
5. Shift him to a hospital immediately if there is no response to the treatment given.

Most asthmatic children have allergies which bring on the attacks, but emotional upsets, temperature changes, pollution, exercise and infection can also bring on attacks. By far the commonest allergy is to domestic house dust — specifically to the house dust mite. Children may also be allergic to grass pollen, pets, feathers in pillows, mould, foods and many other things. The rising pollution levels in metro cities are contributing in a big way to a dangerous increase in Asthmatic patients.

Prevention is the best cure. Avoidance of any known allergic substances is the most obvious starting point, but this can be difficult in practice. Drugs help greatly to prevent attacks and some children can be adequately protected against certain allergies by having a course of desensitising injections. A happy and relaxed family

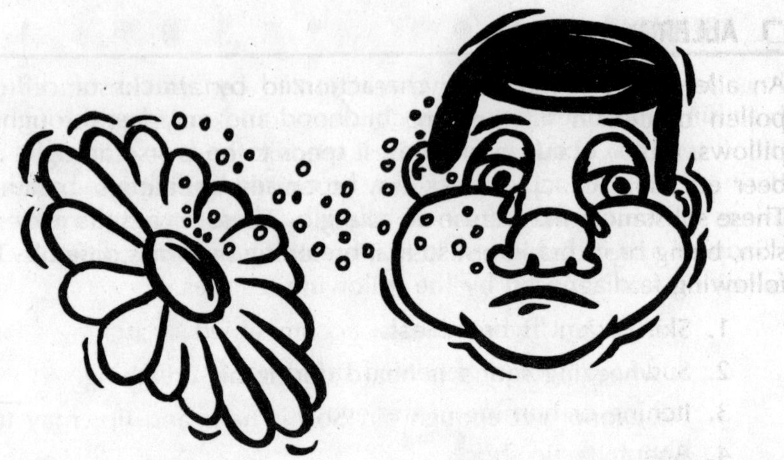

atmosphere and parents who understand the disease make a real difference to the number of attacks a child has.

Most parents get to know when their child is about to have an attack because he becomes pale and lethargic, coughs and has a running nose. If you have any prescribed drugs, use them at this stage and you may abort an attack.

There are four positions in which your child might be more comfortable — see which suits him best during an attack. (1) Lying on one side, slightly rolled forward with the knees bent. The top leg should be in front of the one underneath; (2) lying on one side as in (1), but on a slope of three or four pillows with an extra pillow filling in the gap between waist and armpit; (3) sitting or kneeling forward against a chair, with the upper chest supported by pillows and the back straight; or (4) sitting, leaning forward with a straight back, arms resting on thighs.

Get your child into one of these positions and get him to do diaphragmatic breathing (breathing from waist level rather than from the chest). He will need to be taught this by his doctor or physiotherapist. It is worth practising the breathing with your child everyday so that when he has an attack it may seem natural to him to breathe this way.

Should your child not respond to these simple measures, call your doctor. Do not let the situation get worse because it will then be much more difficult to treat. A very bad attack may mean the child will have to go into hospital.

❐ ALLERGY

An allergy is a hypersensitive reaction to certain substances like pollen of certain flowers and grasses, chicken feathers, feather pillows, moldy blankets or clothes, specific foods — fish, shell fish beer etc., and certain medicines, especially antibiotics or serum. These substances may cause an attack by contact with the patient's skin, being breathed in or eaten. The condition is diagnosed by the following features.

1. Skin rash : hives, wheals, accompanied by itching.
2. Sudden attack of repeated sneezing.
3. Itching or burning of the eyes.
4. Anaphylactic shock.

First-aid

1. Stop the use of the specific substance responsible for the allergy immediately.
2. Apply cold compresses for severe skin itching and burning.
3. Send him to a doctor immediately.

Prevention

1. Avoid contact with substances that precipitate an attack.
2. Send him to a doctor for desensitization therapy.

❐ HICCUPS

Hiccups occur due to spasms of the diaphragm, which divides the abdomen from the chest. They are commonly due to eating or drinking too much or drinking carbonated beverages in large quantities. They can also be due to diseases that irritate the phrenic nerve that supplies the diaphragm. There are so many hiccup remedies. They all work when the hiccups are ready to stop anyhow. Hiccuping lasting for days is exhausting.

First-aid

1. Make the patient lie down and rest.
2. Ask him to drink some water slowly.
3. Ask him to breath in and out of a paper bag fitting tightly over the face.

4. Give half a teaspoonful of sodium carbonate in water for drinking.

❒ CONSTIPATION

Failure to pass stools for 2 or more days is called constipation. It is often due to a diet poor in fiber, e.g. fruits and green vegetables. It may be caused by pregnancy, use of drugs like iron, and tumors of the large intestine.

First-aid

1. Give diet rich in fiber.
2. Give plenty of fluids orally.
3. Give a laxative like isapgol or liquid paraffin at bed time. A glycerin suppository or an enema of soap or liver oil may also be used.
4. Send him to a doctor if these measures fail.

❒ INDIGESTION

It is a condition characterized by a sensation of fullness of the stomach along with belching and upper abdominal pain or discomfort (heartburn). It may be caused by any of the following.

1. Ingestion of lot of food which makes it too difficult to digest.
2. Drinking too much alcohol.
3. Tension and anxiety.

First-aid

1. Place the patient comfortably in bed.
2. Give him some milk to drink.
3. Give him an antacid.
4. Send him to a doctor if these measures fail.

❒ OBSTRUCTED HERNIA

A hernia is an abnormal protrusion of an abdominal organ or a part of an organ through an abnormal opening in the abdominal wall. Various types of hernias are inguinal hernia, umbilical hernia, femoral hernia etc. A baby may be born with a hernia. An elderly person develops an inguinal hernia due to enlargement of his prostate, which makes him strain for passing urine. A hernia may develop in the scar of an abdominal incision too, due to poor healing of the wound. Usually the opening is big enough so that the contents of the hernia can be reduced back into the abdominal cavity. Sometimes this cannot be done. Such a hernia is said to be obstructed. The condition is diagnosed by the following features.

1. There is a history of a reducible lump on the abdominal wall.
2. There is an inability to reduce the lump over the last few days.
3. There may be constipation and vomiting due to intestinal obstruction.
4. There may be severe pain locally due to strangulation of the hernia.

First-aid

1. Do not try to reduce the contents of the hernia back into the abdominal cavity.
2. Do not give him anything orally.
3. Shift him to a hospital immediately.

❐ PILES (HEMORRHOIDS)

These are varicose veins of the rectum. They may be caused by constipation. They feel like little lumps or balls when they prolapse out of the anus during defecation or permanently. They cause bleeding per rectum when passing stools. They are painful when they get thrombosed. When a hemorrhoid begins to bleed, the person develops anemia due to chronic blood loss.

First-aid

1. Give diet rich in fiber.
2. Give plenty of fluids orally.
3. Give a laxative like isapgol or liquid paraffin at bed time. A glycerine suppository or an enema of soap or liver oil may also be used.

4. Give Sitz bath to get relief from pain. Make him sit in a tub filled with warm water to which some potassium permanganate has been added.
5. Send him to a doctor immediately.

❐ RETENTION OF URINE

It is an inability to pass urine collected in the urinary bladder and may be caused by any of the following conditions.

1. Enlargement of prostate in an elderly male.
2. Trauma to the urethra of a male, e.g. after fall astride a hard object.
3. Lying down in bed.
4. Pelvic tumors pressing on the urethra.

First-aid

1. Apply hot water bags over lower part of abdomen.
2. Make him hear sound of running water.
3. Pour some cold water on his penis.
4. Make him sit in a hot water tub.
5. Shift him to a hospital immediately if these measures fail.

❐ MOTION SICKNESS

Motion sickness is an illness characterized by nausea and vomiting due to hypersensitivity to movement. It is due to a disturbance in the equilibrium center. It occurs during travel by ship, plane, bus, car, or train.

First-aid

1. Ask him to avoid eating or drinking too much before or during the journey.
2. Give him an antiemetic before starting the journey.

❐ INSOMNIA

It is a condition characterized by an inability to sleep and may be caused by mental tensions, bad food habits, and excessive tiredness.

First aid

1. Ask him to take adequate exercise during the day.
2. Give a glass of warm milk before going to bed.
3. Ask him to take a warm bath before going to bed.
4. A sleeping pill may be given if prescribed by a doctor.

❐ GLARE IN EYES

It is produced by seeing welding with naked eyes, looking at the sun directly, and looking at reflected light from polished surfaces or ice. The condition is diagnosed by the following features.

1. There is an inability to open eyes in bright light (photophobia).
2. There is pain in the eyes.
3. The eyes are swollen and red.

First aid

1. Give rest to the eyes.
2. Apply cold compresses to the closed eyes.

Prevention

1. Use sunglasses while going out in the sun.
2. Do not look at the sun.
3. Do not look at welding light. Use welding screens to protect your eyes while welding.

❐ PSYCHIATRIC EMERGENCIES

A number of acute psychiatric emergencies may present to the first aider. Agitation, confusion and depression can result from stress.

First aid

1. Approach such a person in a calm, reassuring, and non-threatening manner.
2. Speak softly. Use short and simple sentences when speaking to him.
3. Do not force him to talk about something, if he doesn't want to.

4. Reassure him.
5. Take him to a quiet room to decrease his sensory stimulation.
6. Turn on soothing music if possible.
7. Provide a safe environment, as he may accidentally hurt himself.
8. Do not say something bad about him to anyone else in his presence, as he can still hear and understand what you say about him.
9. Do not allow his family members to answer questions you ask him.
10. Do not be over friendly.
11. Establish a rapport with him and win his confidence.

❐ SUICIDAL PATIENT

Suicidal tendencies may be due to recent loss of a loved one, status, or body integrity, failure in examination, love, or loss of money, employment. They are also seen in certain psychiatric illnesses.

First-aid

1. Reassure the victim.
2. Make him understand the importance of life.
3. Prevent self injury by close observation.
4. Send him to a hospital immediately for expert psychiatric care.

❐ RAPE

It is defined as sexual intercourse with a female by force or under the threat of a force. The victim suffers from the following.

Manifestation	Features
Physical injury	Genital injury, local bleeding, wounds elsewhere on the body inflicted during attempts at resistance, fractures, dislocations.
Phase of disorganization	Fear, anger, humiliation, guilt, self blame.
Phase of resolution	Sleep disturbances, phobias, sexual fear.

First-aid

1. Reduce the emotional trauma of the victim.
2. Reassure her that anxiety is natural and appropriate support will be given to her.
3. Do not leave her alone.
4. Give first aid for injuries.
5. Do not change her clothes or allow her to wash her private parts, as these need to kept undisturbed for examination by a doctor.
6. Send him to a hospital immediately.
7. Inform police.

❐ ALCOHOLIC HALLUCINATIONS

It is an acute toxic state that follows a prolonged heavy drinking. Hallucinations are perceptions of sensations that do not exist. The conditions is diagnosed by the following features.

1. There is anxiety.
2. Irritability is seen.
3. Agitation and insomnia are present.
4. Visual, tactile and auditory hallucinations are present.

First-aid

1. Give the patient adequate sedation and support.
2. Keep him in a place with minimum disturbances.

❐ UNCONSCIOUSNESS

Any disturbance with the normal functioning of the brain and the nerves can bring about unconsciousness. It may be not only due to some disease or injury to the brain, but also of other organs in the body. Various types of unconsciousness are shown in the following table.

Type	Features
Stupor	It is a state of semiconsciousness in which person responds only to external stimuli or loud noise. Pupils of the eyes contract in response to light.
Fainting	It is the temporary loss of consciousness. The person recovers spontaneously.
Somnolence	It is a state when person feels sleepy or drowsy.
Coma	It is a state of complete loss of consciousness. The person does not respond to even painful stimuli. Eye movements are absent. The pupils do not respond to light. It can last for many years even.

Causes of unconsciousness

1. Acute fever
2. Alcohol consumption
3. Brain injuries
4. Convulsions
5. Diabetes or overdose of insulin
6. Epilepsy
7. Fainting
8. Heat stroke or exhaustion
9. Hysteria
10. Metabolic disturbances
11. Severe loss of body fluids.

First-aid

1. Do not try to arouse an unconscious person. Let him lie quietly.
2. Do not pour water on him.
3. Do not move him unnecessarily.
4. Let him have fresh air.
5. Loosen clothes around his neck, chest and waist.

6. Do not give him anything orally.
7. Resuscitate him if he has cardiorespiratory arrest.
8. Keep him in recovery position.
9. Apply specific treatment for the cause of unconsciousness.
10. Send him to a hospital immediately.

❐ FAINTING

It occurs most frequently in healthy young people, especially during very hot weather and mostly occurs on prolonged standing as in heavy crowd or on a parade ground. People who are tired, hungry, fearful or emotionally upset faint more readily. Also induced by an emotional shock or on sight of a horrible scene. The condition is diagnosed by the following features.

1. The person who is about to faint feels giddy and looks pale.
2. Then he collapses.
3. His pulse is weak and slow.
4. The skin becomes cold and clammy.

First-aid

1. Place him flat on the ground and raise his legs to improve the blood flow to his brain.
2. Loosen tight clothes around his neck.
3. Consciousness returns in one to two minutes.
4. Give him a cup of tea or coffee after he recovers consciousness.
5. If he does not recover very soon, send him to a doctor or hospital immediately.

Prevention

If a person feels faint, make him bend forward at his waist, bringing the head down between the knees. Alternatively he may lie down.

❐ CONVULSION

It is a condition characterized by repetitive contraction and relaxation of a group of muscles in the body and is caused by disturbance in the function of the brain. Convulsions are usually followed by loss of consciousness. Various causes of convulsions are as follows.

1. Disease of the brain.
2. Epilepsy.
3. Head injury.
4. High fever (in children below the age of 3 years).
5. Inadequate supply of oxygen to the brain.
6. Low blood sugar.

The condition is diagnosed by the following features.

1. There is a cry.
2. Then there is stiffness of the body (tonic part of a convulsion), the body becomes cyanotic in that phase.
3. It is followed by repetitive convulsive movements (clonic part of a convulsion). The cyanosis passes away. There is frothing at the angle of the mouth.
4. That is followed by the postictal phase in which the person may become unconscious. He recovers from it after a variable interval. He may lose all memory of this event.

First-aid

1. Keep the patient lying down, making no attempt to stop his fit.
2. Make enough space around him.
3. Place a spoon wrapped in a handkerchief or a folded cloth between his teeth to prevent him from biting his own tongue.
4. Send him to a doctor or hospital immediately after the convulsion.

❒ FEBRILE CONVULSIONS IN YOUNG CHILDREN

These develop in children below the age of 3 years. The child has high fever due to some cause. The convulsion is as described before.

First-aid

1. Give first aid as for convulsions in an adult.
2. Give tepid sponging.

3. Place him under a fan for cooling his body.
4. Position pillows or soft padding around the child so that even violent movements will not result in injury.
5. Keep the airway open.
6. Send him to a doctor or hospital immediately.

❒ HYSTERIA

It is a psychiatric disorder in which there is attention seeking and is usually found in women. There are manifestations of different diseases when there is actually no organic disease present. It is due to conversion of her anxiety into physical symptoms. They range from something as minor as giddiness to something as serious as blindness or paralysis. However the symptoms are bizarre and do not fit in any particular disorder.

First-aid

1. Do not pay extra attention to her, because that aggravates her symptoms.
2. Be firm but kind in dealing with her.
3. Try to find out the family environment and personal background so the basic problem can be dealt with.
4. Send her to a psychiatrist for treatment.

❒ STROKE (APOPLEXY)

It is a condition characterized by decreased blood supply to the brain due to formation of a blood clot in its arteries, lodging of an embolus in its artery, or rupture of its artery and hemorrhage from it. It usually occurs in elderly persons, especially if they suffer from high blood pressure. The manifestations of a stroke depend on the site and severity of involvement of the brain. The condition is diagnosed by the following features.

1. There is a sudden and severe headache.
2. The person may become unconscious.
3. There is usually paralysis of right or left half of the body.
4. Bladder and/or bowel control may be lost.
5. Speech may be lost.

First aid

1. If he is unconscious, treat him as described before.
2. If there is cardiorespiratory arrest, resuscitate him.
3. Send him to a doctor or hospital immediately.

❒ HYPOGLYCEMIA

This is characterized by a drop in blood sugar level below normal and occurs in a person suffering from diabetes mellitus, who takes his medication but does not eat as required. The condition is diagnosed by the following features.

1. The person behaves abnormally.
2. There is excessive sweating, weakness, faintness, and tremors.
3. He may become unconscious.

First aid

1. If the patient is conscious, give him glucose in water orally. If that is not available, give him anything sweet orally.
2. If he is unconscious, keep him in recovery position and give him 20 ml of 25% glucose solution intravenously.
3. Send him to a doctor or hospital immediately.
4. Don't panic.

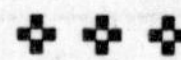

CHAPTER

19

Understanding Emergency Childbirth

In the cities, most babies are born in hospitals or other institutions where professional help from trained nurses and doctors is available. Even in villages, deliveries are conducted in primary health centers by professionals. However sometimes the women cannot get to a hospital and childbirth may take place at home, or on her way to the hospital in a bus, train, taxi, ambulance, or even unplanned on a plane or ship. The first-aider should be able to conduct this delivery properly so that at the end of it there is a healthy mother and a healthy baby. A first-aider may have to give help when a miscarriage occurs.

❐ MISCARRIAGE

It occurs before 28th week of pregnancy, when the woman really does not except to deliver and hence is not ready for it. Then she is even less likely to be in a hospital than at term. She may be distressed and frightened and may be reluctant to confide in a stranger, particularly if that person is a man. Miscarriage is a dangerous event and needs prompt medical attention. It is often accompanied by vaginal bleeding which can be quite severe and sometimes life threatening. Features of a miscarriage are as follows.

1. Pain in lower abdomen and back.
2. Mucoid vaginal discharge.
3. Vaginal bleeding.
4. Loss of fluid vaginally.

First-aid

1. Reassure her.
2. Place her in a reclining position.
3. Give her privacy.
4. Monitor her vital parameters.
5. Keep any expelled material for showing to the doctor.
6. Treat shock.
7. Shift her to a hospital immediately.

❒ CHILDBIRTH

Childbirth is a natural process and one does not have to do too much to see it to completion. But done improperly, there can be serious complications. Majority of births do not threaten the lives of both the mother and the baby. Labor usually lasts several hours, and there is normally adequate time to arrange for a transfer to a hospital. However sometimes a mother presents too late, or is trapped in a place due to natural disasters and cannot reach a hospital. Such a mother may be very anxious when she starts delivering in a place that is not the most ideal place for that purpose.

The stages of childbirth

Stage	Features
First	It extends from the onset of labor to the full dilatation of the birth passage. It lasts for 12 to 14 hours. The woman experiences periodic pains in the lower abdomen and back. There is mucoid vaginal discharge, often mixed with a variable amount of blood. The membranes rupture towards the end of this stage and there is expulsion of a lot of aminotic fluid vaginally.
Second	It extends from full dilatation of the birth passage to the expulsion of the baby. It lasts for up to 2 hours.
Third	It extends from the delivery of the baby to the delivery of the placenta and membranes. It lasts for 30 minutes.
Fourth	It is the 1-hour period after the third stage.

❐ ARTICLES TO KEEP READY FOR A CHILDBIRTH

Minimum requirements

1. A lot of very clean clothes.
2. Alcohol.
3. An antiseptic soap.
4. Clean brush for scrubbing.
5. Clean cotton.
6. New razor blade to cut the umbilical cord.
7. Sterile gauze.
8. Two pieces of sterile, strong thread to tie the umbilical cord.

Additional desirable requirements

1. Antiseptic eye drops for the baby's eyes.
2. Fetoscope or fetal stethoscope for listening to the new born baby's feeble heart sounds.
3. Sterile needle and gut thread for sewing tears in the birth opening.
4. Sterile syringe and needles.
5. Suction bulb for sucking mucus out of the baby's nose and mouth.
6. Two bowls — one for washing hands and the other for catching and examining.
7. Two clamps (hemostats) for clamping the umbilical cord.

❐ INFECTION PREVENTION

When preparing for, and during the delivery it is extremely important to pay strict attention to asepsis and antisepsis because the placental bed is raw and there are a number of areas of injury in the birth passage. These can get infected very readily if microorganisms are allowed to enter it. Measures to prevent infection of the birth passage are as follows.

1. Ask everyone with a cold, cough, or septic spots on the hands to move away from the would-be mother.

2. Wear a face mask. if it is not available, tie a clean handkerchief in its place.
3. Scrub your hands and forearms thoroughly with soap and water for about five minutes.
4. After the delivery, wash your hands thoroughly again.

❒ HOW TO DELIVER A BABY ?

1. Place the woman in left lateral position until the baby starts delivering. Then she can be allowed to roll on to her back and draw her legs up for bearing down.
2. Keep her covered with blankets until the baby starts delivering.
3. Put a clean cloth under her buttock.
4. Place a clean pad over the anus.
5. Moister her lips with water if she feels thirsty.
6. Ask her to push as when passing stools, whenever she gets pains.
7. Tell the mother to stop pushing and pant between pains. When the anus bulges and the baby's head becomes visible, support it from the front as it emerges.
8. When the widest part of the head is through, make pressure with the pad on the anus in the forward direction to deliver the head. Check that there is no membrane covering the baby's face. If present, remove them.
9. Check that the umbilical cord is not around the baby's neck. If it is, slip it off over the baby's head.
10. Deliver the rest of the baby by holding its head.
11. Suck out fluid in the baby's mouth and nose with a rubber bulb.
12. Dry the baby's head and trunk. It is does not cry immediately, stimulate its feet by tapping on them gently.
13. Wrap the baby in a dry towel.
14. Clamp the umbilical cord at two places when its pulsations stop.

15. Cut it between the two clamps with a new razor blade or scissors that have been kept in boiling water for at least 10 minutes.
16. Do not pull on or cut the umbilical cord. When the placenta separates, the cord appears to lengthen and there is some bleeding vaginally. Then pull on the cord and deliver the placenta attached to the other end of the cord.
17. Examine the placenta and membranes to see if any portion of them is left behind. If it is, it needs to be removed or severe hemorrhage may take place.
18. Clean the external genitals of the mother with a hot sponge or a clean cloth. Put one or two cotton pads there.
19. Give her hot tea, coffee or milk.

❒ BLEEDING CONTROL

There is always a little loss of blood when the placenta comes out. If it is more, it must be stopped. Put your hand on her abdomen and massage the uterus that lies below the level of the umbilicus. Shift her to a hospital immediately.

❒ CARE OF THE NEW-BORN

1. Hold the baby's head down so that mucus comes out of his mouth.
2. Keep the baby between the mother's legs, below the level of the uterus until the cord is tied.
3. If the baby does not begin to breathe right away, rub his back or tickle its soles.
4. Perform suction of the baby's mouth and then of its nose using mucus catheter or rubber bulb with a narrow pointed end.
5. Dry the baby's head first and then the rest of its body.
6. Wrap the baby in a clean towel. Then warp it in a blanket to keep it warm.

7. Put the baby to the mother's breast as soon as the mother's condition allows.
8. Put one drop of soframycin or gentamicin eye drops in each eye.
9. Tie the cord with two pieces of strong, clean thread. A cord clip may be applied instead, if available. Apply spirit to the cut end of the cord.

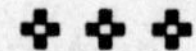

CHAPTER

20

Ensuring Safe and Quick Transportation

❐ GENERAL PRINCIPLES OF TRANSPORTATION ?

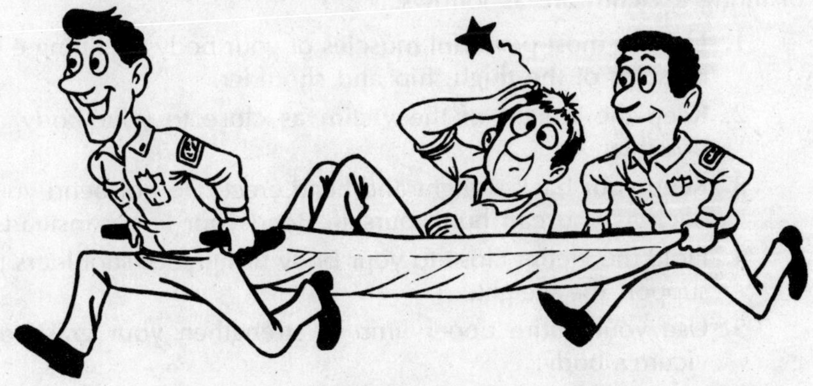

1. The objective of transportation is to enable the victim to reach the destination without deterioration of his condition.
2. Do not move a severely injured or ill person unless there is immediate danger to his life or skilled help is not available. That is because moving a casualty may result in aggravation of his or her injury or condition.
3. Do not presume that a victim can sit or stand without support.
4. If it is possible to wait, it is better to leave the victim undisturbed and send for help. If there is risk of exposure, the victim may be moved to a sheltered place while you wait for help to arrive. If the victim is to be shifted to a hospital, arrange for an ambulance or a suitable vehicle.

5. If there is a risk to your life at the site of the mishap, move the casualty as quickly as, possible without endangering you life.
6. The method of transportation depends on the nature and severity of injury, the distance to be covered, the facilities available, the condition of the road of transportation, and the victim's build.
7. Confirm that everyone involved understands the steps involved in transportation.

❒ HOW TO LIFT A VICTIM ?

If a proper method of lifting is used, even a critical victim can be lifted without undue strain for the first aider. The basic principles of lifting a victim are as follows.

1. Use the most powerful muscles of your body for lifting e.g. muscles of the thigh, hip and shoulder.
2. Keep the weight of the victim as close to your body as possible.
3. Keep your back straight and head erect. Do not bend your back as you can hurt yourself. Bend your knees instead.
4. Hold the victim close to your body using your shoulders to support the weight.
5. Use your entire upper limb to strengthen your grasp on victim's body.
6. If the victim begins to slip from your grip, let him slide slowly and gently to the ground without causing further damage to the injured area. Do not try to hold him up at any cost, because you may injure your own back in that process.

❒ DIFFERENT METHODS OF MANUAL LIFTS AND CARRIES

Method	Features
Carries for one first aider	
Cradle method	It is used when the victim weighs less or is a child. Carry the victim comfortably from below the shoulder and knees with the hands.

Drag method	It involves pulling the victim along the ground without lifting him. It is used when the victim is unable to stand and must be moved quickly from a source of danger. Fold the victim's arms across the chest and crouch behind his shoulders, grasp the armpits, cradle the head on your forearms and drag him along the ground.
Human crutch	It is used to support a conscious victim who is able to walk with support. Stand at the victim's side. Injured side is preferred. Place his nearest arm around your neck and hold it with your free hand. Put your other arm around his waist and grasp his clothes at the hip. Give him a walking stick for additional support.
Fireman's lift	It is used to move a conscious or unconscious child or a lightweight adult when a hand has to be kept free. Help the casualty to stand up. If the casualty is unconscious or unable to stand, turn the casualty face down and stand at the head. Place your arms under his armpits and raise him on to the knees and then the feet. Grasp his right wrist with your left hand. Bend down with your head under his extended right arm so that your shoulder is level with the lower part of his abdomen. Allow him to fall gently across your shoulders. Place your right arm between or around the his legs. Stand up, taking his weight on your right shoulder. Gently pull the victim across both shoulders. Hold his right wrist with your right hand leaving your left hand free.
Pick a back	It is used if the victim is small, light, conscious and able to hold on to you.

Carries for two first-aiders

Four handed seat	This method is used to carry a conscious casualty who can use one or both upper limbs to hold. Stand facing each other behind the victim. Make a seat by grasping your own left wrist with your right hand, and your partner's right wrist with the free hand. Stoop down. Instruct the victim to sit back on to your hands, to place his arms around your necks to steady him.
Two handed seat	This method is used to carry a victim who is unable to assist the bearers in his transportation, e.g. a hand fracture. Squat facing each other on either side of the victim. Pass your hands nearest the victim under and around the back just below his shoulders, grasping each other's wrists or the victim's clothes. Raise the victim's legs slightly, pass your other arms under the middle of his thigh and grasp each other's wrists. Rise together, step off with the outside feet and walk as usual.
Fore and aft carry	It is used when there is no sufficient space for the use of a chair. It is used to move the victim on to a chair. Supporting the victim on both sides, help him to sit up and fold the arms across his chest. Go behind the victim and place the arms through and under his armpits and grasp his wrists. Get the other first aider to remain at the victim's side and place one arm under the thighs. Lift him on to the chair together.
Chair method	It is used when a conscious victim with no serious injuries is to be moved up or down stairs or along a narrow passageway. Place him on a sturdy chair and secure him in position with broad bandages. Stand facing each other, one in front of him and the other

	behind him. Hold the back and the front legs of the chair and carry him.
Blanket lift	It is used when the victim is lying on a blanket or a bed sheet. Fold it on both sides and lift up the victim by holding the corners of the blanket. Place him on a stretcher.
Improvised method	Open the buttons of the victim's shirt. Open the flaps of his shirt and catch their corners. Get other helpers to hold his head and legs. Then lift and carry him to a stretcher.

❐ CARRY CHAIRS

These chairs are usually kept in many schools, workplaces, and shops and are used for moving casualties along passages and up and down stairs.

Method :

1. Unfold the chair.
2. Test it by pushing down the seat, to check that it can support the casualty's weight.
3. Confirm the following things.
   - The canvas seat and back are not showing signs of wear and tear.
   - The wheels move freely.
   - The safety strap is secure.
   - There are no signs of any other damage.
4. Place the casualty in the chair.
5. Secure the safety strap over his arms.
6. Put his feet on the footbar.
7. Get a helper to support the chair's back so that it does not topple backwards along with the casualty.
8. Explain the procedure to the casualty.
9. Tip the chair backwards gently. Push it forwards carefully, maintaining safe speed.
10. Take corners widely to prevent the chair from overbalancing.
11. Do not pull the chair, as it may cause the chair along with the casualty fall towards you.

If there is a step or an immovable object in the way, use the following method.

- Stand behind the chair.
- Face it towards the top of the steps.
- Get your helper to sit a few steps down, facing the chair.
- Tip the chair backwards gently. Push it forwards so that the wheels are on the edge of the steps.
- Ask your helper to squat down and grasp the handles or footrest. Let him control the lift.
- Pick up the chair together, your helper straightening his legs as he lifts the chair.
- If you have to rest in the mid-lift, use the landing rather than the steps.
- If going up the steps, use reverse procedure.

❒ STRETCHERS

A stretcher is used to carry a seriously ill or injured victim. There are a number of stretchers available, e.g. the standard stretcher, the

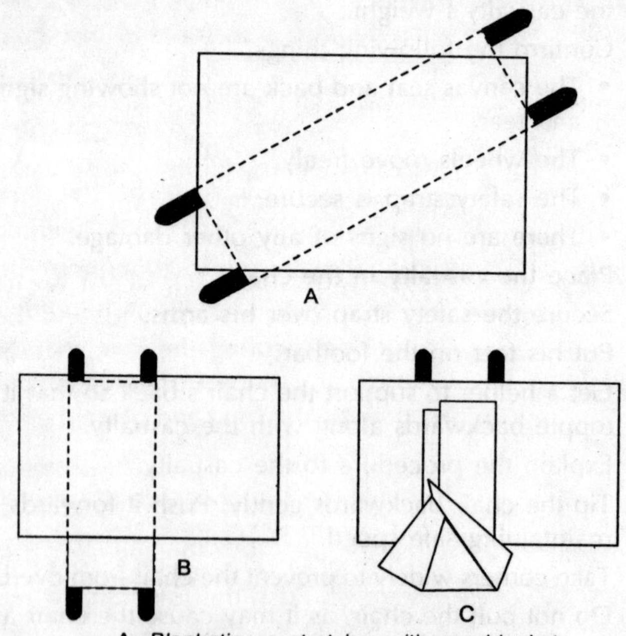

A. *Blanketing a stretcher with one blanket;*
B and C. *Blanketing a stretcher with two blankets.*
PREPARATION OF A STRETCHER

Orthopedic stretcher

pole-and-canvas stretcher, the Utila folding chair, the trolley bed, the Neil Robertson stretcher, and the paraguard stretcher. A stretcher should be rigid enough to carry casualties with suspected spine fracture without having to add boards to it. To ensure that a stretcher is capable of taking the weight of a victim, it should be tested before it is used. A person should lie on it and then others should lift it up, one end at a time first, then both the ends at the same time.

Types of Stretchers

Type	Features
Standard (Furley) stretcher	It consists of a canvas bed, poles, handles, traverses, and runners. The traverses are jointed such that the stretcher can be opened and closed. In closed state the poles lie close together with the canvas bed folded on top. This is then kept in position by two transverse straps. If slings are carried then they are laid along the canvas held by the straps. To open the stretcher place it on its sides with its runners towards you, and the studs or buckles securing the straps uppermost. Unfasten any straps. Push the traverses fully open with your heel and place the stretcher on its runners. To close the stretcher turn the stretcher on its side with its runners towards you and the studs or buckles which secure the straps uppermost. Push the joints of the traverses inwards with your heel to open them. Push

the poles together pulling the canvas out from between them. Fold the canvas over the poles and secure them with the straps.

Folding stretcher — It is a lighter version of the standard stretcher.

It has light metal poles with telescoping handles and a plastic or canvas bed. There are two types available. One folds like the standard stretcher, and the other folds in half in the center and occupies less space.

Pole and canvas stretcher — It is one of the most commonly used stretchers. It consists of a plastic or canvas sheet measuring 200 cm in length and 50 cm in width. There are two long poles. The canvas can be folded and slid under the victim where he lies. The poles are passed through the sleeves of the sheet to form the stretcher. Spacer bars are placed over the ends of the poles to keep them apart and maintain the firmness of the stretcher.

Scoop (orthopedic) stretcher — It is used to transfer a victim to an ambulance in the same position in which he is found, as is required when a fracture of the spine is suspected. Its length can be adjusted to suit any height of the victim.

Place the stretcher to the victim's side and adjust its length. Dismantle the two ends of the stretcher and slip each half under the victim from each side. Join the two sections again. Place the head pad and secure it. Lift up the stretcher with the victim on it and place it in the ambulance. Then dismantle it and remove it from under the patient, if it is required to move other victims. Otherwise it can be kept under the victim until he is taken to a hospital bed.

Trolley bed — It is found in many ambulances. It is a fully adjustable stretcher bed with wheels and is

	made of a light metal. A canvas stretcher is laid on the stretcher bed and two blankets are placed on top.
Neil Robertson stretcher	It is made of bamboo and light canvas. It is caused to lift casualties in the upright position through small hatches like pothole entrances and manholes, or to lower victims from a height in mountain accidents. There is a rope at the base to hold the victim's feet like stirrups and a strap at the top for securing the victims's head. The upper flaps are wrapped around the victim's chest and secured with two short straps. The arms are secured with the long strap. The lower flaps are strapped around the lower limbs. There is a ring at the head end for hoisting the stretcher up. There is a ring at the foot end, to which a rope is attached for guiding the stretcher.
Paraguard stretcher	It is similar to the Neil Robertson stretcher and is used in similar situations. It is lighter, more durable and more convenient to use than the Neil Robertson stretcher. It can be folded up and carried on the back. It can bend in the middle to help negotiate obstacles.
Improvised stretcher	Two poles can be passed through the sleeves of two or three coats turned inside out. Then the coats are buttoned up. The poles may be kept apart by strips of wood tied to the poles at each end of the stretcher.

❐ PREPARING A STRETCHER

1. One blanket method : place a blanket diagonally over the stretcher so that there are two opposing corners at the ends of the stretcher. After placing the victim on the stretcher, bring the point of the top blanket at the foot of the stretcher up over the victim's feet and tuck a small fold between the ankles. Fold the point of the blanket at the head around the head and neck. Bring the right side of the blanket over the casualty and tuck it in. Then repeat the procedure with the lift side of the blanket.

2. Two blanket method : place the first blanket lengthwise across the stretch with one edge covering half the length of the handles at the head end, leaving a little more of it on one side of the stretcher than the other. Fold the other blanket lengthwise into three and place it on the stretcher with the upper edge about one third of the way down the stretcher, leaving adequate length for folding over the feet. After placing the victim on the stretcher bring the fold of the top blanket over the victim's feet and tuck a small fold between his ankles to prevent their rubbing together. Bring the folds of the blanket over the feet and legs and tuck them in. Turn the upper corners of the first blanket in. Bring the shorter side over the victim and tuck it in. Then repeat the procedure with the long side of the blanket.

❒ CARRYING A LOADED STRETCHER

When the casualty has been placed on the stretcher the bearers should take up their positions at each end of the stretcher. At least two trained persons are required. The person in charge of the victim should remain at his head. If bystanders are available they should be asked to help. The general rules for carrying a stretcher are as follows.

1. The head should be kept higher than the feet, unless the victim is in shock.
2. He should always be carried feet first, except in the following situations.
   - When carrying a victim to the side or foot of a bed.
   - When going downstairs or hills when the victim's lower limbs are injured or there is hypothermia.
   - When going upstairs or hills when the lower limbs are not injured.
   - When loading a victim into an ambulance.

Carrying a Stretcher

Situation	Technique
Four bearers	Secure and grasp the handles with their your hands, palms inwards, keeping your backs straight. Rise together when the order 'rise' is given. Hold the stretcher with the arms extended and keeping it level. With the order 'advance' walk simultaneously but out of step to avoid bouncing. On reaching the ambulance lower the stretcher to the ground evenly, with the casualty's head nearest the ambulance. When crossing uneven ground, secure the victim to the stretcher with broad bandages or a harness before you start. Keep the stretcher as level as possible by each bearer adjusting the height of the stretcher individually.
Four bearers, only a short distance to be covered	Stand at the side of the stretcher facing inwards. Grasp the poles with one hand and place the other about 75 cm from the end of the stretcher. Then move sideways.
Four bearers, crossing a wall	Avoid crossing a wall, if possible. If not, place the stretcher on the wall, with the front runners beyond the wall. After the front bearers cross the wall one at a time while the others steady the stretcher, lift it up and advance until the back end of the stretcher is close to the wall. Let the other bearers cross the wall. Then resume carrying the stretcher.
Four bearers, moving from one level to another	Stand on either side of the stretcher facing each other across the stretcher. Lift the stretcher so that it is at level with the top of the elevation. Place its front end on the

	elevation. Let one bearer get up on to the elevation and receive the stretcher while the others pass it forward. Then let another bearer climb up the elevation. Move the stretcher forward until the rear runners are on the bank. Then let the rear bearers climb up the elevation. Resume carrying the stretcher.
Two bearers	Stand in between the two handles of the stretcher at either end of the stretcher. At the order 'lift', lift the stretcher up together, keeping the upper limbs straight. With the order 'advance', start walking simultaneously. While placing it down bend down simultaneously and put it down slowly

❒ HOW TO LOAD AN AMBULANCE

1. A few ambulances have flat built-in beds with grooves to take the runners of a standard stretcher. Four persons should do this together. One person should stand inside the ambulance to guide the stretcher. The other three should stand on both sides and one end to lift the stretcher.
2. If there are two berths to be loaded, always load the left one first.
3. While loading a trolley bed into an ambulance, two bearers should stand at the ends of the trolley bed, raise the trolley bed to the required height, and carry it head first into the ambulance.

❒ HOW TO UNLOAD THE STRETCHER

The victim is unloaded from the stretcher after transportation to the desired place like the hospital or his home. The methods applied for the unloading are the same as of loading, except that the order is reverse.

1. He is picked up by four persons holding the four corners of the bed sheet or blanket on which he is lying, and placed on his bed. Then the sheet is folded in around the person in all sides and drawn out from under him.

2. If he is not lying on a bed sheet or blanket, then he is lifted up with their hands below his head, waist, chest, hips and legs.

❐ HOW TO LABEL A CASUALTY

During emergency, the seriously injured or unconscious persons are carried on stretchers to hospitals for treatment. Labels made up of hard paper are placed on his stretcher and/or his forehead for easy identification. The symbols put on these labels and their interpretation are as shown in the following table.

Labelling the Casualties

Label	Interpretations
C	Contaminated by persistent gas.
H	Severe hemorrhage has occurred.
M	Morphine has been given. The time of administration and dose should be written on the label.
P	Burnt by phosphorus.
R	Radioactive exposure.
T	A tourniquet (constrictive bandage) has been applied. The time of application and subsequent releases should be indicated on the label.
X	Requires urgent removal to a hospital from the accident site and urgent treatment of mainly, but not exclusively for wounds of the chest and abdomen, for internal haemorrhage and for a unconscious victims.
XX	Poisoned by nerve gas or nonpersistent gas.

❐ AMBULANCE SERVICE

If there are multiple casualties, as in a disaster, first aid has to be administered to a large number of victims. In such cases, the ambulance service has to be very good for rapid and efficient transfer to a hospital. The process of triage is used to sort patients according to priority for care and transport. Accordingly the patients are placed in three categories as shown in the following table. Every ambulance and rescue unit should carry tags that can be used during triage phase of disaster operation.

When there are a number of casualties at a time, as in a disaster or a calamity, you have to decide whom to give first aid first, and whom to transport in an ambulance first. This is explained in the following table.

Priority of First Aid Treatment and Transportation

Priority	Conditions
Highest (red tag)	– Respiratory arrest, airway obstruction and severe breathing difficulties.
	– Cardiac arrest.
	– Uncontrolled severe hemorrhage and shock.
	– Severe head injuries.
	– Open chest wounds.
	– Burns involving respiratory tract.
	– Unconsciousness, coma.
	– Heart attack.
	– Poisoning.
	– Open abdominal wounds.
Second (green tag)	– Severe burns.
	– Injuries to spine.
	– Moderate hemorrhage.
	– Multiple fractures.
	– Head injuries, patient conscious.
	– Spinal injury.
Lowest (white tag)	– Minor fractures.
	– Minor bleeding.
	– Moderate or minor burns.

❒ THE AMBULANCE

It should be in perfect condition in all of the following respects.

1. Wheels, engine, and brakes.
2. Doors and windows.

3. Communication equipment.
4. Warning devices.
5. Lights.
6. Fuel.
7. Road worthiness.

When on emergency duty of transporting a patient, an ambulance driver is generally granted the following privileges with respect to speed, passage through traffic, and parking.

1. Exceed the speed limit by 5 to 10 mph as long as life and property of others are not endangered.
2. Pass in no-entry-zones after providing an appropriate signal to other drivers.
3. With the proper caution and signals, disregard the regulations about traffic lights, turning etc.
4. Use sound signals like siren sparingly.

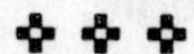

CHAPTER

21

"Dangerous" Effects of Temperature

Our body has some in-built mechanisms to help it adapt to changes in the environmental temperature. However when the changes are extreme and last for long durations, the protective mechanisms may fail, and the person may suffer from illness. The following factors increase risk of adverse effects of extremes of temperature change on the human body.

1. Infants and elderly people.
2. People who are exposed to the sun for prolonged periods, e.g. soldiers, farmers.
3. Individuals with medical disorders like diabetes mellitus, cardiovascular disease, and obesity.
4. Poorly insulated and ventilated homes, congested neighborhoods or slums.
5. Sedentary life styles.
6. Low socio-economic class.

❐ HEART STROKE (SUNSTROKE)

It occurs when the body can no longer control its temperature by sweating as in the following conditions. It can prove to be dangerous.

1. Very high environmental temperature.
2. Prolonged confinement in hot atmosphere.
3. Consumption of alcohol.
4. Illness like malaria.

The conditions is diagnosed by the following features.

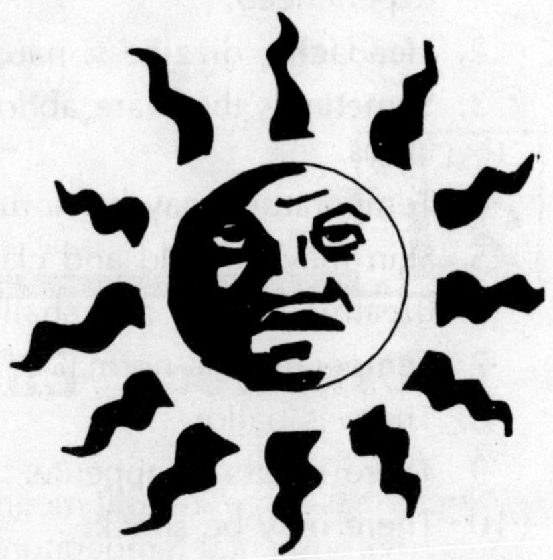

1. There is restlessness, headache, dizziness, and discomfort.
2. The skin is hot, flushed, and dry.
3. The pulse is bounding.
4. The body temperature is 40°C or higher.
5. Breathing is noisy.
6. Muscular cramps may occur.
7. The victim may become unconscious.

First-aid

1. Move the victim to a cool place. Place him in half sitting position with head and shoulders supported if he is conscious, and in recovery position if he is unconscious.
2. Remove his clothing.
3. Sprinkle cold water on his body or wrap him in a thin wet sheet. Start a fan to cool his body.
4. Apply ice cap with ice pieces over the head and neck.
5. A cold water enema can be given.
6. Record his body temperature every 10 minutes. Do not let it fall below 102°F. At that stage wrap him in a dry sheet and keep the fan on so that the temperature does not rise again.
7. Give him cool water to drink. Maintain his hydration.
8. Shift him to a hospital if he does not respond to treatment.

❒ HEAT EXHAUSTION

It occurs in hot and humid environment after heavy and prolonged sweating either due to exposure to the sun or working in a close, hot atmosphere like factories, with failure to replace salt and water. The condition is diagnosed by the following features.

1. Restlessness and exhaustion are present. Faintness may be experienced.
2. Headache, dizziness, nausea, vomiting are present.
3. Sometimes there are abdominal cramps, or cramps in the limbs.
4. Temperature may be normal or subnormal.
5. Skin may be cold and clammy.
6. Breathing is fast and shallow.
7. Temperature is normal or slightly elevated.
8. There is pallor.
9. There is loss of appetite.
10. There may be shock.

First-aid

1. Place the victim in supine position in a cooler place with fresh air.
2. Give plenty of cold water (250 ml every half hour) with salt in it (2 teaspoons in 1 liter of water). Fruit juice may be given too.

❐ HEAT CRAMPS

They occur when one replaces the fluid lost in sweat by drinking water without salt. The conditions is diagnosed by the following features.

1. There are intermittent painful contractions of skeletal muscles in the body.
2. They occur in those muscles that have been involved in strenuous activity, usually those of the legs.
3. Body temperature is normal or low.
4. The cramps last a few minutes and generally disappear spontaneously.

First-aid

1. Replace body sodium with salt tablets or electrolyte solutions.
2. Shift him to a hospital if his condition is severe or does not respond to treatment.

❒ HOW TO PREVENT HEAT INJURIES ?

1. Stay indoors during heat waves. Wear a minimum of clothing that is light in colour, cool and loose fitting.
2. Improve ventilation in the house. use shades and drapes to cut direct sunlight.
3. Limit the strenuous activities to the cooler times of the day.
4. Cook food in the early morning or late evening to avoid heating up the house during the hot part of the day.
5. Use exhaust fans and vents over stoves and ovens to help remove heat from the house.
6. If necessary, expose yourself to hot weather gradually.
7. Use an umbrella or a wide brimmed hat and walk in the shade if you must go out.
8. Take plenty of fluids and salts.

❒ SUNBURN

It occurs after excessive exposure to the blazing sun. It is seen at high altitudes in winter due to exposure to ultraviolet rays. The condition is diagnosed by the following features.

1. There is itching over the burn.
2. The skin is red, swollen and painful.
3. In mild cases there are superficial burns. Severe cases have painful blisters.

First-aid

1. Place the patient in a cool place.
2. Sponge the affected parts with cold water.
3. Apply a soothing cream like a cold cream.
4. Shift a severe case to a hospital.

❒ HYPOTHERMIA

Fall of the body temperature below 35°C is called hypothermia. Mild and moderate cases are reversible, but recovery is unlikely if the body temperature falls below 26-24°C. Hypothermia occurs in the following conditions.

1. Very low environmental temperature without adequate protection in the form of warm clothes, properly heated house etc.
2. Prolonged immersion in cold water.
3. Wearing wet clothes.
4. Exhaustion in cold climate.

Severity varies with age and physical condition of the individual. Consumption of alcohol or drugs and some problems like diabetes mellitus aggravate this condition. It is diagnosed by the following features.

1. The skin is very pale and abnormally cold to touch.
2. There is loss of muscle coordination.
3. Speech is slurred.
4. The victim is irritable, confused, and restless.
5. He may become unconscious.
6. Breathing becomes increasingly difficult.
7. Cardiac activity drops.

First-aid

1. Place the victim in supine position in a warm place. If he is unconscious, place him in recovery position.
2. Cover his body with a woolen blanket.
3. Remove his clothes if wet and replace them with dry, warm clothes.
4. Do not rub or massage the limbs.
5. Do not give him alcohol.
6. Resuscitate if cardiorespiratory arrest develops.
7. Shift him to a hospital immediately.

❒ FROSTBITE

During very cold weather, especially if there is also a strong wind frostbite occurs in the ears, nose, chin, hands and feet. The condition is diagnosed by the following features.

1. Initially there is a white patch on a red face. Then it changes to mottled blue colour.

2. Pickling pain is felt in affected part.
3. The exposed part becomes cold, painful and finally numb.
4. It becomes waxy white in appearance.
5. Prolonged freezing causes irreparable damage.

First-aid

1. Warm the body gradually. Place the injured part in hot water if available. It is better to warm him by dry or radiant heat.
2. Elevate the affected parts to relieve swelling and pan.
3. Take the patient to a closed room.
4. If the frozen part is on the face, cover it with a gloved hand until normal colour and sensation return.
5. Remove his tight gloves, boots, socks, rings etc. in case of frostbite of fingers or toes. The hand may be placed under the clothing in the axilla. Wrap the feet in a warm cloth.
6. Do not rub the frozen part with anything.
7. Give him warm drinks. Do not allow the victim to smoke.
8. Shift him to a doctor or hospital immediately.

❐ TRENCH FOOT

It occurs when there is exposure to temperatures above the critical tissue temperature in presence of moisture over prolonged periods. Predisposing conditions are malnutrition, deficiency of proteins and vitamins, and dehydration. The condition is diagnosed by the following features.

1. There is hyperemia of the part.
2. The affected part feels numb.
3. Pain, itching and tingling, and paresthesia develop.
4. Blisters appear later.
5. Infection may develop locally.

First-aid

1. Rewarm the part gradually.
2. Shift him to a doctor's clinic.

❐ CHILBLAIN

It is an allergic reaction to cold and dampness in susceptible individuals. There is patchy constriction of blood vessels of the skin associated with it. It may progress to trench foot if not treated adequately. The condition is diagnosed by the following features.

1. The toes become red. There is intense itching.
2. Severe pain develops.
3. Blisters and ulcers may develop.

First-aid

1. Warm the part gradually.
2. Shift him to a doctor's clinic.

Safety from cold injuries

1. Dress in warm clothes. Wear several layers of loose, warm clothes rather than a singe thick garment.
2. Cover vulnerable parts well.
3. Apply protective cream to the face prior to exposure.
4. Plan activities carefully to minimize exposure.
5. Avoid vigorous washing of the face and shaving until after the day's work is done rather than early in the morning.
6. Use mittens rather than gloves for hand protection.
7. Do not use excessive heat to thaw frozen tissues.

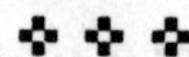

CHAPTER
22

"Painful" Bites and Stings

❒ BEE AND WASP BITES

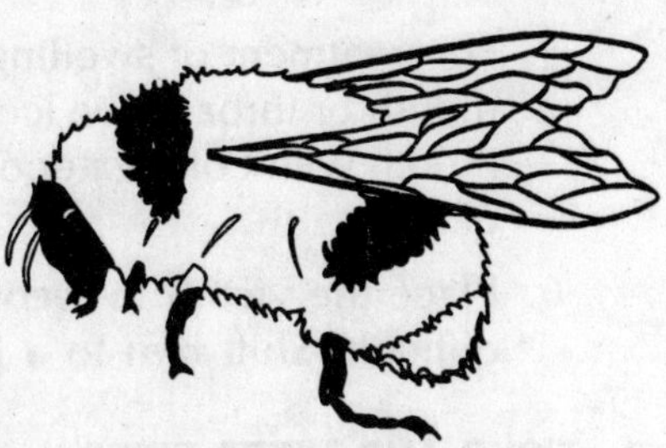

Bee and wasps are the most harmful amongst all insects. Their stings have poison in small quantity. Some people could be very sensitive to this poison and develop severe reaction to it. The condition is diagnosed by the following features.

1. There is severe pain locally.
2. Itching and swelling develop around the central reddened puncture point.
3. Sting may be found in the wound.
4. Persons hypersensitive to the poison in the sting develop severe reaction characterized by fall in blood pressure and respiratory difficulty due to swelling in the throat and contraction of the windpipe. The victim may become unconscious, develop anaphylactic shock and may die if not treated in time.

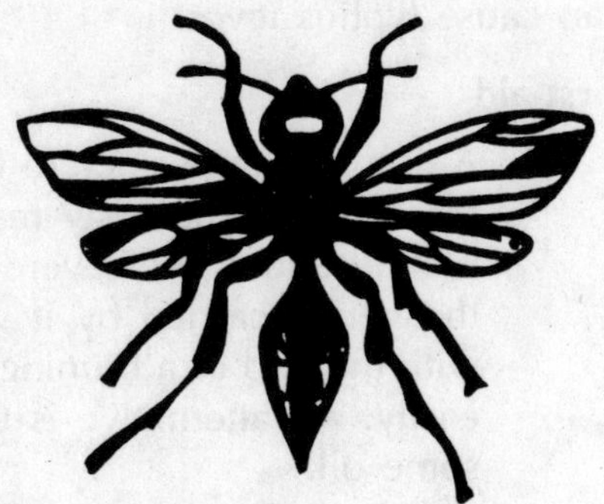

First-aid

1. Remove the sting with tweezers, held as near to the skin as possible. An alternative method is to rub the skin in the affected area gently, so that the skin puncture enlarges a little, and the sting comes out along with the poison around it. Do not squeeze the poison sac because this will force the remaining poison into the skin.
2. Apply ammonia, soda or methylene blue locally as antidote for bee venom.
3. Apply vinegar or lemon juice locally as antidote for wasp venom.
4. Apply a cold compress and spirit locally to relieve the pain and swelling.
5. For treatment of swelling caused by insect stings inside the mouth or throat, give ice to suck. Ask the victim to rinse the mouth with cold water or solution of water and bicarbonate of soda.
6. Place the victim in recovery position if breathing becomes difficult. Shift him to a hospital immediately.

❒ TICKS AND MITES BITES

Ticks are found in jungles. It is a small insect like a bed bug with a great capacity to stick to the body and suck blood. It spreads germs of certain diseases like Rocky mountain spotted fever and tularemia. Mites are found in wood and stored grains. Their bite can cause typhus fever.

First-aid

1. A tick or a mite stuck to the skin should not be pulled out forcefully as that may result in its mouth parts remaining behind and cause severe inflammation. If it gets crushed, the germs carried by it will enter body tissues. Touch it with the end of a burning cigarette. Then it comes off very easily. An alternative is to apply kerosene, turpentine, or some oil.
2. Wash the wound well with soap and apply a dressing to

❐ SCORPION BITE

Generally scorpions can be seen in the moist dark places and in rainy season in villages, farms, and jungles. They are not seriously poisonous. But sometimes person hypersensitive to its poison can develop serious reaction and may even become unconscious. The condition is diagnosed by the following features.

1. There is burning pain at the site of the sting.
2. Itching and swelling develop around the site.
3. Sensation may be altered near the site of bite.
4. There is restlessness.
5. Lacrymation and salivation may develop. Nausea, vomiting, and profuse sweating develop 4-6 hours after bite.

First-aid

1. If the sting is on a limb, apply a tourniquet proximal to the site of the sting. Release it every 20 minutes for 5 minutes to prevent development of gangrene.
2. Apply ice locally to cause constriction of blood vessels and slow the rate of absorption of the scorpion's poison.
3. Apply freshly prepared potassium permanganate solution on the wound.
4. Consult a doctor soon.

❐ SPIDER BITE

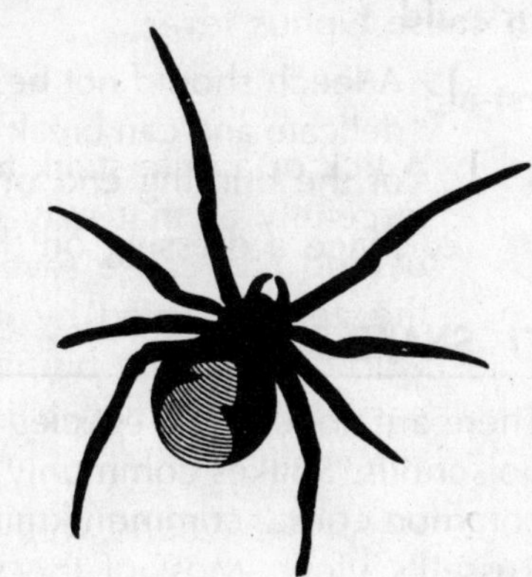

Spiders are generally found in corners of the house, gaps in wood, hollow and dark places. Two types of spiders commonly found are black spider and tarantula. A tarantula is big, hairy and less poisonous, while a black spider is more poisonous. Diagnosis of a spider bite is made by the following features.

1. The victim experiences severe pain locally.
2. Redness and swelling develop at the site of the sting. Small blisters arise locally.
3. The face, hands and legs develop swelling.
4. Stomach cramps develop. Muscles become hard.
5. Breathlessness and shock can develop. Death is rare.

First-aid

1. Place the victim in a comfortable position.
2. Cover him with a blanket or a bed sheet.
3. If the bite is on a limb, tie a tourniquet proximal to the site of bite to prevent absorption of its poison and spread to other parts of the body.
4. Clean and dress the bitten area.
5. Consult a doctor if his condition worsens.

❒ LEECH BITE

Leeches are generally found in water tanks, moist and muddy places, and rivers. Leeches are normally harmless, but they suck blood from the victim. Though a serious condition does not arise with their bite but they suck a lot of blood from the victim. Hence they should be removed quickly.

First-aid

1. A leech should not be pulled off the skin because it is quite delicate and can break if pulled. Remove it by the application of the burning end of a cigarette or stick to its back.
2. Place a dressing on the wound after its removal.

❒ SNAKE BITE

There are about 3000 species of snakes, of which only 250-300 are poisonous. Snakes commonly found in our country are king cobra, common cobra, common krait, common striped krait, pit viper and Russell's viper. Most of the snakes are harmless. Remember, all snake bites are not fatal. Generally people die from fear and not the venom. Most snakes bite only if provoked. Even the bite of a poisonous snake is not always dangerous, because when the snake bites in defense, little or no venom is injected. The snake must be identified because no anti-venom is necessary if it is nonpoisonous. If it is poisonous, its type must be identified so that specific anti-venom can be administered. If the snake cannot be found or cannot be identified, it should be treated as poisonous, and general anti-venom should be given. The differences between poisonous and non-poisonous snakes are as shown below.

Poisonous and Nonpoisonous snakes

Variable	Poisonous	Nonpoisonous
Belly scales	Large, cover entire breadth of the belly.	Small or moderately large, but not covering entire breadth of the belly.
Head scales	Small. In case of vipers large and with : • Conspicuous pit between eye and nostril in pit viper. • Third labial scale touches the eye and nasal shields in cobra, king cobra, and coral. • Central row of scales on back enlarged, the undersurface of mouth with only four infralabials, the fourth being the largest in krait.	Large.
Fangs	Long and grooved or canalized.	Short and solid.
Tail	Compressed.	Not markedly compressed.
Bite	Two fang marks with or without small marks of outer teeth.	A number of small teeth marks in a row.

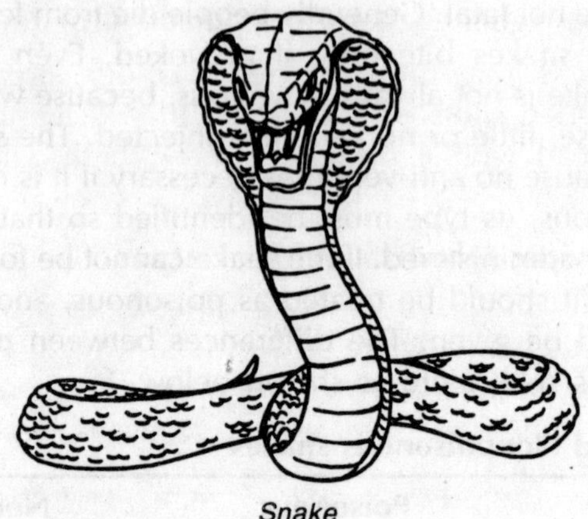

Snake

The main characteristics of common poisonous snakes found in India are given below.

Cobra (naag or kala samp)

1.5 to 2 meters long, black in colour, head of the same width as the trunk, neck has a hood with a spectacle mark, 2 or 3 series of very dark or black belly scales under the neck, and divided tail shields.

King cobra (raj naag or raj samp)

2.5 to 4 meters long, yellow, green, brown or black in colour, white or yellow cross bars on the body, hood without a spectacle mark, tail scales entire proximally and divided distally.

Common krait (manyar, chitti, or kawriya)

1-1.25 meters long, glistening black in colour, single or double white arches across the back, a short distance from the head, creamy white belly, head covered with large shields, tail scales.

Banded krait

2 meters long, alternate black and yellow bands across the back, and other features as of a common krait.

Common green pit viper (bamboo snake or hara phisi)

30-100 cms long, vivid green in colour, body flat and broad, head triangular with a pit between the eye and nostrils, yellowish white line on flanks, tail long with divided scales.

Russell's viper (ghonus, daboia or khadchitro)

1.55 meters long, brown or buff in colour, three series of black diamond-shaped spots on the back, tail with divided shields, flat triangular head with a distinct V mark, belly white with broad plates.

Saw scaled viper (phoorsa, echis or afai)

50-75 cms long, brown, brownish-gray or greenish in colour, triangular head with a white arrow mark, wavy line on each flank, diamond shaped area between the upper curves of the two wavy lines, small head scales, serrated body scales, broad belly plates, tail shields entire.

How is a snake bite diagnosed ?

1. There is a history of snake bite.
2. There are 2 fang marks, a finger's breadth apart.
3. Intense pain is experienced by the victim at the site of the bite of a viper. That area is swollen and blackened. Bleeding might be seen from different places. The patient vomits. Collapse and coma follow.
4. Fifteen minutes to two hours after the bite of a cobra or similar snakes neurotoxic effects are seen e.g. giddiness, lethargy, muscular weakness and spreading paralysis. Breathing becomes slow and labored. After a couple of hours, respiration ceases with or without convulsions, and the heart stops.
5. A bite from a sea snake is felt as a sharp initial prick that subsequently becomes painless. After 1-2 hours, generalized muscular pain and stiffness develop, starting in the neck, shoulders and hips. Urine becomes brown in colour. Respiratory failure may occur.

First-aid

1. Place the person on a flat surface comfortably.
2. Reassure him that all snakes are not poisonous, and the condition is curable.
3. Tie a tourniquet between heart and the bitten area to avoid absorption of the poison into the venous blood. Loosen it for a few seconds every ten minutes.

4. Immobilize the affected limb.
5. Make a 2.5 cm long cut over the bitten area and squeeze out blood mixed liquid from the wound.
6. Wash the wound gently with normal saline.
7. Apply ice packs on the wound if the area is on a limb.
8. Treat shock.
9. Shift the patient to hospital immediately, along with the killed snake, if available for identification.

❒ STING OF JELLYFISH

The effects vary from slight local reaction to large wheals, severe pain and sometimes swift death.

First-aid

1. Apply calamine cream, lotion or paste of sodium bicarbonate in water.
2. Send a severe case to a hospital immediately.

❒ STING OF PORTUGUESE MAN OF WAR

The effects vary from slight stinging to cramps, nausea and difficulty in breathing.

First-aid

1. Swab the area with methylated sprit to which vinegar has been added to acidify it.
2. Do not rub or apply fresh water or sand.
3. Remove any gelatinous strands present in the flesh using cloth or soft paper, once the symptoms subside.
4. Send a severe case to a hospital immediately.

❒ SEA URCHIN STING

The spine of a sea urchin can break off in the skin causing local burning and numbness. The wounds heal slowly and the rate of infection is high.

First-aid

1. Wear gloves while handling the sting.
2. Remove the spine.

3. Cover the wound with dry dressing.
4. Send him to a hospital immediately.

❐ CONE-SHAPED SHELL STING

A snail like creature is found in such shells. It injects a very potent poison through a minute hollow barbed harpoon. It can be fatal and there is no antidote. Such a shell must not be handled.

First-aid

1. Watch the patient's pulse and respiration, and give external cardiac massage and artificial respiration when necessary.
2. Send him to a hospital immediately.

❐ CORAL CUTS

Coral is razor sharp. The cuts are large and deep and get infected readily. They heal slowly and tend to form ulcers.

First-aid

1. Swab the area with methylated spirit.
2. Remove all foreign material from the cuts.
3. Cover the wound with sterile dressing.
4. Send him to a hospital immediately.

❐ DOG BITE

A person may be bitten by a domestic dog or a stray dog. A domestic dog may or may not be immunized against rabies. If it is immunized, there is no risk of rabies in the victim. If it is not immunized, it can contract rabies from a rabid dog, and then its bite is dangerous. Rabies is a viral disease found in dogs, and also in other animals like rat, cat, fox, wolf etc. A human being can get it by bite of any of these animals, and also by licking of a rabid dog, if there is a cut in the area licked. A rabid dog may be restless, barking, and biting or it may be quiet. A quiet dog is more dangerous than a restless

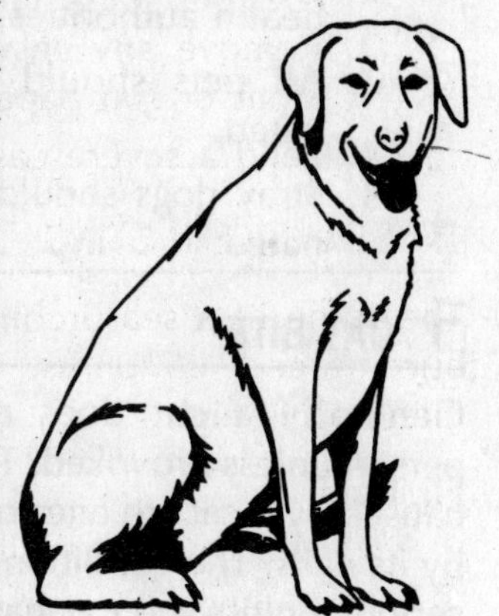

dog, because no illness is suspected in it. Incubation period of the illness is 10 days to 1 year. Untreated victim is likely to develop rabies. Rabies (hydrophobia) is a fatal illness. Features of rabies after a dog bite are as follows.

1. There is a history of bite.
2. Discomfort and pain are present locally.
3. Headache, nausea and vomiting develop soon.
4. Agitation, confusion and hallucination follow.
5. There is an intense fear of drinking water, because that causes spasm of throat muscles and severe pain.
6. There is foaming at the mouth.
7. Respiratory paralysis develops later.

First-aid

1. Wash the wound thoroughly with soap or detergent and water.
2. Shift the patient to hospital immediately for antirabies vaccination and local treatment of the wound.
3. Apply an antiseptic cream locally.
4. The dog should be kept under observation for ten days. If the dog remains healthy then there is no risk to the victim. If the dog gets rabies, the victim is at risk, and needs rabies vaccine.

Prevention of rabies

1. Any case of rabid dog bite to be immediately notified, to health authorities.
2. All pets should be vaccinated.
3. Stray dogs should be eliminated.

❐ CAT BITE

Generally a cat does not bite a person unless provoked. The injuries caused by a cat are bites or scratches by its nails. The condition is not very serious unless the cat has rabies.

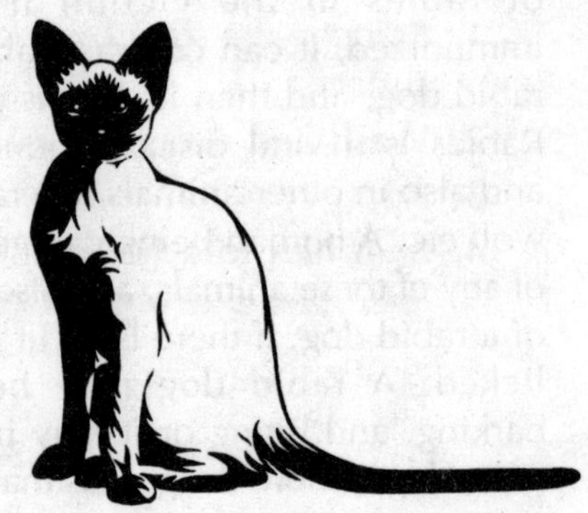

First-aid

1. Wash and dress the wound.
2. Send the victim to a doctor to get an injection of tetanus toxoid for prevention of tetanus.
3. Watch out for features of rabies in the cat.

❐ RAT BITE

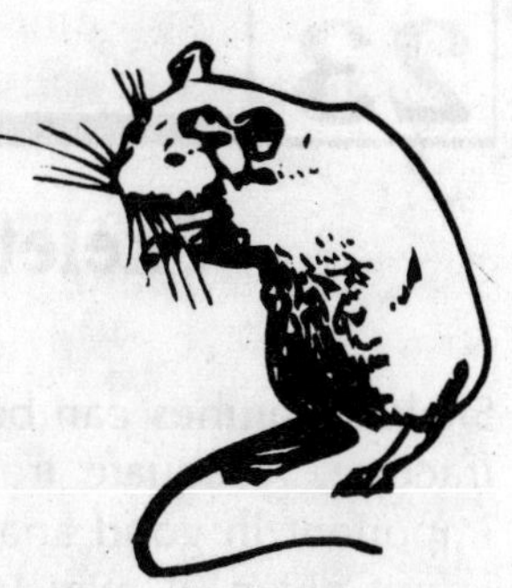

Rats are found in the house, garden, farm, gutter, and jungle. Generally they live in dirty places so the places scratched by them get easily infected. They can spread a dangerous disease called plague. Send the victim of a rat bite to a hospital immediately.

❐ FISH BITES

Jelly fish and sting ray fish can harm the human beings by stinging. Their stings are located on the lower border of their tails. The stings of these fishes are quite painful but never fatal. The condition is diagnosed by the following features.

1. The jelly fish generally stings on the hand or feet.
2. The victim is uneasy.
3. There is local pain.
4. The sting of the fish breaks in the tissues bitten.
5. The local area looks blue or black.

First-aid

1. Remove the sting by scratching the skin, if it is seen on the surface.
2. Wash and dress the wound.
3. Apply cold compress of ammonia and water to relieve pain.
4. Shift him to a hospital immediately if there is no relief in spite of the treatment given.

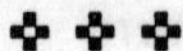

CHAPTER

23

Skeletal Injuries can be Critical

Skeletal injuries can be classified as sprain, strain, dislocation and fracture. Adequate treatment given at the time of injury is very important in good anatomical repair and functional recovery. If it is not given, it may lead to further injury, shock and permanent disabilities, Sprain and strain are joint injuries in which there is no displacement of joint surfaces. In a dislocation there is displacement of bones at the joint. A fracture is partial or complete break in the continuity of a bone (periosteum).

❒ CAUSES OF SKELETAL INJURIES

Most of these injuries are the result of trauma, direct or indirect. A bone can be fractured directly at the point a blow is applied. An indirect force may cause the bone to break away from the spot of application of force (transmission of force from one part of the body to another) e.g. fracture of clavicle after a fall on the outstretched hand. Violent contraction of a group of muscles may pull pieces of bone away from the point where the muscle is attached i.e. fracture of patella by powerful contraction of quadriceps muscles. Wrenching of a joint can cause its ligaments to pull so hard at the bones forming the joint that one of the bones may fracture, e.g. fracture of lower leg bone at the ankle after stumbling. Pathological fracture is caused when the bone may be the seat of a number of diseases, which weaken it, and make it liable to break even with very minor injuries.

How to tell if there is a fracture

1. There is usually (but not always) pain over the fracture bone.

2. There may be swelling and/or bruising.
3. There is loss or severe restriction of use of the area affected.
4. Bone may poke through the skin.
5. There may be obvious deformity, bending angularity, or floppiness of the affected part.

How do I know it is not a fracture ?

You do not. It is often very difficult even for doctors to tell. Sprains can be extremely painful so the degree of pain in nothing to go by Often only an X-ray after careful medical examination will finally clear up the diagnosis.

If in doubt — treat as a fracture.

❑ TYPES OF FRACTURE ?

1. Simple (closed) fracture : the skin surface over the fracture is intact.
2. Compound (open) fracture : the skin surface over the fracture is broken and fracture communicates with outside. There is risk of extensive blood loss and infection.
3. Complicated closed or open fractures : there is injury to nerves and/or blood vessels in addition to the fracture.

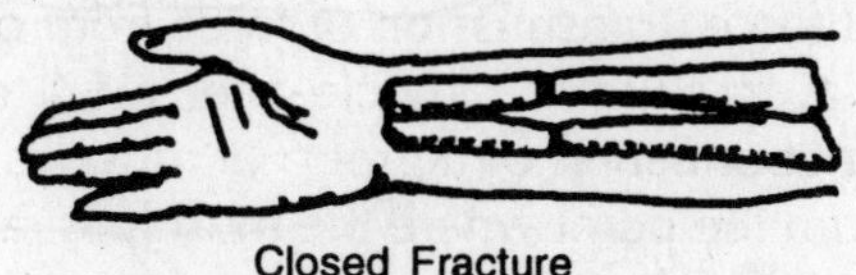

Closed Fracture

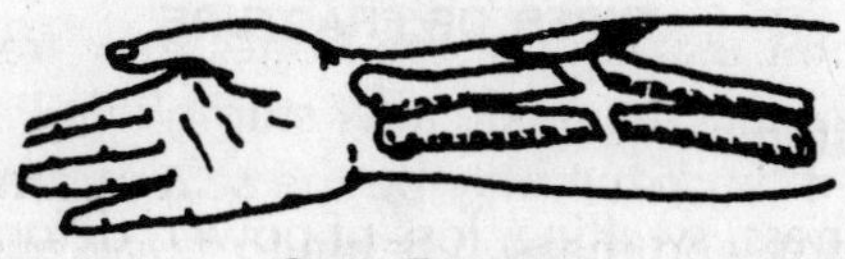

Open Fracture

❐ ANATOMICAL TYPES OF FRACTURE

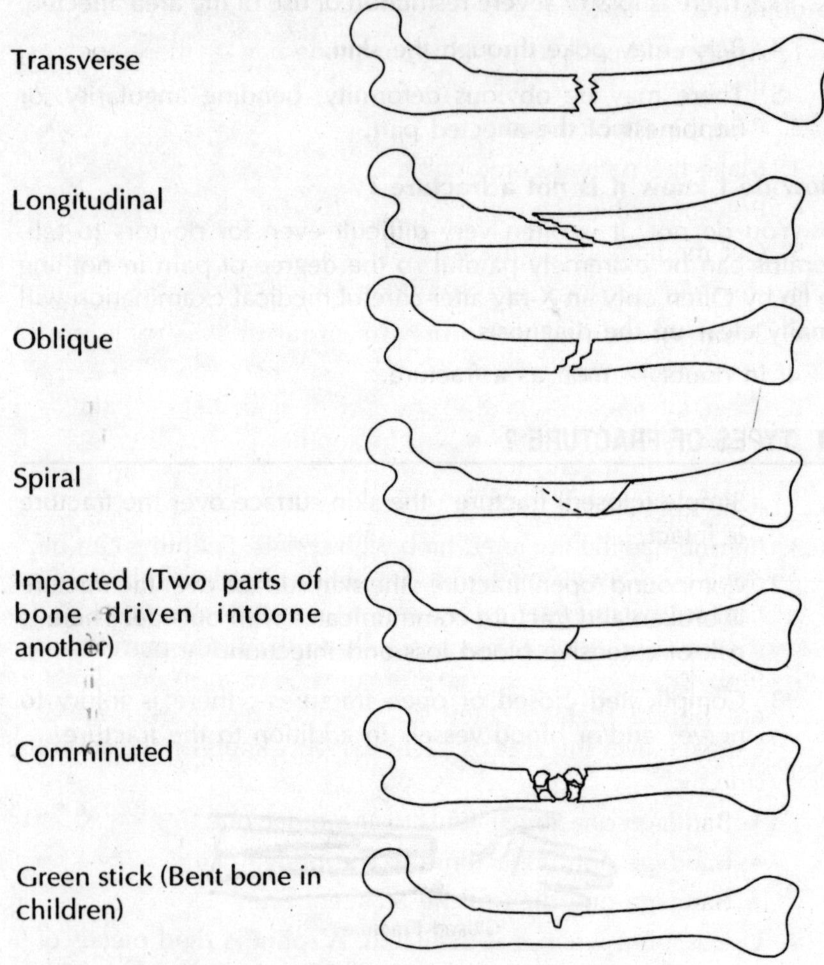

TYPES OF FRACTURE

Signs and Symptoms :

Pain, tenderness, swelling, loss of power, deformity of the limbs, irregularity of the bone, crepitus, abnormal mobility at fracture site, bluish discolouration of skin at site, cyanosis.

❒ FIRST-AID FOR A FRACTURE

The objectives of first-aid are :

1. Apply cold pads or ice in a polythene bag — these soothe the pain.
2. Rest the affected part.
3. Make the patient comfortable.
4. Prevent further damage.
5. Get medical aid at the earliest.

The first aid measures are as follows.

1. Treat bleeding, difficulty in breathing, shock and unconsciousness first.
2. Treat all fractures in the position in which the victim is found rather than move him to another place. This is not possible if there is bad weather or risk to the victim's life if he is left there.
3. Immobilize the fractured limb with splints. Splinting can be done by different methods. The bandaging should be fairly firm so that there is no movement at the fracture site. But it should not cut off blood supply to the distal part of the limb. Place padding material in between so that when limbs are bound together they are comfortable. Never apply bandage over the area of fracture. Apply knots on the sound side.
   - Bandage one lower limb to the other one.
   - Bandage one upper limb to the body.
   - Bandage one digit to the adjacent one.
4. Use a splint when it is available. A splint is rigid pieces of wood, plastic or metal. It should be well padded with cotton or cloth. It is tied to a fractured limb to support it and to prevent movement at the fracture site. Wide splints are better than narrow ones. A splint should extend enough to immobilize the joints above or below the fractured bones.
5. Raise the injured part after immobilizing it to reduce swelling. A rolled up blanket can be used for this purpose.
6. Shift him to a hospital immediately.

❐ SKULL FRACTURE

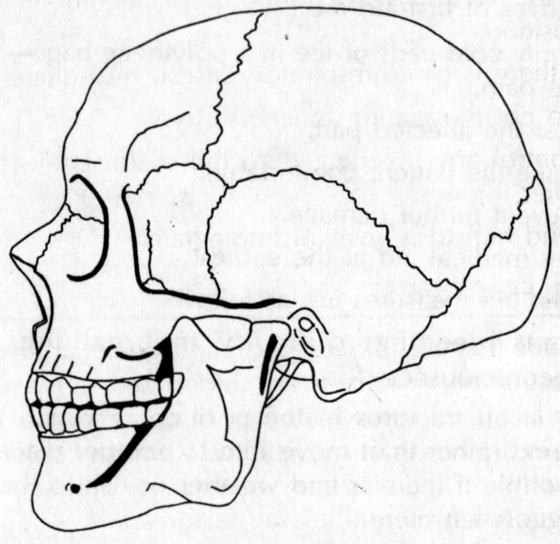

The skull is a closed box made of many bones that are united by immovable joints. It protects the brain. It can be fractured by a direct blow or trauma e.g. falling from a height, landing on the feet. Direct trauma usually fractures the vault of the skull, while indirect trauma fractures the base of the skull and causes injury to the vertebral column. Fracture of the skull is a very serious injury, because it may be associated with brain damage. The brain can be bruised. Or there may be bleeding outside the brain, and the hematoma compresses the brain. The fracture may be linear, depressed, or comminuted. The condition is diagnosed by the following features.

1. There is often a would on the scalp in case of direct trauma to the head.
2. Cerebrospinal fluid may be found leaking from the ear or nose, as clear fluid or watery blood.
3. Unconsciousness that lasts for more than three minutes is suggestive of a fracture of the skull.
4. There is a soft, boggy area or depression under the scalp at the site of the fracture.
5. Features of brain injury are seen, e.g. paralysis, altered sensorium, irritability and convulsions.

First-aid

1. If the victim is unconscious, place him in the recovery position.
2. If there is cardiorespiratory arrest, resuscitate him.
3. Do not move him unnecessarily.
4. Control any bleeding from the scalp. Look for, and treat, other injuries.
5. Send him to a hospital immediately.

❐ FACIAL FRACTURES

These include fractures of the nose, cheekbones or jaw. The airway may be obstructed by loose teeth, blood and saliva, or displaced, swollen or lacerated tissue. Absence or depression of cough reflex may result in aspiration of regurgitated stomach contents into lungs causing asphyxia. Bleeding may be profuse. Fracture of the lower jaw is diagnosed by the following features.

1. There is difficulty in opening mouth and speaking. Attempts at that increase pain.
2. Blood stained spit is present.
3. Irregularity may be felt along the underside of jaw.
4. Irregularity of the teeth alignment may be present.
5. There may be a wound inside the mouth.

First-aid

1. Ensure clear airway to maintain breathing.
2. Make a conscious patient sit up with head well forward to permit drainage of blood and secretions.
3. Clean the mouth.
4. Press the lower jaw upward against the upper jaw with your hand on the chin. Apply a lower jaw bandage.
5. Shift him to a hospital immediately.

❐ FRACTURE OF NASAL BONE

It is due to direct trauma to the nose. It is diagnosed by the presence of bleeding from nose, difficulty in breathing due to airway obstruction.

First-air

1. Treat as for nasal bleeding.
2. Clear the airway.
3. Apply a cold compress locally.
4. Shift him to a hospital immediately.

❐ FRACTURE OF COLLARBONE

The clavicle fractures due to fall on the outstretched hand or on the tip of the shoulder. It is diagnosed by the presence of the following features.

1. Pain and tenderness at the site of injury increased by movement of the upper limb.
2. Reluctance of the victim to move the limb on the injured side.
3. He may be found to be supporting the arm on the injured side at the elbow to relieve pain.

First-aid

1. Place the victim in sitting position, with the limb on the injured side across the chest, the fingertips reaching the opposite shoulder.
2. Place a pad of gauze or cloth between the arm and chest on that side.
3. Support the limb in an elevation sling .
4. Shift him to a hospital.

❐ FRACTURE OF ARM

It is caused by a direct blow but it is much more common, especially in the elderly. It is a stable injury. Hence the victim may walk around for sometime before reporting to a doctor for treatment. It is a difficult fracture to treat as the muscles produce overlapping of ends that are broken and angulation. The condition is diagnosed by the following features.

1. There is pain, increased by movement.
2. Swelling develops rapidly. Bruising may develop more slowly.
3. There is local tenderness, increased by movement.

First-aid

1. Place the victim in sitting position. Place the injured arm across his chest gently, if it is possible to do so.
2. Place soft padding between the arm and chest, and tie a broad-fold bandage around the chest over the sling.
3. Shift him to a hospital immediately.

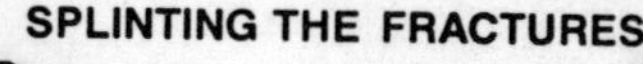

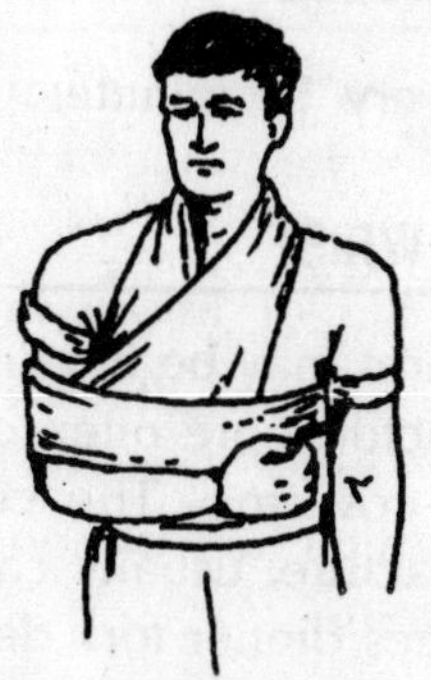

Arm splinting

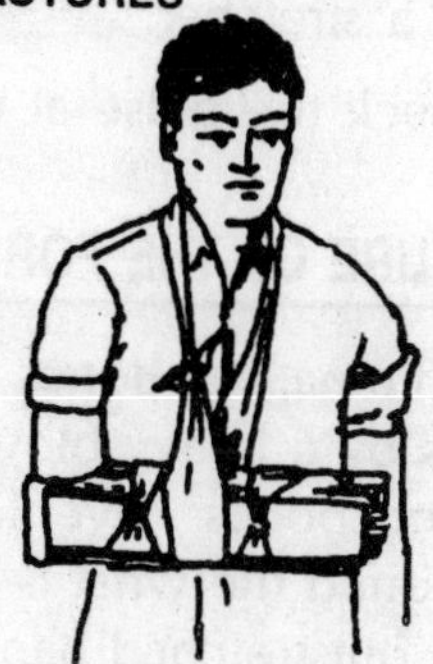

Splinting forearm

❐ FRACTURE OF ELBOW JOINT

These are quite common, resulting from a fall on the outstretched hand. This is an unstable injury. The broken ends of bone may move and damage surrounding blood vessels and nerves. The condition is diagnosed by the following features.

1. There is pain in the elbow, increased by movement.
2. There is tenderness over the site of the fracture.
3. If the head of radius is fractured, the elbow is stiff and it cannot be fully straightened.
4. Circulation in the forearm and hand may be impaired due to vascular injury.
5. There may be anesthesia and motor weakness in the hand due to injury to the nerves.
6. Swelling and bruising may be present.

First-aid

1. If the elbow can be bent, strap arm to the chest and support the forearm in a triangular sling.

2. If the elbow cannot be bent, place the victim in supine position. Place the injured limb by the side of the trunk. Do not attempt to bend the elbow forcibly. Place a soft padding between the injured limb and the body. Tie the injured limb to the body by three broad bandages over the wrist and thighs, around the forearm and trunk, and around the upper arm and trunk. Shift him to a hospital immediately on a stretcher.
3. Check the pulse at the wrist every 10 minutes.

❐ FRACTURE OF THE FOREARM AND WRIST

Radius and ulna, the bones of the forearm may be fractured across their shafts by a heavy blow. These fractures are often compound because the bones have little fleshy covering. The commonest fracture around the wrist is a Colles' fracture, usually caused by a fall on the outstretched hand. It produces dinner fork deformity of the forearm and hand.

First-aid

1. Place the forearm at right angles to the upper arm, and place it across the chest, the palm over the chest and the thumb facing upwards.
2. Roll a magazine or folded newspaper around the forearm and hand.
3. Apply one bandage above the fracture and the other over the wrist.
4 Support the limb by a broad arm sling.

❐ FRACTURES OF THE HAND AND FINGERS

The hand is made up of many small bones with movable joints, which may be injured by direct or indirect trauma. Crush injuries cause multiple fractures in the hand. A fracture of the knuckle between the little finger and the hand may occur due to a misplaced punch. There may be severe bleeding and swelling. Sprains and dislocation may affect any fingers. The thumb is particularly prone to dislocation caused by a fall on to the hand.

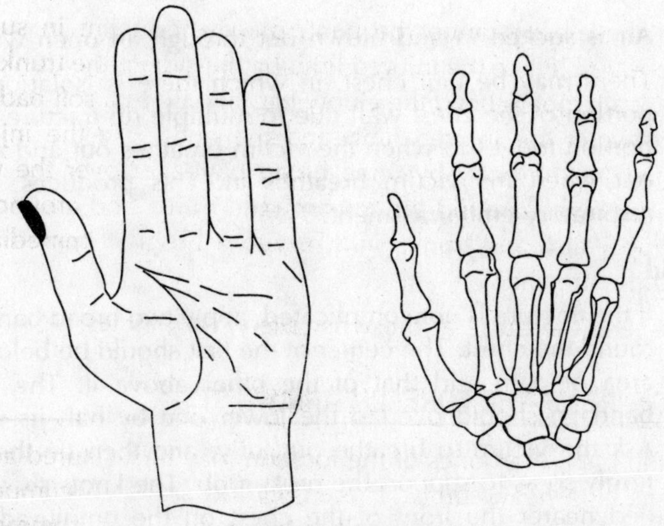

Hand and Figures

First-aid

1. Control bleeding and treat any wounds.
2. Support the affected limb in an elevation sling. Give additional support by applying a broad bandage over the sling. Tie the knot in front of the uninjured side.
3. Shift him to a hospital in sitting position.

❐ FRACTURE OF RIB

Rib fractures may be caused by direct force (a blow, vehicular accidents, or fall on the chest) or by indirect force e.g. compression of the chest from the front and back simultaneously. The condition is diagnosed by the following features.

1. There is pain at the injured area, increased on deep breathing and coughing.
2. The victim takes short and shallow breaths so that the ribs do not move and increase the pain.
3. Crepitus is usually felt.
4. There may be signs of internal bleeding.
5. The patient may be asphyxiated due to entry of air in the pleural cavity from injured lung. He may collapse.

6. Air is sucked in and blown out through an open wound.
7. There may be flail chest, in which there is isolation of a portion of the chest wall due to multiple rib fractures. This portion moves in when the victim breathes out and moves out when the victim breathes in. This produces severe respiratory embarrassment.

First-Aid

1. If the fracture is not complicated, apply two broad bandages round the chest. The center of the first should be below the area of pain and that of the other above it. The upper bandage should overlap the lower one by half its width. Ask the victim to breathe out fully, and then tie the knot firmly so as to support the broken rib. The knots should be tied nearer the front of the chest on the uninjured side. Support the arm on the side of injury in a sling. Shift him to a hospital immediately.
2. If the fracture is complicated, do not apply bandages, except in cases where air is sucked in through an open wound, in the chest. Place the patient with his head and shoulders raised, and turned towards the injured side. Apply sling to the arm in the injured side. Shift him to hospital immediately on a stretcher.

❑ FRACTURE OF SPINE

The spine (vertebral column) is made up of a number of small bones called a vertebrae arranged one above another. The spine is supported by many strong ligaments and the muscles of the trunk. It protects the spinal cord contained within it. The spinal cord is delicate and if damaged, loss of sensation or power can occur in parts of the body below the injured area, e.g. upper limbs, lower limbs. Permanent damage will result if the cord is partially or completely transected.

Fractures of the vertebrae can be caused by both direct and indirect force. Neck and lower back are two areas in spinal column most vulnerable to injuries. If there is a violent forward bending, a backward bending, or a twisting injury of the spine, it is likely to get fractured. Causes of spinal injury are as follows.

1. Awkward fall in gymnastics.
2. Diving into a shallow pool.
3. Fall from a height.
4. Fall from a horse or a motor cycle.
5. Fall of a heavy object on the back e.g. roof-fall.
6. Head-on crash of a motor vehicle.
7. Trauma to the head or face.
8. Whiplash injury.
9. Jarring of spine by a fall on the feet, buttocks or head from a height.

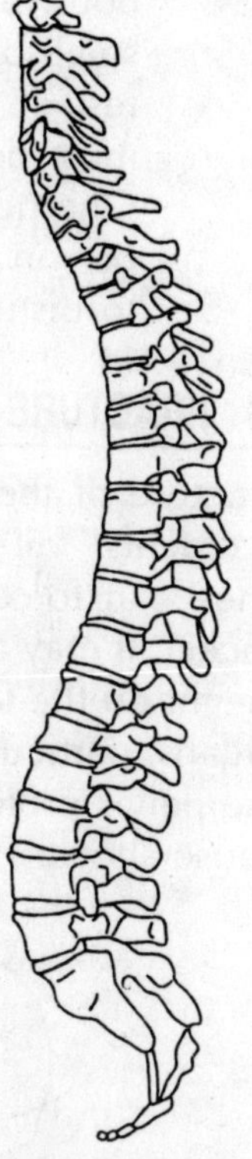

Spinal Column/ Vertibrae

The condition is diagnosed by the following features.

1. Severe pain in back.
2. Irregularity may be felt over the spine.
3. Tenderness on gently feeling the spine.

Features of injury to the spinal cord.

- Loss of sensation of skin below the level of injury.
- Loss of control over limbs.
- Abnormal sensations : tingling or burning, limbs feel heavy, stiff, or clumsy.
- Difficulty in breathing.

First-aid

1. Do not move the victim. Support his head in neutral position.
2. Instruct the victim not to move.
3. In case of suspicion of neck injury, place rolled blankets or other articles around the neck and shoulders to steady the neck and prevent its movement.
4. Shift him to a hospital immediately. Transport on a rigid stretcher with face upwards. The canvas stretcher must be made hard surfaced by short boards placed across the stretcher or a long board itself may be used if a stretcher is

not available. Place small pillows under the neck and the small of the back so that the hollow of neck and the back rest in the normai position. The position of the casualty must not be disturbed when loading on to the stretcher. One person must hold the head firmly but gently. Another person must hold the legs just above the ankles so as not to disturb the trunk.

❐ FRACTURE OF PELVIS

Fracture of the pelvis is mostly due to a direct force, e.g. crush accidents, fall of beams. The impact of a car dashboard on a knee can force out the head of the thigh bone through the hip socket. If may also be due to an indirect force, e.g. fall from a great height on the feet. These may be complicated by injury to internal organs, particularly the urinary bladder and urinary passage which the pelvis protects. Internal hemorrhage may be severe enough to cause shock.

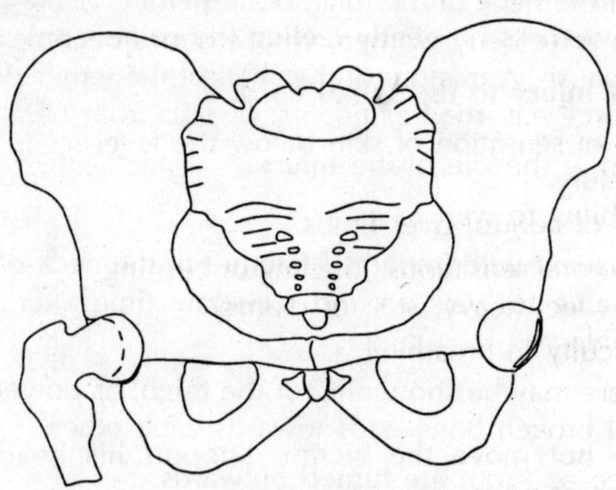

Structure of Pelvis

The condition is diagnosed by the following features.

1. Pain and tenderness in the region of the hip, groin, and/or back, aggravated by movements.
2. Inability to walk or even stand, although the legs appear normal.
3. Difficulty in passing urine.

4. Blood in urine.
5. Signs of internal bleeding and shock.

First-aid

1. Place the victim on the back with legs straight. The knees may be bent a little and a rolled blanket may be placed underneath them if the victim finds that more comfortable.
2. Treat shock, if present.
3. Ask him not to attempt to pass urine.
4. Immobilize his legs by bandaging them together, placing padding between the bony points. But if that causes severe pain, untie them.
5. Shift him to a hospital on a stretcher in the most comfortable position.

❒ FRACTURE OF THIGH BONE

Fractures of the neck of the thigh bone (femur) at the hip joint are common in the elderly women, whose bones become more brittle after menopause. A fracture of the shaft of the femur develops due to severe force e.g. road accidents, or falls from heights.

1. Pain at the site of the injury.
2. Inability to walk.
3. A patient with impacted fracture of the neck of femur may be able to walk around for some time after the fracture develops.
4. There may be shortening of the thigh, as powerful muscles pull broken bone ends towards each other.
5. Knee and foot are turned outwards.
6. Signs of shock may be present.

First-aid

1. Treat shock. Do not raise the legs.
2. Immobilize the thigh by bandaging it to the sound limb up to below the knee. Alternatively a well-padded splint may be applied between the legs from the groin to the foot. Insert padding between the thighs, knees, and ankles. Tie

the feet and ankles to the splint with a figure of eight bandage.

3. Apply a long well-padded splint from axilla to foot, tying 7 bandages at chest, below the arm pits, pelvis, hip joints, thigh, and ankles.
4. Shift him to a hospital immediately.
5. If the victim has to be transported over a long distance, a sturdier support is needed for the leg. A femoral traction splint e.g. Thomas' splint, is ideal. But it can be used only by trained personnel. During transport, keep the foot of the stretcher raised to minimize swelling and shock.

❑ FRACTURE OF THE KNEE JOINT

The knee joint is supported by strong ligaments and muscles. The knee cap lies in front of it. Any of these structures may be injured by direct blow, strain, or violent twist. The condition is diagnosed by the following features.

1. History of a recent trauma to the knee.
2. Pain in the knee joint.
3. Acute pain on attempting to straighten a bent, locked knee.
4. Rapid swelling of the knee joint.

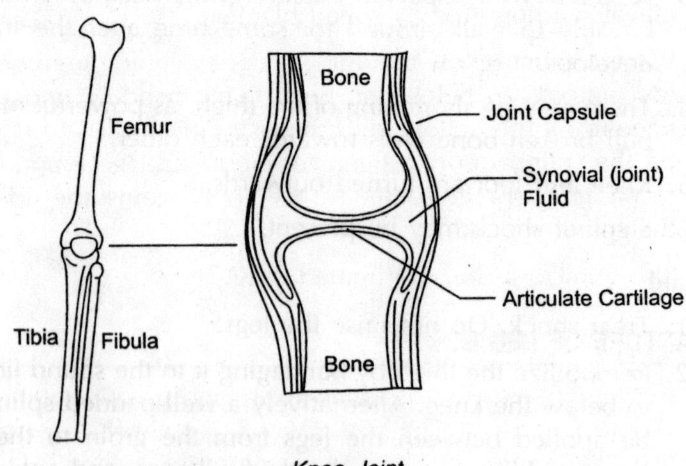

Knee Joint

First-aid

1. Place the victim in supine position, with the knee and leg in the most comfortable position.
2. Bandage a soft padding around the knee.
3. Shift him to a hospital immediately on a stretcher.
4. Do not let the victim walk.
5. Do not attempt to force the knee straight.
6. Do not give the victim anything to eat or drink.

❐ FRACTURE OF KNEE CAP (PATELLA)

It is a small bone in front of the knee joint. It forms the point of attachment of the large muscles of the thigh. It may be fractured from direct blow or as a result of muscular pull. The condition is diagnosed by the following features.

1. Pain on the front of the knee joint.
2. Tenderness at knee.
3. Loss of movements at knee joint.
4. Swelling and bruising at knee.
5. Crepitus over the patella.

First-aid

1. Place the casualty on the back with the head and shoulders elevated, supported by rolled blankets.
2. Place a splint below the injured leg, extending from below the buttocks to below the heel. Place padding under the knee to fill the hollow, and under the heel so as to raise it off the splint. Apply a figure of eight bandage around the ankle, foot and the splint. Tie the knots against the sides of the splint.
3. Shift him to a hospital immediately.

❐ FRACTURE OF LEG BONES

One of the leg bones (tibia) is quite sturdy and usually requires a heavy blow to fracture it. The other (fibula) is thinner and can be broken by twisting force, as during twisting of the ankle. Since the weight-bearing is done by the tibia, a fracture of the fibula does not cause much problem for the victim. The condition is diagnosed by the following features.

1. There is pain in the leg.
2. Swelling and bruising are seen at the site of the fracture.
3. Angulation and twisting of the leg may be present at the site of the fracture.

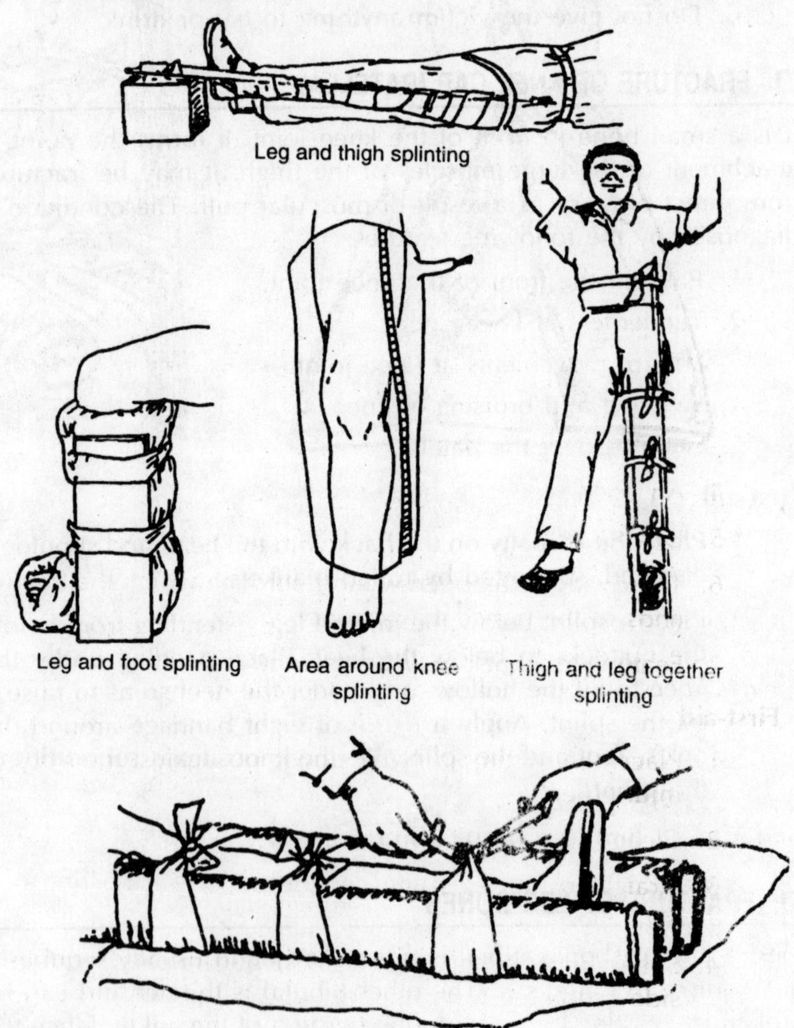

Leg and thigh splinting

Leg and foot splinting

Area around knee splinting

Thigh and leg together splinting

For leg splinting

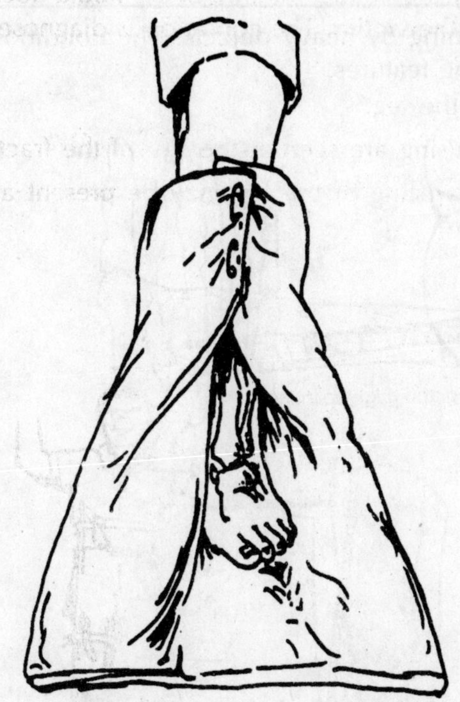

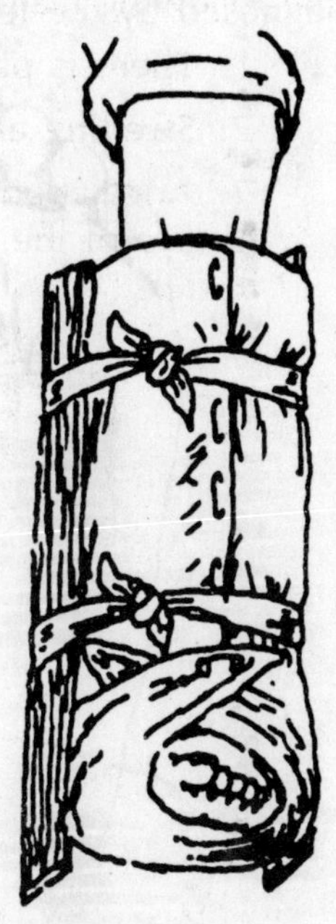

4. An open wound is often present.
5. Unable to walk.
6. There may be an open wound, through which the fractured ends of the bones may project.
7. Features of shock may be present.

First-aid

1. Place the victim in lying down position, supporting the injured leg.
2. Clean and dress the wound.
3. Straighten the leg using gentle traction in the line of the leg.
4. Splint the leg to the other leg. Place extra padding on either side of the leg from upper thigh to the foot.
5. Shift him to a hospital immediately.

❐ FRACTURE OF THE BONES OF THE FOOT

This is due to direct crushing by heavy objects. The condition is diagnosed by the following features.

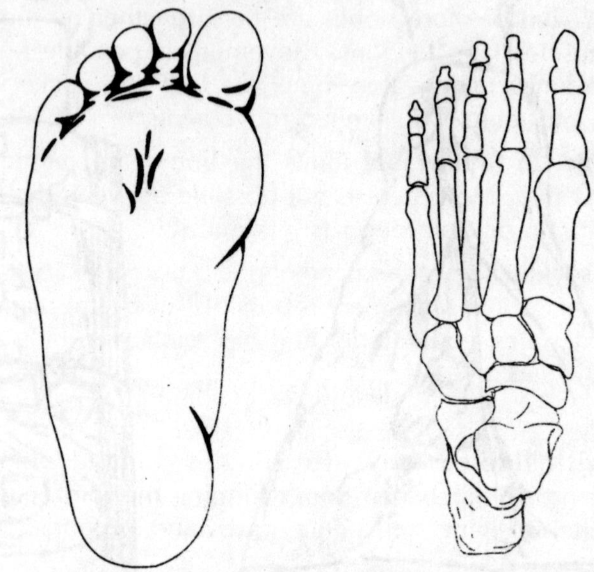

Structure of Foot

1. There is pain in the foot increased by movement.
2. Loss of movement.
3. There is an inability to walk properly.
4. Swelling and bruising are seen at the site of the fracture.
5. Tenderness is present at the site of the fracture.
6. Deformity may be present, e.g. irregularity of the bony arch of the foot.

First-aid

1. Place the victim down in supine position.
2. Gently remove footwear.
3. Control bleeding, if any.
4. Dress wounds, if any.
5. Place a splint on the sole of the foot with adequate padding. Secure is with a figure of eight bandage.
6. Raise and support the injured foot.

❐ INJURIES OF THE JOINTS

A joint is the junction of two or more bones.

Types of Joints

Movable. Two or more bones are held together by means of ligaments, muscles, and tendons. Movement is possible between bones. Three kinds of movable joints are ball and socket joints, hinge joints, and joints with limited movements.

Immovable. In immovable joints the bones are permanently fixed to each other. Movement is not possible between the bones. Chances of sprain or dislocation is minimal.

Ball and socket. The round head of one bone fits in cup-shaped cavity of another bone. Movement is possible in several planes and directions. Examples are shoulder and hip joints.

Hinge. Movement is possible only in one plane, e.g. elbow and knee jóints.

Joints with limited movements. Only limited degree of movement is possible between bones forming the joint, e.g. wrist joint, intervertebral joints and joints of ribs and vertebrae.

Ligaments are tough fibrous structures that bind bones to one another at joints. The remaining part of a joint is covered by fibrous joint capsule. The ends of bones forming the joint are covered by smooth articular cartilage. The joint cavity is lined by smooth membrane (synovial membrane) and filled with lubricating fluid (synovial fluid).

❐ SPRAIN

Sprain is an injury to the ligament(s) and the joint capsule. It is due to sudden movement or twisting of the part involving joint. Ankle is the most commonly sprained joint. The condition is diagnosed by the following features.

1. There is severe pain locally, aggravated by movement at the joint.
2. Bruising and swelling are present around the joint.
3. Local tenderness is present.

❐ DISLOCATION

This is a more severe injury than a sprain. It occurs when a strong force acts directly or indirectly on a joint pulling a bone into an abnormal position. It can occur as a result of sudden muscular contraction too. There is displacement of one or more bones at a joint. There is also tearing of ligaments, joint capsule, and tissues around the joint. Shoulder and hip joints are commonly involved in adults, while elbow, finger, and lower jaw joints are more commonly involved in children. The condition is diagnosed by the following features.

1. There is severe pain at or near the joint.
2. Deformity is seen.
3. Swelling of the joint and late bruising around the joint.
4. There is immobility of the joint.
5. It may be associated with a fracture.

First-aid

1. Place the victim down in supine position.
2. Do not try to reduce the dislocation.
3. Do not give him anything orally.
4. Apply a sling in case of hands.
5. Shift him to a hospital immediately. Use a stretcher in case of dislocation in the lower limb.

❐ DISLOCATION OF SHOULDER

It is caused by a fall on the shoulder or a wrenching force to the upper limb. The condition is diagnosed by the following features.

1. There is severe pain in the shoulder joint.
2. The victim is reluctant to move the upper limb because of the pain. He casually often supports the limb at the elbow by the other hand, and tilts his head on that side.
3. The shoulder appears flat and angular.

First-aid

1. Place the victim is sitting position.
2. Place the affected limb across his chest in a position of minimum pain.
3. Place soft padding between the arm and the chest.

4. Do not try to reduce the dislocation.
5. Do not give him anything orally.
6. Shift him to a hospital immediately.

❐ BACK SPRAIN

The neck and lower back are the most common sites of ligament sprain or muscle strain. They can be caused by prolonged bending forwards. Neck sprain may be caused by the whiplash effect produced in a car accident. The condition is diagnosed by the following features.

1. There is pain in the back or neck, increased by movement.
2. There is spasm of the muscles of the neck or back.
3. Tingling and numbness of the upper limbs may be present due to involvement of nerves supplying them.

First-aid

1. Place the victim in supine position.
2. Ask him not to move the head.
3. Shift him to hospital if the pain does not go away with analgesics and rest.
4. A collar may be applied around the neck to support it.

❐ PROLAPSED INTERVERTEBRAL DISC (SLIPPED DISC)

This occurs when a part of cartilage which separates adjacent vertebrae protrudes backwards into the spinal column. It causes compression of the spinal cord and/or spinal nerve roots. The condition is diagnosed by the following features.

1. There is a sudden, severe pain in the back that may radiate towards the legs.
2. It may be aggravated by movements.
3. There may be tingling and numbness in the limbs, below the level of the disc protrusion.
4. There may be motor paralysis below the level of the disc prolapse.

First-aid

1. Place the casualty flat on a firm surface in the most comfortable position.
2. Shift him to a hospital immediately.

CHAPTER

24

Foreign Bodies Must Be Removed

❐ FOREIGN BODIES IN THE SKIN

Small foreign bodies like shards of glass and wood splinters usually cause small puncture wounds with little or no bleeding. But they are quite painful. Hence they have to be removed early. If a portion of the foreign body is found to be sticking out of the skin, it can be grasped with nails or a small forceps and pulled out. If it is deeply embedded in a wound, attempts at its removal may drive it deeper into the tissues. Such patients should be sent to a doctor. Foreign bodies are often contaminated with dirt and can cause infections including tetanus.

First-Aid

1. Reassure the victim.
2. Clean the area around the foreign body with an antiseptic solution gently, without driving the foreign body into deeper tissues.
3. Pull the foreign body out, if its end is found to be projecting outside the skin surface.
4. Squeeze around the wound to cause loss of a little amount of blood, which drives out dirt too.
5. Put a dressing over the wound.
6. If it is deep, send him to a doctor immediately.
7. Removal of a fish hook from the skin is difficult. It gets driven in further if an attempt is made to just pull it out. Its projecting portion has to be cut before pulling out the rest of the hood. There is no urgency of removing it. The victim should be sent to a doctor for removal of the hook.

❒ FOREIGN BODIES IN THE EAR

Foreign bodies can enter the ear either accidentally (insects) or may be inserted by children during play (peas, buttons, pencils, pins etc.) The condition is diagnosed by the following features.

1. History of insertion of the foreign body may or may not be available. A child may not admit it due to fear.
2. There is pain in the ear.
3. There may be discharge from the ear.
4. On inspection of the ear using a torch light for illumination, the foreign body may be seen in the ear canal.

First-aid

1. Do not try to hook out the foreign body with a hook or any other object, as it may damage the ear drum.
2. If there is an insect in the ear, put olive oil or 2% sodium bicarbonate solution in lukewarm water into the ear.
3. Send him to a doctor's clinic.

❒ FOREIGN BODIES IN THE EYE

Foreign bodies can enter the eye accidentally when there is a strong wind blowing or when one is traveling without protection to the eye, e.g. on a motor cycle. Various foreign bodies that can enter the eye are dust, sand particles, coal particles, small pieces of glass, etc. They are either under the eyelids or in the eyeball. The condition is diagnosed by the following features.

1. History of sudden onset of acute pain in the eye is available.
2. The eye is angry red.
3. There is profuse watering of the eye.
4. On examining the eye by gently retracting the eyelids, the foreign body may be seen in the eye.

First-aid

1. Tell the victim not to rub the eye as that may cause further damage to the eye by the foreign body.
2. Remove a foreign body under the eyelid with the pointed end of a soft handkerchief or a piece of cotton. It is necessary

to wash the hands well before removing the foreign body. An alternative method is to wash the eye with clean water.

3. Pad the eye and send him to a doctor.
4. Shift him to a hospital immediately.
5. Do not try to remove a foreign body on the surface of the eyeball, especially the cornea, as it may cause corneal abrasions, which later get converted into corneal opacities that impair vision.

❒ FOREIGN BODIES IN THE NOSE

A child may insert a foreign body like a seed or a piece of pencil into the nose either accidentally or during play. When it tries to remove it, it gets driven in further. Foreign bodies like seeds absorb water and swell up. Then their removal becomes even more difficult. The condition is diagnosed by the following features.

1. History of insertion of the foreign body may or may not be available. A child may not admit it due to fear.
2. There is pain in the nose.
3. There may be discharge from the nose.
4. On examination of the nose under illumination (by torch etc.) the foreign body may be seem.

First-aid

1. Instruct the victim not to try to sneeze or blow air out of the nose to expel the foreign body.
2. If the end of the foreign body is found sticking out of the nose, grab it and pull it out gently.
3 Shift all other cases to a hospital.

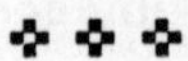

CHAPTER

25

Emergency Medical Aid from Your Kitchen Shelf and Garden : A Boon

This section is particularly useful for the person at home who may not have a handy first-aid kit and wants to give immediate succor and help to a person in distress, since medical aid is not always within reach. To begin with the basic. The first requirement is clean water, whether for drinking, cooking or other domestic purposes. In villages, and often in city homes too, the water we get is not always clean or chlorinated, or at times is downright muddy. The age-old remedy for purifying water was to collect it in a clean container, filtering it through a muslin cloth. The container was often and still is of a particular shape — the *ghara*.

After water is collected the top surface is touched with a 2" piece of *'Alum'* or *'phitkari'* as it is referred to in simple language. This reacts with the ions on the top surface and starts a process by which impurities get precipitated and settle at the bottom. Most of these are organic in nature, but some inorganic ones settle down too. This water is allowed to stand for four to six hours and then the upper clear water is either taken out mug by mug or the whole container tilted and the water collected in another container. The lower part with the impurities gets left behind due to the particular shape of the container. Do not be over enthusiastic and put too much alum, as it changes the taste making it unpalatable and also unfit for making tea, etc.

Another remedy is the use of drumstick seeds. If there is a drumstick tree in your courtyard, collect the seeds and dry them completely. Powder and store. Add a heaped tablespoon of this powder to a bucket full of water and keep aside for two hours. It gets rid of a particularly trouble some pathogen E. Coli responsible for gastrointestinal and urinary tract infections. Recent studies done in Africa and Indonesia show the efficacy to be 98.1% !!

❐ FOLLOWING ARE SOME SPECIFIC REMEDIES FOR SHORT TERM USE FOR SOME COMMON DAY TO DAY CONDITIONS. (INGREDIENTS FOUND IN INDIAN KITCHENS)

Only one treatment should be adopted at any given time. Do not try all of them on a single condition. Depending on the availability try what you will be able to do comfortably, and correctly with least distress to the patient.

When boiling any ingredients for longer periods to get a decoction or soup, avoid using aluminum utensils. A steel or tefal coated vessel or a borosil dish is the best. Even in villages people use steel vessels or silver foil coated vessel.

Juice should be made from freshly washed ingredients chopped into small pieces and either crushed or put through a liquidizer and then strained. A decoction can be made from fresh or dry ingredients by first chopping them into small pieces and crushing them. Half a cupful of this crushed ingredient should then be boiled in four to five times the water and reduced to a quarter. Strain or filter and use. Herbal teas are made by putting the crushed ingredients 1-1½ teaspoon into 2 cups of water and reducing to 1½ cup. For an infusion, soak a cup full of fresh crushed ingredients in 4 cups of hot water. Let it cool to room temperature and then use. Pastes can be made by grinding with a little water, milk or oil as specified. As far as possible, everything should be made just before use unless specified. For children use half the doses specified and for infants a quarter of the adult dose.

❐ ABDOMINAL COMPLAINTS

1. Pain/flatulence/indigestion, etc.

Ajwain : Spasmodic pain in the abdomen related to diarrhoea, dysentery, indigestion, colic, and flatulence gets a measure of relief by eating ajwain. Half to one teaspoon can be ingested with half a glass of warm water. For those who find swallowing this difficult, a decoction can be made by boiling one teaspoon ajwain in a cup of water for five to six minutes. Basically it has a carminative action and helps expel gas from the digestive tract.

Ajwain mixed with dry ginger called *'sonth'* and black salt in a ratio of 1 teaspoon + $\frac{1}{2}$ teaspoon + $\frac{1}{4}$ teaspoon divided into 4-5 doses, taken three times a day with warm water is a good temporary measure for colic. For infants and children this could be boiled in water and a teaspoon of the boiled water given.

Boiled water

Infants	$\frac{1}{2}$ tsp (liquid)	3-4 times a day	(Powder should be less than a pinch)
Children	1 to 2-3 tsp (liquid)	3 times a day	(Powder should be just a pinchful)

Carminative mixture	Coriander seeds	(Dhania)
	Fennel seeds or Aniseed	(Saunf)
	Carom seeds	(Ajwain)
	Cumin seeds	(Jeera)
	Caraway	(Sha jeera)

Half teaspoon of each of the above, boiled together in a cup full of water, made like tea with a little plain milk or sipped after a particularly heavy meal relieves the feeling of indigestion. This is also good for flatulence.

Mint or *pudina tea* or *chutney* made only from its leaves is good for indigestion.

Basil or *tulsi leaves boiled* in water or had as a herbal tea is good for hyperacidity, heart burn, etc.

2. Nausea and vomiting

Add a teaspoon of freshly grated *ginger* to a cup of boiling water. Keep aside for five to six minutes. Strain and add sugar to taste. Sip this frequently. Relieves nausea or vomiting during pregnancy, travel sickness, and indigestion.

Keeping a *clove* in the mouth also gives relief. Drink water in which cloves have been soaked.

Nausea

Cumin seeds/Jeera : Grind them, add a little *lime* and salt to taste. Take a quarter teaspoon a couple of times a day. Relieves nausea and vomiting.

Curry leaves (karhi patta) boiled in water or *butter milk* with a pinch of salt to taste relieves the distress of indigestion, biliousness.

3. Diarrhoea

Diarrhoea is one condition which should never be neglected. Dehydration sets in insidiously. All cases of diarrhoea with or without vomiting must have the lost fluid replaced.

Acacia or *babul* leaves : This tree is also called the kikar tree and grows all over the country in towns and villages. A handful of tender leaves boiled with one teaspoon of *cumin* seeds, made into a tea can be had to replace lost fluids. Helps in relief of watery diarrhoea. This has an astringent action and helps reabsorb water being lost.

Stone apple or *bael* is another fruit free found growing all over the country. This fruit can be eaten half ripe or unripe. (The ripe fruit is useful to relieve constipation). The unripe fruit has an astringent taste. It can be sliced or baked and its pulp mixed with *Jaggery* or sugar and had as *buttermilk* or water beverage. It stimulates the appetite and relieves the discomfort of indigestion. A decoction can also be made by boiling the half-ripe or unripe fruit in a glass of water.

Nutmeg or *jaiphal* can be grated or quarter to half teaspoon of the powder mixed with mashed banana is a good remedy for indigestion/diarrhoea. Infants can be given a bit of the liquid with a little water (not more than half teaspoon). This will have just a few strands of *nutmeg.* This has sedative properties and so relieves stomach cramps and colic in infants, but too much can have adverse effects of addiction and other problems.

One tablespoon of Isabgol *husk* with half a cup of curd is good for constipation.

Barley water (jau), *arrowroot, rice* and *oats* can also be cooked as thin gruels or broth to be given as nutrition when a person cannot retain solids. A few slices of *onion* or *onion leaves* can be boiled with the gruel but then fished out. *Buttermilk* or *fresh yogurt* is a time honoured remedy.

Other remedies are :

- Grind to a paste and boil fresh, tender *guava leaves.* Strain this and give a couple of teaspoons thrice a day.

- Tender fresh *pomegranate seeds* ground and mixed with *curd* or *buttermilk* help control indigestion, diarrhoea and dysentery. Make a powder from the fruit skin. Two teaspoons with fresh buttermilk three times a day for five days or its fruit juice (60 ml or a quarter cup) three or four times a day can be given. Even the flowers and tender leaves of the plant can be used. Make a paste of these with a few drops of water, and take a couple of teaspoons thrice a day.
- Boil and strain a handful of bits of *neem* bark in one glass of water for 10-15 minutes. A cup full of this water should be taken twice a day for three days.

❐ CONSTIPATION

- Drinking plenty of water during the day ensures regular bowel movements. More specifically, a glass of water at bedtime and on getting out of bed, a brisk walk in the garden or walking around in the house helps peristaltic movements.
- Regular intake of ripe fruits like *ripe bael, apricots, guava, papaya, grapes, dates, bananas* are good for the digestion.
- *Anwla* chutneys, or murabas (jelly/jam).
- Dried *prunes* with hot milk.
- *Hot milk* with *honey* at bedtime.
- *Sat Isabgol* (2 tablespoons) or *wheat bran* (4 tablespoons) with hot milk.
- Have plenty of green leafy vegetables specially *spinach, cooked bathua* or *raw spinach juice, beetroot, lettuce* and *raw cabbage salad.*
- Six teaspoons of fresh raw *chulai ka sag* with *Jaggery* taken with warm water at bedtime is a sure remedy.
- Powder *liquorice* (*mullethi/jastimudh*). Half a teaspoon mixed with *jaggery* or sugar, to be had with warm water.
- *Tamarind* pulp mixed with *dates* (1 oz each) taken with water or a glass of hot *milk*. It is difficult to drink but is a popular household remedy in the south.

❐ INDIGESTION

A teaspoon of fresh *ginger* juice, a teaspoon of fresh *lemon* juice, a pinch of salt taken after meals twice daily for a week or chewing on a small piece of ginger with salt before meals helps.

❐ ULCERS IN THE MOUTH

- Local application of *glycerine* on ulcers causes intense salivation and gives relief from pain.
- Gargles with *alum* water (2-3 grams to a cup of water) removes soreness.
- *Catechu* or *katha* powder found in Indian homes as an ingredient for *paan* or *betel* leaf preparation — a paste made with a few drops of water and applied locally soothes the ulcer.
- If there is a *banyan* tree in your garden, grind a little piece of the bark with few drops of water or break a leaf/stem and apply a drop of the sap and then gargle with fresh water. It relieves the pain.
- A few drops of raw *papaya* juice applied on the ulcer surface digests the inflamed mucous membrane and heals. Just a drop or two mixed with a little milk should be used twice or thrice a day for a maximum of two days.
- A paste of *fresh guava* leaves can be applied on the ulcer for two to three minutes and then gargling, leaves a soothe coat on the ulcer which masks pain. If a few fresh, tender guava leaves are chewed before taking your meal these coat the ulcer and eating food does not cause pain or burning of the ulcer.

❐ FEVER

The following remedies may be tried for a fever.

- *Tulsi* (basil) tea with cardamom, milk and sugar to taste.
- *Tamarind* extract made into a sherbet with *dates, cardamom* and *sugar*. Can be had 3-4 times a day.
- *Black pepper, tulsi leaves* and *dried ginger* can be brewed as a *weak* tea. Sweeten with sugar. Useful in seasonal fevers.

- A tea made with *methi* (fenugreek) seeds.
- *Lemon grass* tea.
- *Bael* fruit sherbet.
- *Neem, cinnamon* and *clove* tea.
- *Conjee* — rice water with *lime* juice and sugar.
- A teaspoon of fresh *turmeric* powder in a cup of hot *milk* thrice a day for 5-7 days in case of seasonal cold with fever.
- A teaspoon of *turmeric powder* in a cup of *hot milk* taken thrice a day brings down fever due to seasonal colds and changes of weather.
- Fever due to exertion, heavy manual labour or heat can be brought down by drinking water prepared by soaking four to five *Hibiscus* flowers in a glass of cold water (only the five petal shoe flower variety). It is soothing and cooling.
- Application of cool *sandalwood* paste on the forehead is soothing and helps bring down fever.

❐ COUGHS, COLDS, SORE THROAT, ASTHMA AND BRONCHITIS

- All the *herbal* teas mentioned earlier are helpful in chest conditions especially *ajwain* tea.
- *Tulsi* tea with or without *pepper,* or with a pinch of *ground cloves* and a stick of cinnamon.
- Tea made with *methi seeds* and *amla* leaves.
- *Liquorice* can be used as a lozenge.
- Fresh juice
  — *red cabbage*
  — *grape fruit*
  — *Carrot juice*
- *Raw cabbage,* its juice, or even cooked is excellent for asthma. As soon as a chronic asthmatic feels the asthma coming up, he should eat raw cabbage or have its juice.

- Fresh *garlic* eaten raw or in food.
- Make a decoction with *barley, honey* and *lemon* and grind to a paste.
- Steam inhalations thrice a day.
- Apply *eucalyptus* oil with normal bath massage oil on chest.
- Large dried grapes called *munakha* (the seedless variety) — one or two slowly chewed relieves a coughing bout and chronic asthmatic wheeze. In the case of chronic asthmatics this remedy should be continued for 2-3 months. The raisins are slowly chewed throughout the day. It gets a bit irritating to do it 3-4 times a day.
- Hot *milk* with some pure ground *turmeric.* One glass milk, with one level teaspoon of turmeric powder and sugar added to taste is a soothing cough relieving drink specially at night.
- *Black pepper, cloves,* and dried *ginger* all can be ground separately and a pinch of each mixed with *honey* can be had thrice a day for 3-4 days with warm water.
- One teaspoon of fresh *ginger* juice with one teaspoon of *honey* can be had thrice a day for a week with warm water.
- Soak a teaspoon of grated dried *pomegranate* peel in a cup of hot boiling water for a few minutes. Cool till it comes down to a warm comfortable temperature. Use this for gargling. Relieves an unpleasant sore throat.
- Boil 5-6 *eucalyptus* leaves and 5-6 cloves in a glass of water for 5-6 minutes. Add a little lemon juice, sweeten with honey and drink. Helps in giving relief to a bronchial cough.
- For asthma and respiratory tract disorders, eliminating or reducing the intake of white starches — white flour or maida, macaroni, noodles, sweets, pastries, cakes, white sugar — helps.

❒ ARTHRITIS

- Fresh *celery* : A cup of juice a day is good for arthritis. Celery soups and salads also have a beneficial effect.

- *Foods* : Celery, parsley, bitter gourd, beetroot, asparagus, yeast, wheat germs.
- *Fruits* : Banana, pecan, grapes, raisins, cherry, strawberry, guava and musk melon.
- *Fresh vegetable juice* : Carrot, spinach, beetroot and cucumber. A combination of vegetable juice is better than having one only for arthritic conditions.
- Warm a leaf of the *castor* plant and place it over a painful joint. Change frequently.
- *Turmeric* paste application over a painful joint is soothing.
- *Fenugreek, i.e. methi seeds,* are specially recommended for arthritis. One teaspoon of seeds taken with water early morning, or methi seeds ground into a chutney or soaked for a few hours/ overnight and made into a main dish preparation are helpful.
- Saffron soaked in hot milk.
- Use *apple cider vinegar* instead of synthetic vinegar.

❒ FOR PAINFUL SWELLING OF JOINTS

- Fresh *tamarind* leaves crushed and ground into a paste can be locally applied as a poultice for a few hours.
- *Lemon grass* crushed and mixed with coconut oil for local application.
- Crushed *garlic* mixed with warm *mustard oil* for local application.
- Ground *pepper* added to warm *sesame oil* as a liniment.
- A few grams of *camphor* mixed in warm *mustard oil,* apply locally for sprain.

Caution : Do not massage vigorously. The technique of massaging should be learnt as an incorrect method can do more damage than good.

Wounds/burns/scalds/brits/whitlow/eczema : All these effected areas must be washed with clean water

❑ WOUNDS

Remember first to wash your hands with soap and water before rendering this first aid.

Betel leaves

Crush a handful of betel leaves and extract fresh juice. Pour this over the wound, cover with another washed, cleaned, dried betel leaf and bandage. The juice has certain ingredients that arrest bleeding.

Garlic

Its juice has wound cleaning and healing properties. One part of fresh garlic juice to three parts of water can be used to clean a wound and a few drops of diluted garlic juice applied as a base for dressing also stops bleeding.

Ginger

A piece of fresh ginger peeled and ground into a paste with a little sugar can be applied to a fresh cut or wound and bandaged. Now keep the bandaged area absolutely dry for three to five days. Remove after five days. The wound heals. This is only possible on small wounds. Large wounds will bleed and till the bleeding stops they are difficult to heal.

Parsley

– Suppurating wounds can be cleansed by pouring a slightly warm infusion of parsley leaves. Freshly washed, bruised parsley can be applied to dress a wound. This dressing should be changed every two to three hours as it soaks up the pus.

– Fresh juice of a fresh *turmeric* root makes a good antiseptic dressing. In the absence of a fresh root, home ground, clean, washed and dried *turmeric* root powder can be used.

Liquorice

A bit of liquorice powder mixed with pure ghee and a few drops of *honey* to make a paste is another helpful remedy.

Fresh cactus

Cutting a fresh cactus stalk or succulent leaf will have juice flowing out from the cut edge. Let this juice be dropped directly on a fresh wound. It helps to clean the wound especially in the absence of clean water. It also helps the small cut blood vessels in the area to contract and controlling the bleeding. Now slice a fresh piece of the cactus taking care the prickly hair/thorns are removed and place the cut surface on the wound and bandage. Remove after two to three hours. The bleeding would have been controlled. The wound can later be cleaned and dressed the normal way.

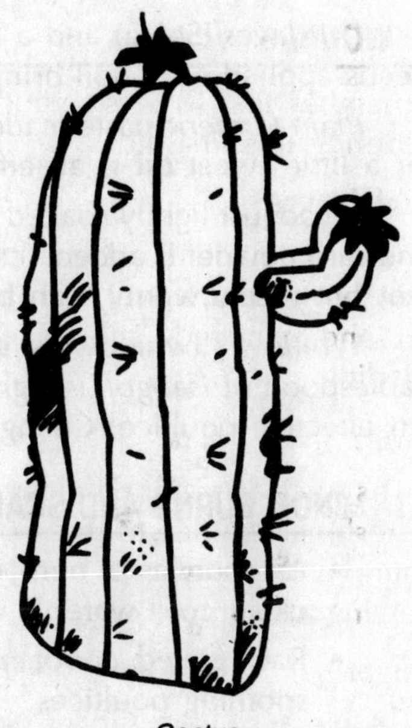

Cactus

– On a fresh wound the pulp of *Aloe* leaf obtained by splitting open the leaf and applying twice daily on the injured area helps in good healing. Alternately, cut a leaf into two, sprinkle fresh turmeric powder and apply this to the wound and bandage.

– The *lajwanti* plant or mimosa grows wildly in a garden — its leaves crushed and applied twice daily too can be used.

❐ BOILS

Betel leaf

Gently warm a betel leaf over a flame, coat it with castor oil on one side. Place it on the boil which has not yet come to a head and bandage lightly. Repeat this every few hours with a fresh leaf. This helps the boil to come to a head and rupture. Once that happens express the collected pus out by putting pressure from the periphery inwards and then apply a clean dressing. The leaf does not stick to the boil and is easy to remove.

Parsley leaves

Place a handful of freshly washed parsley leaves in boiling water. Use the water to wash the boil area and place the leaves on the boil. Cover with a bandage. Repeat every few hours till the boil ruptures, express pus out and dress.

Dill laves (Sowa) and a *turmeric paste* or ground black cumin seeds applied on a boil brings it to a head and helps it to rupture.

Plain turmeric paste made with fresh turmeric powder and water or a little sweet oil is an effective poultice.

Bread just lightly soaked in boiling water to which fresh ground mustard powder is added, (check warmth — should not be scalding hot but nicely warm), can be applied as a poultice.

Whitlow (whitlow is swelling at the base of a nail) — A tablespoon of *isabgol* (ispaghula) made into a paste with *vinegar* is an effective poultice. Change every three hours.

❒ MINOR BURNS AND SCALDS

- As soon as a burn or scald occurs, wash with plenty of clean cold water.
- Raw grated *carrot, potato* or crushed *cabbage* leaves are soothing poultices.
- Pure *honey* used on its own is a soothing salve.
- *Betel* leaves make a good dressing for burns.
- *Calendula flowers* pounded and mixed with *olive oil* makes a healing unguent.
- In a warm pot place tender leaves of the *Tamarind* tree and turn over till they are dry and a little burnt. Grind these into a paste with *til oil*. Can be applied on the burnt skin surface, prevents swelling and helps growth of healing skin.
- Steamed and cooled *banana leaves* applied on minor burns and scalds are very soothing.

❒ SUNBURN

- Fresh cool *cucumber juice*, or both *yogurt* and *buttermilk* are soothing for sunburn.

❒ CONJUNCTIVITIS AND WATERING OF EYES

- Wash eyes with water in which *babul* (keekar) leaves have been boiled. Add a handful of leaves to a litre of water. Boil till only half the water remains. Strain and use the water either lukewarm or cool to wash eyes with.

- To clean eyes which are matted with discharge — boil a glass of water to which a pinch of salt has been added. Take clean cotton swabs or piece of clean cloth. Soak cotton in this water and wipe the eyes gently, taking the discharge away from nose end to the ear side. For each stroke, wash the piece of cloth or use a fresh swab. Do not let the dirty water fall back into the eyes.
- A *grain* or two of *alum* added to a cup of water can be used to wash sore eyes.

❒ SCABIES

- If there is a localized scabies infection, dry and powder *neem* leaves. Half a teaspoon of this powder can be taken as a morning drink in a glass of hot water with sugar added to taste for ten days.
- A decoction made from *neem* leaves, *neem* tree bark can be used to wash the effected area.
- A *paste of neem leaves* with an equal amount of *turmeric* powder mixed with a little mustard oil can be applied over the area. Leave it for 45 minutes to an hour. Wash the area. Continue the process for a week.
- Alternatively, the bark of the *neem* tree dried and burnt to make washes, mixed with a little *coconut oil* to make paste and applied on the affected area after a bath, morning and evening, gets rid of the condition.

❒ JAUNDICE

Once jaundice presents, it implies that there is an underlying disordered state which needs urgent medical attention. However, in most cases, domiciliary care, which means giving the correct nutrition, is of paramount importance.

- Fresh s*ugarcane* juice is the ideal nourishment during the acute phase.
- Eating fruits like *grapes, water melon, papaya* is helpful.
- Fresh *coconut* water.
- *Radish, beetroot* and *carrots* as salads or the juices.

- Tea made with *mint*, or methi leaves.
- Since there is loss of appetite, *onions* peeled and cut into small bits with *fresh lemon juice* and a little *roasted ground cumin powder* is effective both as an appetite stimulant and therapeutic measure.
- *Bhuin awla* — which botanists refer to an phyllanthus amarus has proven present studies of efficacy in jaundice. The plant is such that any part of it is useful. Make a paste and take a teaspoon full thrice a day with half a cup of milk for ten days to three weeks. This fruit is a smaller version of the amla one uses in chutneys and murabbas. The fruits are slightly larger than mustard seeds. The leaves of the amla and bhuin awla plant are similar.
- Take two teaspoons full of the pulp of the *aloe* leaf with *honey* or one thrice a day for 10-20 days.

❒ URINARY COMPLAINTS

Drinking plenty of water two to four times a day is the remedy for most urinary tract problems, e.g. a burning sensation while passing urine. However, in case the patient is having difficulty in passing urine and the bladder is obviously full or if there is swelling of the feet/body and retention or scanty urine, it is best to restrict fluid intake and consult a doctor immediately.

For burning in urine, drink plenty of

- Fresh *coconut* water.
- Make a decoction of *barley* and drink several times a day.
- Fresh *Strawberry juice* with plenty of water.
- Boil kidney beans — called *'kulth ki dal'* and have this soup several times a day.
- Parsley tea can be made by placing freshly-washed parsley leaves in a jar and pouring boiling water over them. When the water cools down, strain and drink regularly if prone to kidney problems.
- Boil *washed potatoes* and drink the water in which they have been boiled.

- *Corn silk* — the silky tassels on a fresh young corn cob, can be boiled to make tea. It is soothing for the entire urinary tract.
- *Lemon juice* and *lemon peel* boiled in warm water may be had as a drink.
- A few small strips of the *outer fibre* of the *banana tree* boiled in water or an infusion made from them can be had two to three times a day.

Fruits and vegetables

Eating cherries, awla, asparagus, grapes, figs, lettuce, runner beans and boiled bhindi (lady's finger) is good for clearing out urinary tract infections.

Pumpkin and its seeds are excellent for kidney infections and stones, and for those who have prostatic problem too. *Rice* bran is a preventive for stone formation.

❒ WORM INFESTATIONS

When a person has worms, the doctor prescribe a deworming dose. However, in practice it is often seen that a child/person does not get rid of worm infestations with one deworming dose. Repeated doses have their own hazards.

Practitioners of traditional medicine — vaids/hakims — in rural areas have time-tested remedies which have actually formed an integral part of our traditional practices of which we are unaware.

Pumpkin seeds are considered very efficacious in removing tapeworm — an infestation which even allopaths find difficult to treat. The seeds crushed into a coarse powder and taken with *milk* and *honey* at bedtime for three to five days or alternately having *walnuts* with warm water at bedtime is effective. *Garlic* eaten regularly or a quarter cup of *cabbage juice* every morning for three days helps. Another remedy is to powder the dry ripe skin of a *pomegranate* and have a teaspoon with water every morning and evening for three days. A teaspoon of *neem leaf powder* twice a day with milk or hot water for a week generally sanitizes the intestional tract. Give a break of a week to 10 days and repeat. This is specially good for thread worm infestation and may be had by the entire family.

Papaya is a good fruit to eat when ripe but unripe is helpful in treating roundworm infestations too. A home remedy is a tablespoon of green fruit mashed and mixed with an equal amount of honey — as the green fruit is awful to taste. Add half a cup of hot water and drink it followed by a tablespoon of *castor oil*. Alternately, crush two or three *papaya* seeds, mix in a glass of warm *milk* and drink. Repeat next day.

A small *betel nut*, powdered (not more than 1 teaspoon full) and had with *milk* on an empty stomach gets rid of tapeworms. People in Assam, i.e. marshy moist lands and humid weather with heavy rainfall would have worm infestations but for their habit of eating betel nuts. However, too much betel nut can lead to oral cancer. The tradition of eating pan/supari — a little but after the main meal every day was probably to help the digestive tract remain free from worm infestation.

A recipe for a relishing chutney follows for children but to be had only once a week. Take an ounce of fresh *neem flowers*, or of tender sweet neem leaves, quarter teaspoon of *ajwain*, a few *black pepper seeds*, a little dried or fresh ginger and a teaspoon of *saunf*. Fry these in pure ghee and grind to a paste and serve with main meal. A little *jaggery* can be added. This will ensure a good appetite, no constipation, indigestion, flatulence, worms or phlegm in the chest.

❐ HEADACHE

- Herbal teas made with *tulsi, jheera, mint* or *thyme*.
- Half a teaspoon of *black pepper powder* taken with *honey*.
- Hot *honey* and *lemon water* drink.
- *Ginger* paste applied on the forehead relieves a headache.
- *Coconut* hair oil massage.

❐ TOOTHACHE AND DENTAL CONDITIONS

- Place a crushed *clove* in your mouth where the tooth hurts.
- To one and a half tablespoon of *mustard oil add* a teaspoon of *salt*. Massage your gums daily with this twice a day followed by warm water gargles. This keeps the gums healthy and teeth intact.

- *Mint leaf tea, tulsi tea, cherry juice, turnip leaf juice, raw spinach* and *carrot juice* make for healthy teeth and gums.
- Eat *guavas* and *apples* and chew on dried *anwla.* Drink *buttermilk* and have fresh yogurt regularly.

❐ PAIN AND DISCOMFORT DURING MENSTRUATION

Herbal teas made of *saunf* (fennel), *parsley, mint,* and *liquorice.* These actually cause diuresis which gets rid of the water retention in the pelvic organs thus relieving the bloated feeling.

❐ INSOMNIA

A glass of hot milk at bedtime flavoured with *saffron, nutmeg* and *cardamom* is ideal to ensure a peaceful relaxing sleep. However, don't make the addition of nutmeg a 'habit'. It can be addictive and constipating.

❐ HIGH BLOOD PRESSURE

A teaspoonfull of fresh juice or paste of *yellow drumstick leaves* taken after meals, or a teaspoon of *fresh ginger juice* with a teaspoon of *cumin* seed powder and *honey* helps keep blood pressure under control. This is probably due to the high natural fibre content or cholesterol lowering properties of these ingredients! Our traditional diets had a regular intake of curds, raw onion, garlic, and turmeric used liberally for seasoning of curries and vegetables — all of which are good for lowering blood pressure.

❐ DIABETES

- Dry and powder jamun seeds. Add a teaspoon to a glass of hot water, keep aside for a while and then strain it. Drink this water every day.
- *Fenugreek* (methi) seeds : Two teaspoons of powdered fenugreek can be had everyday with milk or broth. You could soak these overnight and swallow them whole or just drink the water they have been soaked in. The efficacy of this has been proved by modern scientific methods.

❐ HANDY HERBAL INGREDIENTS IN THE KITCHEN

- Ajwain, anise, hing, betelnut, black pepper, caraway, cardamom, cinnamon, coriander, dill seeds, fenugreek, mustard, nutmeg, poppy.
- Alum, camphor, catechu, honey, isabgol, salt, turmeric, sandalwood, dried ginger, liquorice, tamarind, walnuts.
- Barley, rice, castor oil, mustard oil, linseed oil and til oil.
- Milk, buttermilk, yogurt.

❐ USEFUL KITCHEN GARDEN AND COURTYARD TREES

- Acacia, amla, bael, country fig, country gooseberry, lime, neem, papaya, pineapple, plantain, pomegranate, sapota (peach).
- Betel leaf, capsicum, coriander leaves, dill leaves, edible hibiscus (shoeflower), bhindi, fresh ginger rhizome, fenugreek leaves, garlic, tulsi, parsley, lemon grass, mint, spinach, lettuce, bathua, chaulai, amaranth, while pumpkin.
- Trees — neem, peepal, sesame, tamarind, drumstick, plantain, guava, papaya, citrus.

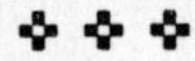

CHAPTER

26

Common Occupational Diseases and First-Aid

❒ COMMON OCCUPATIONAL DISEASES DUE TO LEAD

Signs/Symptoms

Lassitude, insomnia, colic, anaemia, lead line, lead palsy with wrist drop, vomiting.

First-Aid

- Eye irrigation.
- Soap wash for skin.
- Artificial respiration if breathing is disturbed.
- Vomiting in case of swallowing.
- Medical attention.

❒ COMMON OCCUPATIONAL DISEASES DUE TO LEAD TETRAETHYL

Signs/Symptoms

Irritation of eye, dermatitis, headache, dizziness, restlessness, disorientation, convulsions, tremors, coma.

First-Aid

- Eye irrigation.
- Soap wash for skin contamination.
- Water vomiting in case of swallowing.
- Medical attention.

❐ COMMON OCCUPATIONAL DISEASES DUE TO PHOSPHORUS

Signs/Symptoms

Marked thirst, restlessness, shock, petechial haemorrhage, jaundice, oliguria, anuria, "Phossy-Jaw".

First-Aid

- Eye irrigation.
- Water wash for skin.
- 0.2% solution of copper sulphate orally for vomiting.
- Gastric lavage with 0.1% potassium permanganate.
- Immediate medical attention.

❐ COMMON OCCUPATIONAL DISEASES DUE TO PHOSPHORUS COMPOUNDS

Signs/Symptoms

Irritation of eye; Skin burns, dizziness, headache, chest pain.

First-Aid

- Eye irrigation.
- Wash skin with 5% solution of copper sulphate then with soap.
- Oxygen therapy.
- Medical attention.

❐ COMMON OCCUPATIONAL DISEASES DUE TO PHOSGENE

Signs/Symptoms

Conjunctivitis, corneal turbidity, skin irritation, headache, rapid respiration, chest pain, dyspnea, nausea, vomiting, shock, pulmonary oedema.

First-Aid

- Oxygen with positive pressure breathing apparatus.
- Artificial respiration.
- Irrigation of eye.
- Water wash of skin.
- No vomiting induction.

❒ COMMON OCCUPATIONAL DISEASES DUE TO MERCURY

Signs/Symptoms

Burning in mouth, thirst, shock, nausea, vomiting, abdominal pain, salivation, dyspnea, chest tightness, insomnia.

First-Aid

- Water to vomit.
- Gastric lavage if swallowed with 5% solution of formaldehyde, sulfoxylate, then with 2% solution of sodium bicarbonate.
- Irrigation of eye.
- Soap wash for skin.
- Artificial respiration if needed.

❒ COMMON OCCUPATIONAL DISEASES DUE TO MANGANESE

Signs/Symptoms

Papulo-erythematous dermatitis, metal fume fever, dry throat, cough, tight chest, vomiting, back pain, nervousness, vertigo, gait disturbances.

First-Aid

- Artificial respiration.
- Water vomiting.
- Gastric Lavage.

❒ COMMON OCCUPATIONAL DISEASES DUE TO ARSENIC

Signs/Symptoms

Industrial poisoning is due to inhalation of arsenic. Headache, garlic odour of breath, numbness, tingling of hand and feet, chest pain, nausea, abdominal cramp, pulmonary oedema, haematuria, dermatitis (Bronze skin).

First-Aid

- Artificial respiration.
- Immediate medical attention.

❐ COMMON OCCUPATIONAL DISEASES DUE TO NITROUS FUMES

Signs/Symptoms

Dry imitating cough, tightness of chest, pain, choking of throat, canary yellow sputum, cyanosis, pulmonary oedema.

First-Aid

- Irrigation of Eye.
- Skin (contaminated) should be washed with soap.
- Artificial respiration.
- Water.
- No vomit.

❐ COMMON OCCUPATIONAL DISEASES DUE TO CARBON-DISULPHIDE

Signs/Symptoms

Headache, dizziness, nausea, vomiting, abdominal pain, conjunctivitis, sensory disturbances, atherosclerotic changes, ocular changes, chronic gastritis, anorexia.

First-Aid

- Artificial respiration.
- Eye irrigation.
- Soap wash for skin (contaminated).
- Water vomit.
- Vit. B_1 and B_{12}.

❐ COMMON OCCUPATIONAL DISEASES DUE TO BENZENE

Signs/Symptoms

Euphoria, irritation of eye and upper respiratory tract, headache, nausea, vomiting with burning pain in stomach, giddiness, air hunger and frequent urination, palpitation, unconsciousness, coma.

First-Aid

- Eye irrigation.
- Soap water wash of skin (contaminated).

- Artificial respiration.
- No vomit.

❒ COMMON OCCUPATIONAL DISEASES DUE TO CHROME ULCERATION (Chromium compounds)

Signs/Symptoms

Eczymatous dermatitis, loss of finger nails, ulcer on hand, feet, fingers (chrome hole), similar ulcer on nose, perforation of nasal septum, rhinitis, bronchitis, gastritis, conjunctivitis.

First-Aid

- Irrigation of Eye immediately.
- Soap wash for skin (contaminated).
- Artificial respiration.
- Water vomit if ingested.

❒ COMMON OCCUPATIONAL DISEASES DUE TO ANTHRAX

Signs/Symptoms

Pimple with area of redness, swelling, oedema, lymph glands enlarged and tender, toxemia, headache, joint pain, nausea, vomiting, pneumonia with frothy blood stained sputum.

First-Aid

- Eye irrigation.
- Soap wash for the contaminated area.

❒ COMMON OCCUPATIONAL DISEASES DUE TO SILICOSIS

Signs/Symptoms

Dyspnea, cough, tightness of chest, emphysema, pneumoconiosis develops.

First-Aid

- Irrigation of eye and removal of dust.
- Water wash for skin.

COMMON OCCUPATIONAL DISEASES DUE TO HALOGENS AND DERIVATIVES OF HYDROCARBONS :

❒ (a) CHLORINE

Signs/Symptoms

Irritation of eyes, nose, mouth, lacrimation, cough, tightness in chest, frothy-pink sputum, nausea, vomiting, syncope, suffocation.

First-Aid

- Irrigation of eye.
- Water wash for skin (contaminated)
- Artificial respiration if needed.

❒ (b) TRICHLOROETHYLENE

Signs/Symptoms

Dizziness, nausea, headache, vomiting, confusion, stupor, staggering gait, unconsciousness.

First-Aid

- Irrigation of eye.
- Soap water wash of skin.
- Artificial respiration if needed.
- Salt water vomiting.

❒ (c) CARBON TETRACHLORIDE

Signs/Symptoms

Dizziness, lack of co-ordination, nausea, vomiting, dermatitis, loss of appetite, enlargement of liver.

First-Aid

- Irrigation of eye.
- Soap water wash of skin.
- Artificial respiration if needed.
- Induce vomiting by salt water.

❒ COMMON OCCUPATIONAL DISEASES DUE TO RADIO-ACTIVE SUBSTANCES AND X-RAY

Signs/Symptoms

Anaemia, leukaemia, bone destruction, dry inelastic skin, fissured, cracked and brittle nails, painful wart like growths, skin burn, sterility.

First-Aid

- Management similar to that of skin burns.
- Decontamination.
- Medical attention.

❒ COMMON OCCUPATIONAL DISEASES DUE TO PRIMARY EPITHELIOMATOUS CANCER OF SKIN (Arsenic pitch, Bitumen, Mineral Oil, Tar, Soot, Cresote, X-ray)

Signs/Symptoms

Oil acne, epitheliomata of scrotum, conjunctivitis, corneal damage, papulovesicular skin eruption, hyperpigmentation, nausea, vomiting, headache, giddiness.

First-Aid

- Irrigation of eye.
- Soap wash of the skin.
- Give water to induce vomiting.
- Artificial respiration if inhaled.

❒ COMMON OCCUPATIONAL DISEASES DUE TO TOXIC ANAEMIA (Benzene, Xylene, Toluene, Naphtha, Carbon tetrachloride, lead, etc.

Signs/Symptoms

Loss of appetite, fatigue, depression, dyspnea, haemoglobin less than 70%, cyanosis, bleeding nose and gums, blue line on gum etc., abnormal W.B.C. count, dyshaemopoiesis.

First-Aid

- Eye irrigation.
- Soap water wash of skin.

- No vomiting induction.
- Artificial respiration if necessary.

❒ COMMON OCCUPATIONAL DISEASES DUE TO TOXIC JAUNDICE
(Aromatic hydrocarbons, chlorinated hydrocarbons)

Signs/Symptoms

Headache, nausea, exhaustion, dizziness, loss of appetite, vomiting, liver function tests abnormal.

First-Aid

- Eye irrigation.
- Soap wash of the skin.
- Artificial respiration if needed.

❒ COMMON OCCUPATIONAL DISEASES DUE TO MINERAL OIL DERMATITIS

Signs/Symptoms

Oil ache usually in areas contaminated by mineral oil. Nausea, vomiting, pain in abdomen epitheliomata of scrotum may result.

First-Aid

- Eye irrigation.
- Soap water wash.
- No vomiting.

❒ COMMON OCCUPATIONAL DISEASES DUE TO BYSSINOSIS
(Cotton dust)

Signs/Symptoms

Tightness of chest, breathlessness, cough, headache, dizziness.

First-Aid

- Eye irrigation.
- Water wash and change of clothing.
- Artificial respiration.

❒ COMMON OCCUPATIONAL DISEASES DUE TO ASBESTOSIS
(Asbestos fibres)

Signs/Symptoms

Breathlessness, pain in chest, anaemia, clubbing, cough.

First-Aid

- Eye irrigation.
- Artificial respiration if needed.

❒ COMMON OCCUPATIONAL DISEASES DUE TO CONTACT DERMATITIS

Signs/Symptoms

Dermatitis; Urticarea

First-Aid

- Soap water wash of skin.

❒ COMMON OCCUPATIONAL DISEASES DUE TO NOISE

Signs/Symptoms

Disturbances of speech communication, tinitus, headache, gait disturbance, high B.P., syncope.

First-Aid

- Alienate from the noisy area.
- Systemic and supportive.
- Complete rest in peace.

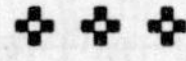

CHAPTER

27

General Chemicals and First-Aid : Everyone Must Know

❐ CHEMICAL : ACETIC ACID

Signs/Symptoms

Skin and hand blackish, hyperkeratotic, fissured, erosion of teeth, conjunctivitis, iritis, vomiting, haematesis, diarrhoea, blood in stools.

First-Aid

- Eye irrigation.
- Soap water washing of skin.
- Water, no vomit.
- Gastric lavage with lime water if ingested.
- Artificial respiration if needed.

❐ CHEMICAL : ACROLEIN

Signs/Symptoms

Irritation of eye, skin burn, bronchitis, pulmonary oedema, nausea, vomiting, unconsciousness.

First-Aid

- Eye irrigation.
- Soap water washing of skin.
- Salt water vomit.
- Artificial respiration.

❐ CHEMICAL : ALDRIN

Signs/Symptoms

Headache, dizziness, nausea, vomiting, convulsion, coma, azotemia.

First-Aid

- Eye irrigation.
- Soap water washing of skin.
- Water, vomit.
- Artificial respiration.

❐ CHEMICAL : AMMONIA

Signs/Symptoms

Irritation of eye, skin and throat, dyspnea, bronchospasm, chest pain, pink frothy sputum, skin burn.

First-Aid

- Eye irrigation.
- Water wash for skin.
- No vomit.
- Artificial respiration.

❐ CHEMICAL : ANILINE

Signs/Symptoms

Headache, vertigo, nervousness, chest pain, palpitation, dyspnea, nausea, abdominal pain, syncope.

First-Aid

- Eliminate exposure.
- Remove all clothings.
- Wash and scrape total body surface with soap.
- Eye irrigation.
- Water, vomit.
- Artificial respiration.

❒ CHEMICAL : ANISIDINE

Signs/Symptoms

Headache, dizziness, cyanosis, heavy body.

First-Aid

- Eye irrigation.
- Soap wash of skin.
- Water, vomit.
- Artificial respiration.

❒ CHEMICAL : BROMINE

Signs/Symptoms

Dizziness, headache, cough, corneal ulcer, skin burn, brownish discolouration of tongue, nausea, chest pain.

First-Aid

- Eye irrigation.
- Soap water washing of skin.
- Milk/water, no vomit.
- Artificial respiration.

❒ CHEMICAL : 2-BUTANONE

Signs/Symptoms

Irritation of eye, nose, headache, dizziness, vomiting.

First-Aid

- Eye irrigation.
- Water washing of skin.
- Fresh air.
- Salt water, vomit.

❒ CHEMICAL : BUTYL ACETATE

Signs/Symptoms

Headache, drowsiness, irritation of eye, dryness of mouth and throat, cough, irritation of respiratory system.

First-Aid

- Eye irrigation.
- Water washing of skin.
- Salt water, vomiting.
- Artificial respiration.

❐ CHEMICAL : SEC./TERT. BUTYL ACETATE

Signs/Symptoms

Irrigation of eyes, headache, drowsiness, itching, dryness and irritation of respiratory system, dry skin, dermatitis.

First-Aid

- Eye irrigation.
- Water wash for skin.
- Salt water, vomit.
- Artificial respiration.

❐ CHEMICAL : CADMIUM-DUST AND SALT

Signs/Symptoms

Irritation of nose, throat, cough, metallic taste, tightness and pain in chest, dyspnea, chills, headache, dizziness, nausea, vomiting.

First-Aid

- Eye irrigation.
- Soap water wash for skin.
- Water, vomit.
- Gastric lavage.
- Artificial respiration.

❐ CHEMICAL : CALCIUM OXIDE

Signs/Symptoms

Irritation of eye, conjuctivitis, dermatitis, perforation and ulcer of nasal septum, burns.

First-Aid

- Eye irrigation.
- Soap water washing of skin.
- Water, no vomit.
- Artificial respiration.

❐ CHEMICAL : CARBOFURAN

Signs/Symptoms

Irritation of eye, dermatitis, headache, dyspnea, tremors.

First-Aid

- Eye irrigation.
- Soap water washing of skin.
- Water, vomit.
- Artificial respiration.

❐ CHEMICAL : CHLORDANE

Signs/Symptoms

Blurring of vision, confusion, delirium, cough, pain in abdomen, nausea, vomiting, convulsion, tremors.

First-Aid

- Eye irrigation.
- Soap water washing of skin.
- Water, vomit.
- Artificial respiration.

❐ CHEMICAL : CHLOROBENZENE

Signs/Symptoms

Irritation of eye, headache, dizziness, nausea, vomiting, swelling of hands and feet, jaundice, dermatitis, granulocytopenia, muscle spasm, cyanosis.

First-Aid

- Eye irrigation.
- Soap water washing of skin.

- No vomit.
- Gastric lavage.
- Artificial respiration.

❐ CHEMICAL : CHLORINE

Signs/Symptoms

Irritation of eye, corneal burn, dyspnea, cough, retrosternal pain, nausea, vomiting, cyanosis, pulmonary oedema.

First-Aid

- Eye irrigation
- Water wash for skin.
- Artificial respiration and oxygen.

❐ CHEMICAL : BIS.CHLOROMETHYL ETHER

Signs/Symptoms

Irritation of eyes, skin burns, pulmonary oedema, bronchitis, irritation of throat.

First-Aid

- Eye irrigation.
- Soap water wash for skin with due care for burns.
- Artificial respiration if needed, oxygen.

❐ CHEMICAL : CHROMIC ACID AND CHROMATES

Signs/Symptoms

Irritation of throat, nasal septum, dermatitis, leukopenia eye injury.

First-Aid

- Irrigation of eye.
- Soap water wash of skin.
- Water, vomit.
- Artificial respiration.

❐ CHEMICAL : CHROMIUM

Signs/Symptoms

Dermatitis, fibrosis of lungs, irritation of eyes.

First-Aid

- Eye irrigation.
- Soap water washing of skin.
- Water, vomit.
- Artificial respiration.

❐ CHEMICAL : COPPER FUME

Signs/Symptoms

Irrigation of eye, nose, perforation of nasal septum, dermatitis, nausea, vomiting, jaundice, metallic taste.

First-Aid

- Irrigation of eyes.
- Artificial respiration.
- Gastric lavage.

❐ CHEMICAL : COTTON DUST

Signs/Symptoms

Tightness in chest, cough, breathlessness, upper respiratory tract infection.

First-Aid

- Eye irrigation.
- Fresh air breathing.
- Changing clothes.

❐ CHEMICAL : CRESOL

Signs/Symptoms

Conjunctival burn, corneal necrosis, dermatitis, nausea, vomiting, pain in abdomen, convulsion, confusion, irregular rapid respiration.

First-Aid

- Eye irrigation.
- Soap water wash for skin.
- Water, vomit.
- Artificial respiration.

❐ CHEMICAL : CYANIDES

Signs/Symptoms

Eye and skin irritation, slow gasping respiration, nausea, vomiting, headache, asphyxia-death may occur.

First-Aid

- Eye irrigation immediately.
- Soap water wash of skin immediately.
- Water, vomit.
- Artificial respiration.
- Use AMYL NITRATE PEARLS.
- Immediate hospitalisation.

❐ CHEMICAL : CYANOGEN

Signs/Symptoms

Headache, dizziness, hyperpnea, rapid pulse, nausea, vomiting, convulsion, unconsciousness, death may occur.

First-Aid

- Remove from exposure.
- Eye irrigation.
- Soap water wash for skin.
- Artificial respiration and oxygen.
- Use AMYL NITRATE PEARLS.
- Immediate hospitalisation.

❐ CHEMICAL : D.D.T.

Signs/Symptoms

Headache, dizziness, nausea, vomiting, insomnia, irritability, inco-ordination, tremors, convulsions, coma.

First-Aid

- Eye irrigation.
- Soap water washing of skin, remove clothings.
- Water, vomit.
- Artificial respiration.

❐ CHEMICAL : DEMETON

Signs/Symptoms

Headache, dizziness, agitation, congestion, ataxia, substernal tightness, resp. depression, convulsion, cardiac arrhythmias, pulmonary oedema, coma.

First-Aid

- Eye irrigation.
- Removal of all clothings.
- Soap water wash of skin.
- Artificial respiration and oxygen.

❐ CHEMICAL : DIAZINON

Signs/Symptoms

Headache, dizziness, abdominal cramp, blurred vision, trembling, speech disturbance, pulmonary oedema, coma.

First-Aid

- Eye irrigation.
- Artificial respiration and oxygen.

❐ CHEMICAL : DIBUTYL PHTHALATE

Signs/Symptoms

Conjunctivitis, corneal erosion, nasal irritation, dizziness, nausea, Eczema.

First-Aid

- Eye irrigation.
- Soap water washing of skin.

- Salt water, vomit.
- Artificial respiration.

❐ CHEMICAL : DIELDRIN

Signs/Symptoms

Headache, dizziness, nausea, vomiting, clonic and tonic convulsion, coma.

First-Aid

- Eye irrigation.
- Soap water washing of skin.
- Water vomit.
- Artificial respiration.

❐ CHEMICAL : DINITROBENZENE

Signs/Symptoms

Anorexia, visual disturbance, bad taste, burning mouth, dry throat, yellowing hair, eyes, skin, anaemia.

First-Aid

- Eye irrigation.
- Soap water wash for skin.
- Water, vomit.
- Artificial respiration.

❐ CHEMICAL : DINITROTOLUENE

Signs/Symptoms

Anorexia, anaemia, jaundice, cyanosis.

First-Aid

- irrigation of eye.
- Soap water washing for skin.
- Water, vomit.
- Artificial respiration.

❐ CHEMICAL : DIPHENYL

Signs/Symptoms

Irritation of eyes, nose, skin and respiratory tract anorexia, nausea, vomiting.

First-Aid

- Eye irrigation.
- Water wash.
- No vomit.
- Artificial respiration.

❐ CHEMICAL : ENDOSULFAN

Signs/Symptoms

Nausea, vomiting, stomach pain, headache, dizziness, ataxia, tremor, convulsion, elevated body temperature, unconsciousness, death.

First-Aid

- Eye irrigation.
- Soap water wash for skin.
- Gastric lavage, water vomit.
- Artificial respiration and oxygen.
- Hospitalisation.

❐ CHEMICAL : ELDRIN

Signs/Symptoms

Headache, dizziness, convulsion, epileptic fits, nausea, vomiting, lethargy.

First-Aid

- Irrigation of eye.
- Soap water wash of skin.
- Water vomit.
- Artificial respiration.

❐ CHEMICAL : ETHYL ACETATE

Signs/Symptoms

Conjuctivitis, irritation of respiratory tract, dermatitis.

First-Aid

- Eye irrigation.
- Water wash of skin.
- Salt water, vomit.
- Artificial respiration.

❐ CHEMICAL : ETHYL ALCOHOL

Signs/Symptoms

Irritation of eyes, respiratory tract, defatigation, dermatitis, headaches, dizziness, drowsiness, nausea.

First-Aid

- Eye irrigation.
- Water wash of skin.
- Water vomit,.
- Gastric lavage.
- Artificial respiration.

❐ CHEMICAL : ETHYL AMINE

Signs/Symptoms

Irritation of eyes, skin burn, dermatitis, respiratory irritation.

First-Aid

- Eye irrigation.
- Water wash for skin.
- Water, vomit.
- Artificial respiration.

❐ CHEMICAL : FLUORIDES

Signs/Symptoms

Anorexia, nausea, vomiting, cough, backache, stiffness of joints, fluorosis, dermatitis.

First-Aid

- Eye irrigation.
- Water wash of skin.
- Artificial respiration.

❐ CHEMICAL : HYDROGEN-CYANIDE

Signs/Symptoms

Nausea, vomiting, tachycardia, slow respiration, gasping, asphyxia, coma, death may occur.

First-Aid

- Eye irrigation.
- Water wash of skin.
- Water, vomit.
- Artificial respiration.

❐ CHEMICAL : IRON OXIDE FUME

Signs/Symptoms

Conjuctivitis, cough, bronchitis, benign pneumoconiosis.

First-Aid

- Eye irrigation.
- Artificial respiration if needed.

❐ CHEMICAL : ISOAMYL ACETATE

Signs/Symptoms

Eye irritation, irritation to nose, throat, dermatitis.

First-Aid

- Eye irrigation.
- Water wash of skin.
- Salt water, vomit.
- Artificial respiration.

❒ CHEMICAL : ISOAMYL ALCOHOL

Signs/Symptoms

Irritation to eyes, nose, throat, headache, dizziness, dyspnea, nausea, vomiting, dermatitis.

First-Aid

- Eye irrigation.
- Water wash of skin.
- Salt water, vomit.
- Artificial respiration.

❒ CHEMICAL : ISOBUTYL ALCOHOL

Signs/Symptoms

Irritation of eyes, skin, throat, headache, drowsiness, aching.

First-Aid

- Eye irrigation.
- Water wash of skin.
- Salt water, vomit.
- Artificial respiration.

❒ CHEMICAL : LINDANE

Signs/Symptoms

Irritation of eyes, nose, throat, headache, nausea, vomiting, aplastic amaemia, muscle spasm.

First-Aid

- Eye irrigation.
- Soap water wash of skin.
- Water, vomit.
- Artificial respiration.

❒ CHEMICAL : MALATHION

Signs/Symptoms

Miosis, eyes and skin irritation, headache, tightness in chest, salivation, nausea, abdominal cramp, ataxia.

First-Aid

- Eye irrigation.
- Soap water wash of skin.
- Water, vomit.
- Artificial respiration.

❐ CHEMICAL : METHYL ALCOHOL

Signs/Symptoms

Headache, drowsiness, nausea, vomiting, visual disturbances, eye burns, failure of vision.

First-Aid

- Eye irrigation.
- Water wash of skin.
- Salt water, vomit.
- Artificial respiration.

❐ CHEMICAL : METHYL ISOBUTYL KETONE

Signs/Symptoms

Irritation of eyes and respiratory tract, headache, nausea, dermatitis.

First-Aid

- Eye irrigation.
- Soap water wash of skin.
- Salt water, vomit.
- Artificial respiration.

❐ CHEMICAL : NAPTHALENE

Signs/Symptoms

Conjunctivitis, headache, nausea, vomiting, abdominal pain, parotitis, jaundice, Haemolysis, mental excitement, coma, oliguria, dermatitis.

First-Aid

- Eye irrigation.
- Soap water wash for skin.
- No vomit.
- Artificial respiration.

❒ CHEMICAL : NICKEL CARBONYL

Signs/Symptoms

Headache, dizziness, nausea, vomiting, cough, tightness of chest, sweating, hoarseness, dyspnea, hemoptysis, dermatitis.

First-Aid

- Eye irrigation.
- Soap water wash of skin.
- Water, vomit.
- Artificial respiration and oxygen.

❒ CHEMICAL : NITRIC ACID

Signs/Symptoms

Irritation of eyes and mucous membrane, dermatitis, pulmonary oedema, dental erosion.

First-Aid

- Eye irrigation.
- Water wash.
- No vomit.
- Artificial respiration.

❒ CHEMICAL : NITRIC OXIDE

Signs/Symptoms

Irritation of eye, skin, throat, drowsiness, unconsciousness.

First-Aid

- Eye irrigation.
- Water wash of skin.
- Artificial respiration.

❐ CHEMICAL : PARATHION

Signs/Symptoms

Headache, chest pain, salivation, anorexia, nausea, abdominal pain, sweating ataxia, convulsion, conjunctival and skin irritation.

First-Aid

- Eye irrigation.
- Soap water wash of skin.
- Water, vomit.
- Artificial respiration.

❐ CHEMICAL : PHENOL

Signs/Symptoms

Irritation of eye, nose, throat and skin, anorexia, pain, dark urine, tremor, convulsion.

First-Aid

- Eye irrigation.
- Soap water wash.
- Water, vomit.
- Artificial respiration.

❐ CHEMICAL : PHORATE

Signs/Symptoms

Nausea, vomiting, stomach pain, headache, dizziness, ataxia, tremor, convulsion, elevated body temperature, apnoea, collapse, unconsiousness, death.

First-Aid

- Eye irrigation.
- Soap water wash for skin.
- Gastric lavage.
- Water, vomit.
- Artificial respiration and oxygen.
- Hospitalisation.

❐ CHEMICAL : PICRIC ACID

Signs/Symptoms

Irritation of eye, dermatitis, yellow stain of hair, teeth, mylgia, anuria, hepatitis, nephritis.

First-Aid

- Eye irrigation.
- Soap wash for skin.
- Water vomit.
- Artificial respiration.

❐ CHEMICAL : PYRIDINE

Signs/Symptoms

Headache, nervousness, dizziness, insomnia, nausea, vomiting, increased frequency of urination, dermatitis, eye irrigation.

First-Aid

- Eye irrigation.
- Water wash for skin.
- Water, vomit.
- Artificial respiration.

❐ CHEMICAL : SILANE

Signs/Symptoms

Conjunctivitis, irritation of respiratory tract.

First-Aid

- Eye irrigation.

❐ CHEMICAL : STYRENE

Signs/Symptoms

Conjunctivitis, Anorexia, vomiting, drowsiness, dermatitis, anxiety.

First-Aid

- Eye irrigation.
- Soap water wash for skin with care for burns.
- Gastric lavage.
- Artificial respiration.

❒ CHEMICAL : SULPHUR-DIOXIDE

Signs/Symptoms

Irritation of eye, skin and throat, choking, cough, skin burn.

First-Aid

- Eye irrigation.
- Water washing of skin.
- Artificial respiration.

❒ CHEMICAL : SULPHURIC ACID

Signs/Symptoms

Irritation of eye, skin and throat, pulmonary oedema, emphysema, conjunctivitis, stomatitis, dental erosion, skin, eye burn.

First-Aid

- Eye irrigation.
- Water wash for skin.
- Water no vomit.
- Artificial respiration.

❒ CHEMICAL : TOLUENE

Signs/Symptoms

Conjunctivitis, corneal burns, keratitis, dermatitis, bronchitis, anorexia, nausea, vomiting, headache, dizziness, irritability, mental confusion, narcosis.

First-Aid

- Eye irrigation.
- Soap water wash of skin.

- No vomit.
- Artificial respiration.

❐ CHEMICAL : O-TOLUDINE

Signs/Symptoms

Anorexia, headache, cyanosis, dizziness, drowsiness, hematuria.

First-Aid

- Eye irrigation.
- Soap water wash for skin.
- Water, vomit.
- Artificial respiration.

❐ CHEMICAL : TRICHLORO-ETHYLENE

Signs/Symptoms

Headache, vertigo, visual disturbance, tremor, nausea, vomiting, irritation of eyes.

First-Aid

- Eye irrigation.
- Soap water wash for skin.
- Salt water, vomit.
- Artificial respiration.

❐ CHEMICAL : VINYL CHLORIDE

Signs/Symptoms

Headache, dizziness, conjunctivitis, paraesthesias of extremities, dermatitis, narcosis, anaemia, aero-ostcolysis.

First-Aid

- Irrigation of eye.
- Soap water wash of skin.
- No vomit.
- Artificial respiration.

❐ CHEMICAL : XYENE

Signs/Symptoms

Conjunctivitis, dermatitis, dyspnea, anorexia, nausea, vomiting, headache, dizziness, incoordination, anaemia.

First-Aid

- Eye irrigation.
- Soap water wash for skin.
- Artificial respiration and oxygen.
- No vomit.

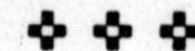